Anatomy--Head and Neck

Andrew Zbar

Anatomy--Head and Neck

A Pocket Book for the Clinician

Springer

Andrew Zbar
Department of Neuroscience and Anatomy
University of Melbourne
University Of Melbourne, VIC, Australia

ISBN 978-3-031-69537-7 ISBN 978-3-031-69538-4 (eBook)
https://doi.org/10.1007/978-3-031-69538-4

This Springer imprint is published by the registered company Springer Nature Switzerland AG
The registered company address is: Gewerbestrasse 11, 6330 Cham, Switzerland

To the spirit of Santiago Ramón y Cajal (1852–1934), artist, histopathologist and Nobel laureate (1906). When pathologists and anatomists could only display their findings through meticulous dissection and their own drawings, he decoded the complexity of the neural forest by painstakingly tracing by hand the dendritic ramifications of single neurons. Through his revolutionary images, art became science and science became art.

Preface

The idea of an anatomical *vade mecum* is not new. We think of it now as somewhat old-fashioned, but it is a book specifically designed to function for ready reference, perhaps to be kept in the pocket and even to be consulted by the bedside. In essence, such a reference defines the very role of anatomy as a living subject that influences clinical practice.

But anatomy is neither taught nor considered in this way by most students and even by its teachers. The study and teaching of anatomy has traditionally been relegated to the early years of medical, dental and veterinary schools and for these students the subject is taught in a manner that is frequently entirely devoid of any clinical context. Anatomy is dreaded by many, appearing as collections of lists which unsurprisingly fail to resonate and where their recall continually needs reinforcement.

In theory at least, anatomy should be one of the simplest subjects to teach and yet it is one of the hardest to learn or to be stamped into the memory. Given this, it is just possible that we should consider learning and teaching it differently.

As a discipline the finite limits of the visible macroscopic (what we call the *gross*) anatomy were pretty well defined through dissection of the cadaver by the middle of the nineteenth century and the publication by Henry Gray (1827–1861) of his great textbook *Gray's Anatomy: Descriptive and Surgical* in 1858 was propitiously timed to coincide with this broad fact. But unlike his predecessors in the field, Gray deliberately chose his illustrator from amongst the medical ranks. Other anatomists before had landed on skilled (and even famous) painters to portray the anatomy at dissection, but Gray's choice of fellow surgeon and resident artist Henry Vandyke Carter (1831–1897) was a masterstroke. Both men understood the learning imperatives that anatomy imposed and Carter's response was to invent a schematic no-frills (some might say dispassionate) style of illustration which set the standard from then on. These iconic images invoked a particular realism in the representations of anatomical dissections that has now been supported by a range of learning options each acting as surrogates for dissection itself. Imagine then, if we transplanted a sixteenth century dissector from his anatomy halls to a modern anatomy lab. All of these alternative methods designed to explain human anatomy (mannikins, plastinated specimens, computer-generated images, 3D-printed models and the progeny of the Visible Human Project) [1] would be learning and understanding tools that to him would be alien. The one thing such a Renaissance dissector could relate to, however, would be the cadaver and each of its surrogates is there to tell him (in a sense) what he already knew.

So if anatomy is largely conceptual, we are forced to ask two discrete questions. When we see it, hear about it, read about it, watch or assist at an operation or dissect a cadaver for ourselves: (1) Do we understand and appreciate what we have just observed? and (2) Can we acknowledge its significance?

Put very simply, in our study of anatomy, do we understand what is the meaning of what we have just observed and why it matters?

Now these two questions may not seem the most obvious things to ask ourselves in anatomy, but some reflection would suggest that they are critical when a conceptual subject is being mastered. Anatomy is relational. It is like being strapped to the front of a train and seeing the branching road ahead running under bridges and through tunnels. If we would be asked to describe such a journey, we could not do so either out of sequence or by ignoring the relative space through which we had just travelled. Understanding this relational anatomy is of course vital if we want to be able to examine our patients, or for the conduct of surgery, in radiology access and in the interpretation of pathology at an autopsy. In short, our anatomical knowledge impacts our ability to be doctors (if that is what you are using it for) or our capabilities in a whole range of other professions where anatomy is part of an integrated programme of diagnosis and care. Without it, we will always be limited.

Anatomy Is Also Contextual

Can you remember your high school days, and for some like me at any rate, the struggle to understand mathematics, physics or chemistry? Today I can readily recall the formula for a quadratic equation or the basis of logarithms, but it is not something that resonates [2]. If my teachers had taught these things to me in a way which explained their meaning and equally importantly how they might have utility in my adult life, then I am certain that these key subjects would be better assimilated into my thinking than they are. It is not only the subject, but its relevance and the way in which it is taught that is important.

As a subject, anatomy has been relegated in our universities; a process which began worldwide (much to its detriment in my view) in the mid- to late 1980s. Vying with all of the other subjects competing for the precious time of the student, universities and colleges across the world decided that the hours spent on anatomy teaching could be sacrificed. Time spent with the cadaver dissecting it and discussing it (the traditional motif of the university medical school) was ceded to other subjects regarded as of equivalent or greater value [3]. There are indeed many medical schools which now no longer teach anatomy at all, their anatomical specimens in some cases part of hidden collections or destined either for burial or cremation [4]. The social implications of relinquishing standards of anatomy knowledge remain unknown. Will our doctors be less proficient in patient examination and diagnosis? Will removal from the medical schools of the cadaver experience (effectively the first patient the student encounters before they are let loose on the real thing) affect their expertise, competence or compassion? [5].

Anatomy Is Historical

The curriculum for how to dissect a cadaver did not come from nowhere. The conduct of a human dissection today is an accumulation of techniques which have been developed and honed over the last millennium. Although often contentious, anatomy is a field of discovery and is in part the story of its discoverers [6]. For anatomy tutors, there are many teaching environments which decry or even censure discussion of its history even when other faculties revel in their historical narratives. If teachers in a Philosophy Department would be subject to such constraints, there would indeed be little to teach about and yet few of our students appreciate the battles fought amongst anatomists over the *terra incognita* of the human body. The art of anatomy (which is an entirely different subject worthy of a book) is historical even if the principal subject itself is considered ahistorical and inviolate. The modern art that currently describes anatomy today may well be formulaic, but it is still embedded in time. Future generations may look upon it perhaps as archaic, but there are elements of the art which reflect that it is a product of its era. We do not, however, consider anatomy in the same way.

Anatomy Is Embryology

I would maintain that if you know a little relevant embryology, you know (or will understand) a lot of anatomy [7]. Embryology is as a discipline a rather young subject and although also conceptual (particularly the earlier foetal development) is for many students frequently confusing. In the past, anatomists cut their teeth dissecting lower animal (and even invertebrate) species and they were relatively expert in the field of comparative anatomy. It is important to return to conveying to our students the relevant developmental anatomy they should know that could improve their appreciation of human anatomy and which would assist in cementing an understanding of important anatomical variations. Study of the normal inherently means an applicative wisdom for the abnormal.

With this series of books, I want to shift focus a little on how we learn and retain our anatomy. The conceptual side of anatomy that we have determined above is supplemented by simple line drawings that I wish the student to practice. When we examine the more complex (and certainly more beautiful) anatomy atlases, the imagery although spectacular at times frequently does not get its anatomical point across. If the student can draw the area of interest, it will stick in the mind and improve understanding. Paradoxically, the simpler the image the more useful it becomes [8]. One of the difficult areas for many of our students are the plexi (brachial, cervical, lumbar, sacral) and in the relevant texts these diagrams will be built up from scratch so that drawing and understanding them will become second nature. In this case, an appreciation of the components of the brachial plexus for example has particular utility during the examination of someone with a plexus injury and defines those cases which are potentially reparable. The approach must then be a fusion of the conceptual and the contextual skills to ensure that students appreciate what they are seeing and why it matters.

Each of the books is divided into component units. This is not to suggest that the parts under consideration are not connected but more to convey quanta of data. In fact, the approach in the upper and lower limbs, for instance, is deliberately comparative. In this case, understanding the homology between the limbs makes study and remembering of the limb compartments easier even if it means that we need to understand a little about how the limbs develop in order to recognize their structural similarities.

You can support your reading in this series with the Open Access anatomy podcast ANATOPOD which has already been recorded and published free of charge. ANATOPOD was commenced in November 2020 after the beginnings of the COVID-19 pandemic with the view that some of our teaching institutions were relatively unprepared with a sufficient digital presence. ANATOPOD was my response to ensure that a basic but comprehensive quantum of anatomical information could be put out there with the view that this was the level of expected knowledge. It is appreciated that the levels will differ for what we artificially regard as undergraduates (when compared with postgraduates) and that this difference extends into other disciplines. Nevertheless, in my opinion a higher standard of clinically relevant packaged data is better than something that for some of our readers would be deficient.

Each unit in this series will include relevant historical aspects that enhance understanding. Embryology that pertains to the field of interest and that will improve static anatomical understanding is added where necessary and where some embryological remnant or sequel influences a clinical presentation and its surgery. Unlike many anatomy texts, there is a short but pertinent bibliography and references are included that the student can analyse. These references are designed to enhance understanding by incorporating anatomy research and by enlivening an appreciation of important anatomical variations that potentially influence surgery or radiology. Diagrams are there for the reader to try and reproduce (or trace) and each has been created to augment a three-dimensional appreciation of the relevant anatomy. In some cases, there are progressive drawings designed to create a complex structure. If you can simply draw it, you will understand it. Each unit is completed by a short multi-choice quiz and answers.

I would recommend whilst studying this series that other anatomy books should be consulted in tandem, gleaning from one what another may not provide. Anatomical understanding relies on such information synthesis. This is no different to looking at a number of cadaveric, prosected specimens where minor differences can be noted that enhance understanding. Cadavers are all a little bit different just as patients and operations are each unique. Try to use all of the resources available on the internet and the video platforms in order to supplement this conceptual approach. If the bronchopulmonary segments have been mastered, for example, go and look at a video of a bronchoscopy (or better yet ask your colleagues if you can attend one at your local hospital). Such synthesis brings the anatomy alive. Once the concepts are in your head, this is one of the best ways to animate them. When studying osteology, access to the individual bones and to an articulated skeleton is vital. Examination of a real human talus allows you to feel its texture, assess its articular surfaces, and see how it fits into the formation of a subtalar joint and contributes to the dynamic stability of the foot. The presence of the sustentaculum tali and the need for the flexor hallucis longus to swerve around it and groove its under surface confirms the central role this muscle plays in stance biomechanics, the constitution and preservation of the medial foot arch and in propulsion.

Don't worry. All will be explained when you get there. Do not forget to use any access you have to plastinated specimens and good prosections or to use these books as you dissect the cadaver or when you have just seen some living anatomy in the operating room. The aim is to improve your conceptual understanding of this living approach. I hope that as readers (and students), you find this series of Anatomy Primers a novel and fun way to study and that together we can change how we come to value and understand this beautiful subject.

References

1. The Visible Human Project (VHP) was realized in 1995 at the US National Library Medicine when the first man was frozen in blue gelatin at −70 °C and then cut into 4 mm slices with a cryogenic microtome and then scanned and photographed as a digital 15GB anatomic archive. There is also a digitized Singapore brain, a University of Michigan digitized pelvis, a Korean head and University of Pennsylvania knee. The pathologist Gunther von Hagens developed plastination a process where the body is immersed in acetone and where the water content is replaced by a vacuum impregnation of polymers with gas curing after dissection or body posturing.
2. It was only when I was Professor of Surgery at the University of the West Indies that I realized the value of the Nernst equation we were taught in high school chemistry. The lowering of the redox potential in the soft-tissues is critical in permitting the growth of anaerobic organisms and in the expansion of synergistic gangrene. In this part of the world, the high prevalence of diabetes, hypertension, hyperlipidaemia and obesity each contribute to a virtual 'epidemic' of macro- and microvascular disease and peripheral neuropathy.

3. The Raven Department of Education at the Royal College of Surgeons Edinburgh has voiced concerns in recent years regarding the level of undergraduate and postgraduate anatomy knowledge suggesting that it has fallen below acceptably safe standards.
4. I would refer readers to Paul Weindling's article 'Cleansing' anatomical collections: The politics of removing specimens from German anatomical and medical collections 1988–1992. Ann Anat. 2012;194(3):237–42.
5. See Singh R, Yadav N, Pandey M, Gareth Jones D. Is inadequate anatomical knowledge on the part of physicians hazardous for successful clinical practice? Surg Radiol Anat. 2022;44(1):83–92.
6. As Jaclyn Duffin, a Canadian haematologist has asserted 'the body is not simply a human continent waiting to be explored'. Quote in Duffin J. History of medicine: a scandalously short introduction. University of Toronto Press; 1999.
7. Unfortunately this does not work the other way around.
8. I do not claim to be an artist but an ability to draw what one is talking about cements a three-dimensional relational construct in the mind. A study by Fernandes et al. has shown drawing to be superior as a mnemonic strategy to reading or writing in boosting memory and is independent of individual artistic talent. See Fernandes MA, Wammes JD, Meade ME. The surprisingly powerful influence of drawing on memory. Curr Dir Psychol Sci. 2018;27(5):302–8.

Melbourne, VIC, Australia Andrew Zbar

Acknowledgments

For the last 200 years, the boundaries of the visible human anatomy have largely been well defined. The task of teaching this inviolable anatomical canon has been how best to transmit great swathes of data in a meaningful way. Today, we are supported by a whole variety of cadaveric surrogates, each designed to supplant the time spent at the side of the corpse engaged in personal dissection. Radiological scans, 3D computer-generated reconstructions, the NIH Human Anatomy Project, the plastination and dehydration of human corpses and AI-generated images and simulations are all designed to replace this close encounter of a cadaveric kind and to obey that first principle of anatomy, namely, to convey the canon.

The discipline of anatomy for trainee doctors, dentists, paramedical staff and ancillary bio-zoologists is no longer a symbol of university study, and its ready access is becoming more and more limited. Worldwide, faculties are less committed than they were (perhaps two generations ago) to anatomy, and its teaching and specialist colleges cannot agree on a basic core set of anatomical knowledge considered essential for effective and safe clinical practice. But they can agree that their data shows that a familiarity with anatomy that governs diagnosis and radiological referral has fallen below acceptable standards. The advent of the COVID-19 pandemic imposed for some anatomy departments a veritable *coup de grâce* to anatomical teaching. There were at many universities a limited digital readiness of an established curriculum and a reliance on distance learning of a practical and tactile discipline that often was not particularly successful.

In this milieu, I felt the need to start a podcast on anatomy that recognized that the limitations imposed could potentially be reversed by contextualizing what was taught to clinical situations. It seemed relatively obvious that students might better appreciate the nuances of an anatomy dataset in a very practical way if the anatomy taught had clinical meaning and value. But the restrictions imposed by podcasting (even though it provided information to students on what I considered a basic and acceptable level of knowledge) still needed an approach to imagery.

With cadaveric surrogates replacing 'by the slab' learning, it seemed that the beautiful complexity of the computer-generated images was not readily conveying the relevant information. Students needed to interpret the relational anatomy of these intricate pictures, and somewhat paradoxically, the more elaborate the image, the more difficult the transmission of that information quantum. Why not simplify images to provide answers to one or two specific questions and make them sufficiently schematic that the students themselves could easily reproduce them? There remains surprisingly little data out there that confirms whether someone learns and retains spatial information if they themselves can draw it as opposed to being able to just relate it orally. Memory is different for different people, but the limited information would suggest that people can draw situations they have never even seen or experienced more readily than they can describe or recall lists attached to the characteristics of such hypothetical situations. In short, will students understand and remember anatomy better if they can draw it? This question requires a whole lot more research, but every anatomy teacher and student knows that concepts are easier to teach, explain and retain when they are drawn.

Some 20 years ago, I tried to begin an operative surgical head and neck video dissection series that expanded on the undergraduate approach adopted by the plastic surgeon Robert Acland (1941–2016); however, it increasingly became apparent that privacy issues surrounding the anatomy rooms made that dream impossible. Nevertheless, the ideas of changing the way we learn and retain anatomy continued to percolate in my brain over time. As international interest in the podcast grew since the pandemic, there was a need to re-examine how we could combine contextualized anatomy with simple line drawings. With this series of books, we shall soon enough see.

In this approach, I am particularly indebted to people who encouraged me within our own department and beyond. I appreciate very much the input of Professors Chris Briggs, Norm Eizenberg and Jason Ivanusic. Each has been a good sounding board. I would also like to thank Matt Farrow and my fellow tutors (some now passed sadly) who inspired me, including Wilf Brooke, Hugh Weaver, Mahendra Menon, Yusuf Sadeghi, Rex Barton-Smith and many more. I now appreciate the passion of my university anatomy professor Ken Russell (1911–1987), who engendered fear in us poor medical students throughout the 1970s; however, it is only now, 50 years on, that I and others had sadly misread him. As it turns out, Professor Russell was unwaveringly devoted not only to the canon but also to its glittering history. I would also like to extend my gratitude to Claudia Corti, who took the time to show me the anatomy of the masterpiece *Venerinas*, among the most intricate and breathtaking wax models of dissected anatomy crafted by Clemente Susini (1754–1814) and so artfully displayed in the *La Specola* museum in Florence, Italy.

To my tireless executive editor at Springer Verlag, Melissa Morton, for her continued support over three decades and to her exceptional production team, my gratitude. I am also indebted to my students over the years for their enthusiasm for this subject and its history. Salutation also to the readers of these books, in the hope that they may glean some benefit from this labour of love.

Melbourne, VIC, Australia — Andrew Zbar
November 2024

Contents

1 Introduction 1

2 The Cervical Fasciae and the Triangles and Spaces of the Neck 3

3 The Neck Viscera: Thyroid, Parathyroids and Salivary Glands 33

4 The Prevertebral Muscles and the Cervical Plexus 73

5 The Autonomic Nervous System of the Head and Neck 91

6 The Skull and Its Foraminae 111

7 The Cranial Nerves and Their Central Connexions 137

8 The Infratemporal and Pterygopalatine Fossae 169

9 The Arterial Circulation 187

10 The Venous Drainage and Sinuses 209

11 The Orbit 231

12 The Nose and Paranasal Sinuses 257

13 The Mouth and Palate 277

14 The Pharynx 299

15 The Larynx 309

16 The Ear 327

17 Relevant Developmental Embryology: An Overview 345

18 Closing Remarks and Introduction to Volume 2 357

Index 359

1 Introduction

Study of the anatomy of the head and neck is perhaps the most daunting of all the compartmentalized anatomical studies. The approach to this complicated region may primarily be somewhat different (or at least differently focused) if there is a dental, oral surgeon, faciomaxillary or plastic reconstructive audience but I hope in this series to include with the anatomy aspects of the discussion an approach that appeals to these separate groups. I think firstly that we need in very broad terms to agree to achieve particular targets even though in areas for example like the autonomic innervation there will be overlapping discussions. In studying the anatomy of the head and neck, both students and teachers alike can often feel at various points that the issue is becoming too disconnected; namely that it is just degenerating into a disconnected series of facts and lists. We should be reminded that areas will overlap (such as the component parts of the cervical plexus, the fascial arrangements around the salivary glands, the foraminae of the skull, the branches of the Vagus nerve, particular aspects of individual cranial nerves and so on).

As assiduously as some students may try to avoid it, embryology will come into play in our study, perhaps no more so than with the anatomy of the head and neck. It appears for example in the formation of Meckel's cartilage and in the pharyngeal arches and their compartmental nerves and vessels, in the anatomy of the styloid apparatus, the hyoid musculature and the muscles of mas-

A. Zbar, *Anatomy--Head and Neck*,
https://doi.org/10.1007/978-3-031-69538-4_1

tication, in the branchial arches and in the development of the thyroid and parathyroid glands. Knowledge of useful and relevant embryology will assist us in appreciating the anatomical approach to the thyroid and thyroglossal masses and fistulae and in locating aberrant parathyroid glands in hyperparathyroidism. The anatomy we learn must have surgical and clinical relevance and these will be discussed in the relevant sections. Try not to be either surprised or dismayed if embryology intermittently pops up in the discussions to reinforce anatomical points and anatomical variations.

In this first volume of the Head and Neck, it is proposed that an understanding of seven discrete areas will suffice for an adequate anatomical knowledge. It is recognized that this regional approach is artificial, however, it improves the level of understanding over a systems approach which for example examines the vascular, neurological or endocrinological systems in isolation. Here I would propose that we understand the neck fasciae (and its triangles), the viscera of the neck, the arterial and venous systems (including the dural venous sinuses), the foraminae of the skull, the pharynx and larynx, the orbit and the autonomic nervous system of the head and neck. There are of course many other areas to examine but this approach will assist in arranging this complex anatomy into a workable system. Therefore, I have deliberately tackled the Head and Neck first because of its complexity and with the aim of reducing it into practical elements.

The Cervical Fasciae and the Triangles and Spaces of the Neck

2

Contents

Triangles of the Neck 7
Submandibular (Digastric) Triangle 8
Carotid Triangle 11
The Muscular Triangle 13
Submental Triangle 13
Posterior Triangle of the Neck 14
Occipital Triangle 15
Supraclavicular Triangle 16
Clinical Significance of This Triangle 17
Scalene Triangle 18
The Cervical Fasciae: The Fasciae of the Head and Neck 18
Clinical Relevance of This Area 26
Q and A: Chap. 2 (Answers at the End of This Chapter) 28
Answers 29
References 30

Please note that the diagrams attached to each chapter have been designed to be simple and reproducible. Each one has been specifically selected to demonstrate a particular point of anatomy and has been designed to assist your understanding of this region. Do try and copy them.

A. Zbar, *Anatomy--Head and Neck*,
https://doi.org/10.1007/978-3-031-69538-4_2

In this chapter we cover the triangles of the neck by which I mean the division of the neck into an anterior and posterior triangle and then subdivisions into a digastric, submandibular, submental, carotid, jugulo-omohyoid (supraclavicular), muscular and occipital triangle. I include these divisions in Diagrams 2.1 and 2.2. These neck triangles are of prime importance in clinical medicine for the purpose of defining the likely origin of neck lumps. In general, a neck mass has specific features (size, shape, consistency, the presence of pulsation or fluctuance, tenderness, fixity, associated draining lymph nodes and so on). The principal feature suggestive of the origin of a neck mass, however, is its location (or site). We can further use this basic neck classification in order to examine the supra and infrahyoid regions. This division in particular is used with various types (and modifications) of

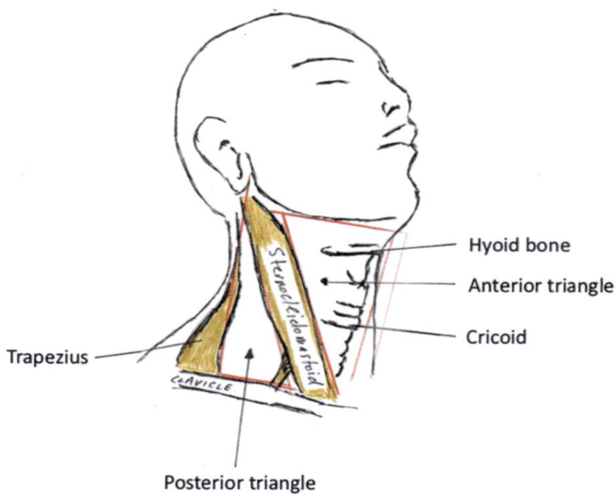

Diagram 2.1 Division of the neck into anterior and posterior triangles
The sternocleidomastoid and the trapezius muscles separate the neck into simple anterior and posterior triangles. Posterior triangle neck masses are usually lymph nodes whereas anterior masses depend on conformation (thyroid, parotid), movement with swallowing by attachment to the pretracheal fascia, high site (branchial cyst, submandibular gland) etc

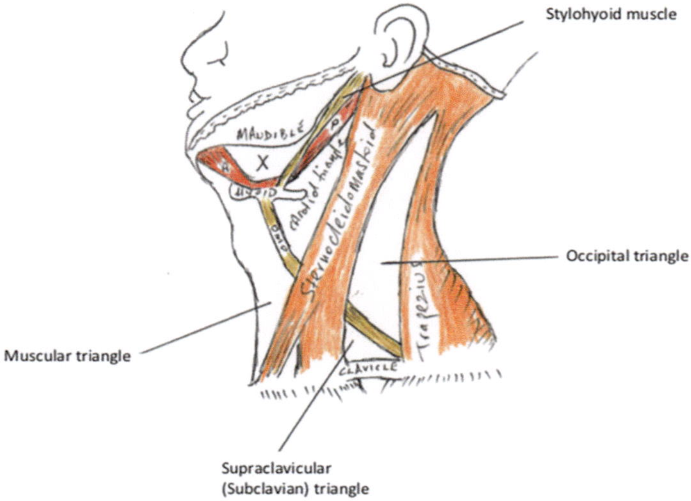

Diagram 2.2 Divisional triangles of the neck
The position of the superior belly of the omohyoid muscle creates sub-triangles forming a subclavian (supraclavicular), occipital, carotid and muscular triangle. The anterior and posterior bellies of the digastric muscle (as shown) with the sternohyoid muscle splitting around the posterior belly of the digastric delineates a submandibular triangle. A digastric triangle under the angle of the mandible can also be defined between the anterior and posterior muscle bellies and the mandible. Even though they are called digastric, both muscles have a separate embryological origin and hence a separate innervation (see main text). A submental triangle can also be formed between the midline mandible, the midline skin and the anterior belly of the digastric muscle. This is the site of lymph nodes draining the floor of the mouth and the tip of the tongue
Legend: A = Anterior belly digastric muscle, P = Posterior belly digastric muscle, X = Submandibular triangle

radical neck dissections that are performed for oropharyngeal squamous carcinomas metastatic to the neck lymph nodes (Diagram 2.3).

Lymph node dissection can broadly divide dissections into suprahyoid (Level 1 and Level II) dissections and infrahyoid (Levels III-VI) dissections. Level 1 dissections remove lymph

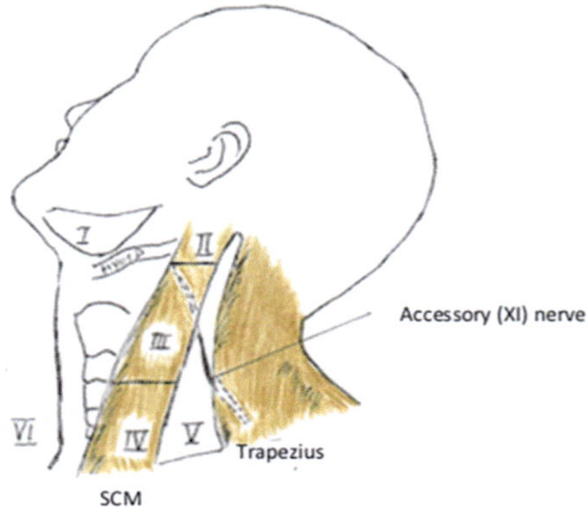

Diagram 2.3 Levels of lymphadenectomy for a radical or modified radical neck dissection. Level I and II are suprahyoid dissections. A level IIA dissection (upper jugular nodes) lies above and anterior to the spinal accessory (XIth cranial nerve) and Level IIB (middle jugular nodes) lie below and posterior to the nerve. Level VA lies above the omohyoid and Level VB is below the muscle. Level VI removes central compartment nodes

nodes from the submandibular [1B] and submental [1A] regions with Level II dissections clearing the top of the sternocleidomastoid (SCM) muscle and upper jugular nodes above the spinal accessory nerve (IIA) and below the nerve but clearing the digastric triangle (Level IIB). The infrahyoid region includes the middle jugular nodes around the internal jugular vein and above the superior belly of the omohyoid muscle (a Level III dissection), the lower jugular nodes down to the supraclavicular triangle (a Level IV dissection), the posterior triangle (Level V) above the omohyoid (Level VA) or below the muscle (Level VB) and the anterior pretracheal region of central compartment nodes (a Level VI dissection). These dissections are increasingly being used as modified radical neck dissections[1] which aim to preserve the internal jugular vein (IJV), the spinal Accessory (XIth Cranial) nerve and the

[1] Modifications of these radical neck dissections are often generically referred to as Bocca dissections after the original descriptor, Italian surgeon Ettore Bocca in 1967 and also by the ENT surgeon Ozvaldo Suarez of Argentina.

sternocleidomastoid muscle. The advantage of the latter is to provide coverage of the carotid vessels should there be wound breakdown or if there is the need for associated radiotherapy (see later).

Triangles of the Neck

The neck itself is limited by the inferior margin of the mandible down to the superior border of the clavicle with extension from the midline to the border posteriorly of the trapezius. The fascia of the chest (which extends in the infraclavicular space as the **clavipectoral fascia**) splits around the clavicle and runs into the neck where it splits around the trapezius posteriorly and the sternocleidomastoid (SCM) muscle anteriorly as the **investing layer of deep cervical fascia**. This fascia then runs past the angle of the mandible and extends to the mastoid process splitting around the substance of the parotid gland as the **parotid fascia**.

In general, the simplest division into anterior and posterior triangles is for the purposes of description of a neck lump as well as for the organization (and communication) of a radical (or modified radical) neck dissection of lymph nodes. The broadest assessment of neck lumps is location-based (although of course there is size, consistency, fluctuance, and a range of parameters). The common lumps such as a thyroid mass are designated based upon its shape, its movement with swallowing (by virtue of its attachment to the **pretracheal fascia**) and of course its locale. The posterior triangle for example has few masses (mostly lymph nodes from lymphoma and Rubella in children).

The anterior triangle of the neck is bounded by the midline and extends to the anterior border or margin of the SCM [1]. This triangle is subdivided into three paired triangles (the submandibular or digastric triangle, the carotid and the muscular triangles) and one paired triangle (the submental triangle). These divisions are created by the trajectory of the omohyoid muscle which attaches to the lower lateral border of the hyoid bone and which runs backwards in its own fascial sleeve across the posterior triangle of the neck and which then continues as the inferior belly of the omohyoid muscle to insert into the upper part of the scapula just lateral to the suprascapular notch.

Submandibular (Digastric) Triangle

The anterior and the posterior borders of this triangle are the anterior and the posterior bellies of the digastric muscle with the base being the inferior border of the mandible. The floor of this triangle is formed by the mylohyoid muscle which attaches inferiorly on to the mandible in front and more superiorly at the rear. These points create a particular complexity. The simpler aspect of this is that the mylohyoid forms an oral diaphragm by running downwards, forwards and medially to join to its fellow on the opposite side as a fibrous raphe which extends from the symphysis menti down to the top of the body of the hyoid bone. The effect is the creation of a *diaphragma oris* similar to the disposition of the levator ani or pelvic diaphragm in the pelvis. The other point here is our appreciation of the embryology of this triangle in that the name of the digastric is a misnomer. The anterior belly of the digastric is a small muscle that develops with the muscles of the first branchial arch and which along with the mylohyoid is innervated by the nerve to the mylohyoid (a part of the motor innervation of the mandibular division of the trigeminal nerve, also referred to as the V3 division or simply V3). The little muscle the anterior belly of the digastric which inserts into a small depression on the lower margin of the mandible (called the digastric fossa) sits on top of the mylohyoid and is also innervated by the nerve to mylohyoid (it does not have a separate nerve name).

By contrast, the posterior belly of the digastric (which inserts into the base of the mastoid process) is derived embryologically with the muscles of the second branchial arch whose compartmental nerve is the facial (VII cranial) nerve and which is combined with other muscles in the region that are innervated by VII including the stylohyoid muscle which splits around the posterior belly of the digastric and attaches to the body of the hyoid bone (in front of the lesser horn). As a consequence, the anterior and the posterior bellies are two separate muscles and fundamentally different parts of the branchial arch formation (first and second arch) and are consequently not part of the same muscle explaining why they have discretely different nerve supplies. Moreover, the difference in the orientation of the mylohyoid (anterior and inferior attachment versus posterior and superior mandibular attachment) means that an infection here (within a wisdom tooth for example) spreads below the mylohyoid and into the submandibular space. Infections confined to the mylohyoid space represent a greater risk to occlusion of the airway and are typically referred to as Ludwig's angina.[2] Within this triangle: are the marginal mandibular branch (MMB) of VII, the facial and the lingual arteries, the submandibular gland, the nerve to mylohyoid, the hypoglossal cranial nerve (XII) and the lower pole of the parotid gland. The surgical point of relevance here is for submandibular gland excision (for stones or less commonly with tumours of the submandibular gland or as part of a suprahyoid neck dissection), taking account of the fact that the MMB of VII lies above a point 2 cm below the mandibular margin. If the incision is continued down on to the fascia overlying the submandibular gland and that layer created is then reflected upwards, the MMB is not injured [2].

Within this submandibular or digastric triangle there is a further subdivision. Diagram 2.4 confirms the main landmarks of this triangle: the lower border of the mandible, the posterior free border of the mylohyoid muscle and the XII running on the surface of the hyoglossus muscle (which is deep to the mylohyoid). Several other small triangles can be identified anatomically in this region. Lesser's triangle (also called the lingual triangle) is a small triangle bounded by the anterior and posterior bellies of the digastric and by the hypoglossal nerve (Diagram 2.5a).[3] The triangle marks the course of the lingual artery with the floor of the triangle being the hyoglossus muscle (the lingual artery lies deep to this muscle). If the triangle is poorly formed or even absent (which occurs in about 10% of the population) the XII cranial nerve may course at a lower level than normal and well below the digastric muscle. This can have implications in the operation of carotid endarterectomy since the XII nerve runs in front of the carotid bifurcation. Pirogov's triangle (also called the hypoglossal

---

[2]First described by Wilhelm Friedrich von Ludwig, (1790–1865) a German physician in 1836.

[3]Named for the German surgeon Ladislaus Lesser (1846–1925).

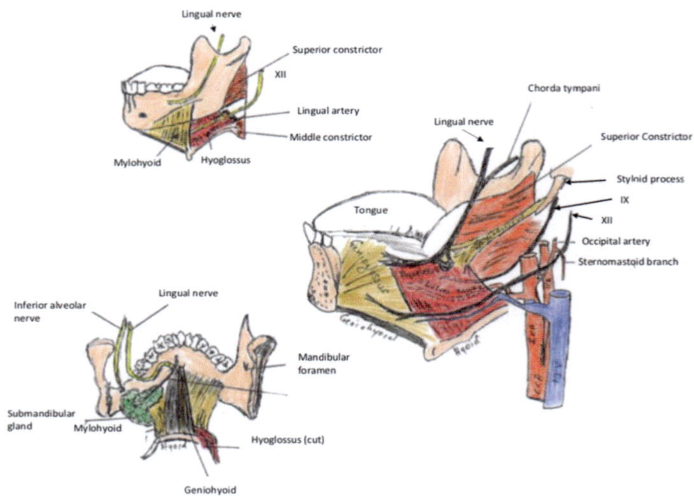

Diagram 2.4 Anatomy of the submandibular triangle
Shows the inner anatomy of the submandibular triangle. The top left sketch shows the free posterior margin of the mylohyoid muscle under which runs the XIIth nerve on top of the hyoglossus. The middle sketch confirms that the hyoglossus separates the XIIth nerve and the lingual artery. Deep to the hyoglossus lies the genioglossus forming the bulk of the tongue. The lingual nerve runs in the same plane as the hypoglossal nerve but at a much higher level. The lingual nerve is attached to the submandibular ganglion transmitting parasympathetic secretomotor (sudomotor) fibres to the submandibular and sublingual salivary glands. The lower left sketch shows how the deep part of the submandibular gland embraces the posterior (free) edge of the mylohyoid and runs deep on top of the hyoglossus. The attachment of the mylohyoid is seen to the mylohyoid line of the mandible
The submandibular duct (Wharton's duct) has the lingual nerve wrapping around initially being superficial but then lying deep to the duct. The relationship is of relevance in excision of the submandibular gland for stones or tumour. Thomas Wharton (1614–1673), English anatomist
IJV Internal Jugular Vein; *ECA* External Carotid Artery; *ICA* Internal Carotid Artery

triangle or Pinaud's triangle) is bound by the XII nerve superiorly, the intermediate tendon of the digastric inferiorly and by the free posterior border of the mylohyoid.[4] Beclard's triangle (Diagram

[4]Named for the Russian surgeon Nikolai Pirogov (1810–1881). This little

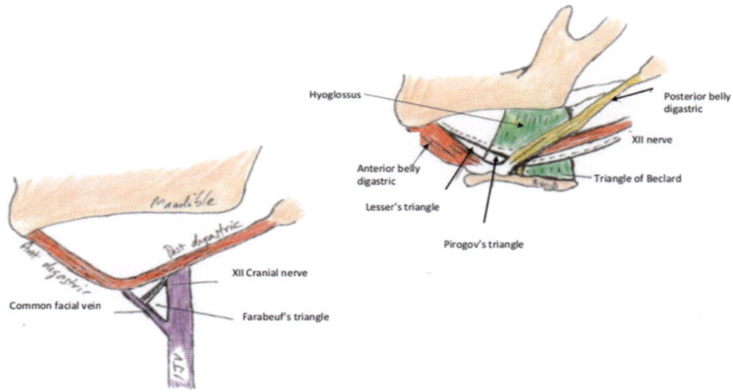

Diagram 2.5 Subtriangles of the neck. (**a**) shows Farabeuf's triangle. (b) shows the Lesser, Pirogov and Beclard subtriangles
Legend: IJV Internal jugular vein

2.5a) is bound by the posterior belly of the digastric, the posterior border of the hyoglossus muscle and the greater horn of the hyoid bone.[5]

Carotid Triangle

The carotid triangle is bordered by the posterior belly of the digastric muscle, the superior belly of the omohyoid and the anterior border of the SCM. The floor of this triangle includes the hyoglossus, the thyrohyoid muscle and the pharyngeal constrictor muscles (the inferior and the middle). The bottom end of this triangle is at the carotid (Chassaignac's tubercle)[6] which is the anterior tubercle of C6 where the common carotid artery (CCA)can be palpated. The level of the carotid bifurcation is normally at the

triangle is really just the posterior part of Lesser's triangle but it is the landmark for a microvascular facial artery anastomosis.

[5]Named after the French anatomist Pierre Beclard (1785–1825).

[6]Named after Édouard-Pierre-Marie Chassaignac (1805–1879), French physician one of the first to use drain tubes in surgery.

C3/4 vertebra. This is important because on occasion the bifurcation is overly high and this can make access in a carotid endarterectomy difficult since the clamp on the internal carotid artery (ICA) becomes difficult to place. In this case if the artery bifurcates high this area can be approached by dividing the posterior belly of the digastric muscle or by expanding the space against the side of the pharynx by blindly pushing and fracturing the styloid process. The only other way of getting into this space is by partially dislocating (or subluxing) the temporomandibular joint (TMJ) on that side.

The external carotid artery (ECA) is the only artery here with branches and is an important identifier of the ICA which tends to lie at a slightly deeper and more medial level as it lies directly against the pharyngeal wall. The branches of the ECA in this triangle include the superior thyroid, the lingual and the facial and posteriorly the occipital. The ascending pharyngeal artery (which by some is regarded as the first branch of the ECA rather than the superior thyroid artery), comes off the inner border of the ECA. The XII cranial nerve travels directly across the bifurcation of the CCA with its component parts of the ansa cervicalis (part of the cervical plexus which innervates the infrahyoid muscles, the thyrohyoid, the sternohyoid and the sternothyroid) and which carries fibres from C1 along with XII to the geniohyoid muscle. Both the external laryngeal branch and the internal laryngeal branch of the superior laryngeal nerve (a branch of the Xth cranial nerve, the Vagus) are in this triangle and these are both identified arising from X medial to the ECA just below the hyoid bone. (These nerves are considered in the next chapter on the neck viscera and in Chap. 15 on the larynx).

In small print we also notice a separate small sub-triangle in the carotid triangle called Farabeuf's triangle (Diagram 2.5b)[7] which includes the boundaries of the internal jugular vein (IJV), the common facial vein and XII with the base of this triangle directed superiorly [3]. The relationship of the common facial vein can thus be either above or below the common carotid bifur-

[7]Named for the French surgeon Louis-Hubert Farabeuf (1841–1910).

cation (again of clinical importance in the approach to the ICA in a carotid endarterectomy, or in neck trauma, or the approach to a carotid body tumour). This point is also the location of a jugulodigastric node which can on occasion be the clinical presentation of a carcinoma of either the palate or the palatine tonsil. The common facial vein needs formal ligation in a radical neck dissection that preserves the IJV.

The Muscular Triangle

The anterior border of this triangle is the midline running from the hyoid bone down to the sternum. The posterior border is the anterior edge of the SCM and the posterosuperior border is the superior belly of the omohyoid muscle. The triangle includes the infrahyoid muscles, the sternohyoid (the round-shaped muscle at the front) and the sternothyroid (the flatter deeper muscle often adherent to the pretracheal fascia overlying the thyroid gland) as well as the omohyoid (more laterally) and the thyrohyoid muscle (more superiorly). The superior thyroid artery, the anterior jugular veins (and frequently a connecting vein between both sides called the jugular arch) along with a leash of delicate inferior thyroid veins are all located in this muscular triangle as are small branches of the ansa cervicalis. These veins are important as they are sometimes in the way (and require ligation) when performing a tracheostomy (which can be on occasion an emergency procedure). Lymph nodes in this muscular triangle include the anterior cervical, infrahyoid, prelaryngeal, thyroid, Delphian, pretracheal and paratracheal nodes, none of which are really separately identifiable but which are positionally named [4]. The most medial part of this triangle includes the cervical trachea, the cervical oesophagus, the thyroid gland and part of the larynx.

Submental Triangle

This is a triangle located at the floor of the mouth and bound by the anterior bellies of the digastric on both sides and by the body of the hyoid bone. The floor of this triangle is the floor of the mouth, (notably the mylohyoid muscle) and this small region contains the submental group of lymph nodes which drain the mental region, the apex of the tongue (where carcinomas drain bilaterally), the lower lip and the incisor teeth. The anterior jugular veins form in this area and there is also a submental branch of the facial artery that traverses this region. If the anterior belly of the digastric is vestigial or absent, then infections of the central and/or lateral incisor teeth can drain directly into this area across the mentalis muscle.

Posterior Triangle of the Neck

This triangle is broadly bound by the posterior border of the SCM anteriorly, the anterior border of the trapezius muscle posteriorly and the middle third of the clavicle inferiorly. The floor is the prevertebral muscles and the area is covered by the investing layer of the deep cervical fascia (*see below*). From below upwards the muscles visible are the scalenus anterior, the levator scapulae, the splenius and the semispinalis. The posterior triangle is subdivided into the occipital and the supraclavicular (subclavian) triangles [5]. The divider of this region is the omohyoid muscle. This triangle contains the spinal accessory nerve (XI), the inferior deep and transverse cervical nodes, the suprascapular and subclavian arteries and more superficially the external jugular vein (EJV) along with components of the cervical plexus (the great auricular nerve, the transverse cervical nerve and the medial, intermediate and lateral branches of the supraclavicular nerves). In this territory we also encounter branches of the thyrocervical trunk (arising from the first portion of the subclavian artery) which include the transverse cervical, the inferior thyroid and the suprascapular artery. The Inferior thyroid artery can be considered the compartment artery of this region of the neck as it is the principal blood supply of the cervical trachea and oesophagus. It is a critical vessel to preserve in a cervical oesophageal anastomosis, since it is the main anastomotic blood supply.

Prior to accurate fine-needle aspiration cytology (FNAC) for neck masses, biopsy of a posterior triangle node used to be a common procedure left on operating lists to junior doctors and was associated with a significant incidence of XI nerve injury. The landmark for this nerve is that it runs under the investing layer of deep cervical fascia from the junction of the top 1/3 and the lower 2/3 of the SCM to the lower 1/3 and the upper 2/3 of the trapezius. In 3D, one can imagine it running in the line drawn from the tip of the mastoid to the tip of the shoulder [6]. Anatomical structures encountered in this region include the common facial vein, the IJV (and its tributaries here, the middle thyroid vein and the superior thyroid vein), the XIth cranial nerve, the transverse cervical nerve, the XIIth cranial nerve and the ansa cervicalis. Location of the junction of the middle thyroid vein with the IJV is the first vessel that needs to be ligated in a thyroidectomy so that the thyroid lobe can lifted up and mobilized.

Occipital Triangle

This subtriangle is in the superior part of the posterior triangle with the inferior border as the inferior belly of the omohyoid. The floor of this triangle is as already stated, the prevertebral muscles including the levator scapulae, the splenius capitis, the semispinalis capitis (very high up) and more inferiorly the scalenus posterior and the scalenus medius. The XI nerve runs on the surface of the levator scapulae with cutaneous (and muscular) branches of the cervical plexus appearing like the spokes of a wheel coming from the back of the SCM. Superficially, the spokes of the cervical plexus include the supraclavicular, transverse cervical, great auricular and lesser occipital nerves (Diagram 2.6). This is strictly slightly different from Erb's point[8] where the C5 and C6 trunks

[8]A point located halfway along the posterior border of the sternocleidomastoid where the cutaneous branches of the cervical plexus (greater auricular—C2,3, transverse cutaneous nerve of the neck—C2,3, lesser occipital -C2 and supraclavicular nerves -C3,4) radiate out like the spokes of a wheel. Wilhelm Heinrich Erb (1840–1921), German neurologist.

join to form the upper trunk of the brachial plexus and which is just above where these trunks divide into anterior and posterior divisions [7]. A brachial plexus injury at or beyond this point is potentially reparable and may be tested by ascertaining whether branches from the nerve roots (the dorsal scapular nerve supplying the rhomboids, the long thoracic nerve to the serratus anterior muscle and the connection to the paravertebral sympathetic chain) are intact [8].

Supraclavicular Triangle

This triangle has relevance in vascular trauma as well as in subclavian vascular disease and the surgical approach towards supraclavicular lymph nodes which can be a sign of metastatic carcinoma (the so-called Virchow's node[9] or Troisier's sign[10]). In this triangle the superior border is the inferior margin of the inferior belly of the omohyoid. This area (also referred to as the supraclavicular fossa) contains the subclavian artery and vein and the supraclavicular part of the brachial plexus providing the roots and trunks (before it forms anterior and posterior divisions behind the clavicle). This region also includes the termination of the external jugular vein (EJV) as it enters the subclavian vein and posteriorly there are the suprascapular vessels. The phrenic nerve (the motor component of the cervical plexus) passes here behind the prevertebral fascia from the lateral to the medial aspect of the scalenus anterior muscle in the base of this triangle. Importantly, this triangle may contain the accessory phrenic nerve (APN) which can run anteriorly near the subclavian vein and which can arise from the delicate ansa cervicalis complex or directly from the nerve to subclavius [9]. This APN typically lies lateral to the phrenic nerve and somewhat posteriorly, however, it can run in front of the subclavian vein (or even through it) and can be injured during subclavian vein puncture. It will, when present, usually communicate

[9]Named after Rudolf Virchow (1821–1902) the father of German pathology.

[10]Named after Charles-Emile Troisier (1844–1919) Professor Medicine, Paris.

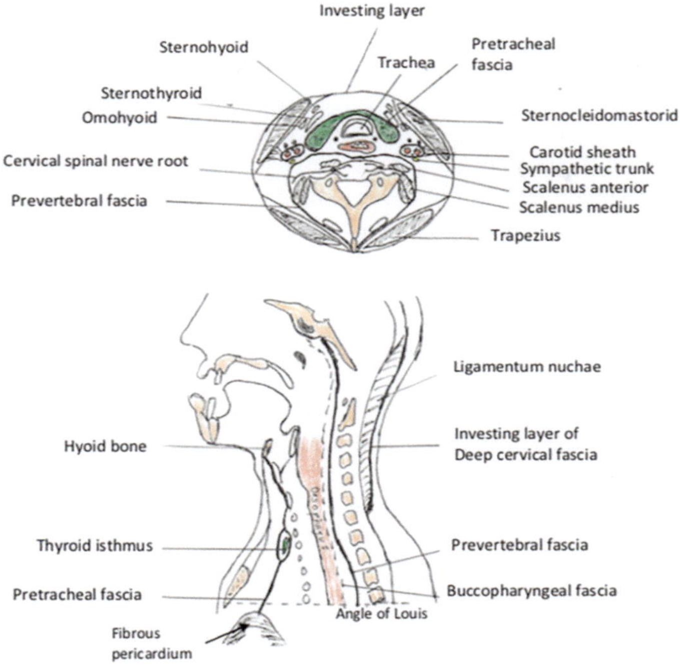

Diagram 2.6 Axial and sagittal views of the cardinal neck fasciae

with the main phrenic nerve in the thorax. The lymph nodes of the supraclavicular triangle drain the inferior larynx, the thyroid gland and even the back of the scalp as the inferior deep cervical nodes.

Clinical Significance of This Triangle

The presence of the Virchow node may be a sign of an intra-abdominal cancer (usually the stomach or the pancreas but also occasionally of the lung, oesophagus and ovary). The supraclavicular triangle can be a site for diseases of the scalp, neck, pectoral and brachial areas as well as the mediastinum, diaphragm, parotid and breast so that it covers a massive area.

Scalene Triangle

The boundaries of this triangle are the lateral border of the scalenus anterior (medially), the medial border of the scalenus medius (laterally) and the first rib inferiorly. This little area critically contains the brachial plexus and the third part of the subclavian artery. There may be neurovascular compressive symptoms which depend on the precise anatomy of this potential space and the presence of a small related muscle the scalenus minimus in the variable presentation of a thoracic outlet syndrome.

Three areas may contribute to this syndrome; namely, the costoclavicular space, the scalene triangle and the pectoralis minor space (also called the retropectoralis minor space or the subpectoralis minor space). This latter space is the lateral most part traversed by the brachial plexus and the adjacent axillary artery and vein passing from the axilla to the thorax. It is a triangle when viewed laterally with its anterior surface the deep part of the pectoralis minor, the posterior wall the subscapularis muscle, the apex the clavicle and the floor the second rib [10]. This area is discussed in Volume 2 of this series on the Upper Limb. In practical terms the expansion of a scalenus minimus muscle, fusion of the scalenus anterior and medius, a fracture of the first rib (which is not an isolated or common feature), an anatomical anomaly such as a cervical rib and a fused first and cervical rib can all result in a thoracic outlet syndrome generated from this region with attendant pressure on the subclavian vessels and the brachial plexus [11].

The Cervical Fasciae: The Fasciae of the Head and Neck

In broad terms the side of the neck is bounded by the clavicle below and above by the lower border of the mandible and extending backwards by the mastoid process of the temporal bone and the superior nuchal line of the occipital bone. Posteriorly this is the origin of the trapezius muscle which then leads back to the posterior triangle of the neck. The upper 3–4 cervical vertebrae are overlapped anteriorly by the facial skeleton. This means that C1 is at the level of the tip of the mastoid process (also at the level of the hard palate) with C2 at the level of the oral cavity and C3 at the level of the junction of the halves of the mandible.

The *investing layer of deep cervical fascia* is an important fascial sleeve that encloses the trapezius muscle and the sternocleidomastoid covering the posterior triangle superficially. The deeper posterior compartment incorporates the vertebral column and the prevertebral muscles as the second cardinal neck fascia, the *prevertebral fascia*. Laterally, this prevertebral fascia covers these muscles forming the deep surface of the posterior triangle and ultimately extending to the erector spinae muscle. This leaves a smaller anterior compartment which houses the pharynx, larynx, upper oesophagus, trachea and the associated muscles (the infrahyoid muscles attached to the hyoid bone, the larynx and the sternum) with on each side the vertical neurovascular bundle of the neck forming the third cardinal cervical fascia—the *carotid sheath* which contains the carotid arteries, (common, internal and external) the internal jugular vein and the Xth cranial nerve (Vagus). This area is innervated by the cervical nerves which supply the skin and muscles of the neck and which form embryologically with the muscles of the tongue. This explains why the XIIth cranial nerve (the hypoglossal) and the cervical plexus are aligned and why parts of C1 transmit nerve fibres to the geniohoid and thyrohyoid muscles and the remainder of the cervical plexus innervates the infrahyoid muscles (which develop with the occipital somites).

The investing layer of deep cervical fascia (which I will refer to from now on as the i*nvesting fascia*) is the homologue of Scarpa's fascia on the thorax and abdomen or of the deep fascia of the limbs. In the neck, the investing fascia does what is says by splitting around the sternomastoid and the trapezius although it is frequently relatively deficient between these muscles as recently shown by Zhang et al. [12]. It attaches to all of the intervening bones along with the ligamentum nuchae and the hyoid bone, creating the dewlap and attaching to the trapezius origin at the external occipital protuberance and thence along the curve of the superior nuchal line to the tip of the mastoid process. The area between the angle of the mandible and the tip of the mastoid process becomes complicated splitting to form the capsule of the parotid gland, with the superficial part of this fascia attached to the zygomatic arch and here as part of the thick *parotid fascia*. The deep part of the parotid capsule so formed extends deep to the parotid gland itself by attaching to the styloid process and creating a specialized part of the fascia called the stylomandibular ligament which connects to the angle of the mandible. Some anatomy texts have also described a thickened continuation of this fascia between the angle of the mandible and the anterior margin of the sternomastoid which has been called the mandibulostylohyoid ligament and which can be traced down to the lower part of the stylohyoid ligament. The thickened parotid fascia confines any form of suppurative parotitis to the parotid gland and prevents such infection spreading to the neck.

Below, the investing layer extends into the pectoral fascia and becomes the *clavipectoral fascia* below the clavicle, attaching posteriorly to the spine of the scapula. Fascia over the sternomastoid also attaches to the clavicle and the manubrium of the sternum. Across the midline this houses the suprasternal notch and space which encloses the anterior jugular veins and the anastomosis between these, the jugular arch. Above the clavicle between the trapezius and the sternomastoid the fascia splits around the inferior belly of the omohyoid muscle binding this intermediate tendon area down to the clavicle and extending behind the clavicle to embrace the subclavius muscle where it is pierced by the external jugular vein (EJV).

The *prevertebral fascia* is as it sounds, a tough membrane that limits the prevertebral muscles and which extends from the base of the skull to the front of the longus capitis and rectus capitis lateralis muscles high in the deep anterior neck down to the limit of the longus colli muscle at the bottom of the third thoracic vertebra. One might not normally be interested in this fascia except that it was the limitation of a prevertebral abscess which originated in the thoracic spine from a chronic thoracic vertebral osteomyelitis. In this sense the definition of the prevertebral fascia is historical. This was the site of chronic tuberculous osteomyelitis also referred to as Pott's disease[11] which was extensively described in the eighteenth and nineteenth centuries and which was relatively common in presentation with the limit of a paraspinal abscess defined by the limits of this fascial sleeve. The prevertebral fascia extends laterally across the scalenus muscles (sc. anterior, medius and posterior) and over the levator scapulae fading out under the trapezius muscle. Further into the posterior triangle the prevertebral fascia attaches to the anterior tubercles of the cervical vertebrae which means that the rami of the brachial plexus lie deep to this fascial sleeve with the regional lymph nodes and the XIth cranial nerve (the spinal accessory nerve) lying superficial to this fascia. The fascia is prolonged over the subclavian vessels as the axillary sheath with the subclavian artery deep and the subclavian vein superficial until these become the axillary vessels (by definition) at the outer border of the first rib. This fascia is pierced by all of the cutaneous branches of the cervical plexus (the greater auricular, the transverse cervical, the lesser occipital and the supraclavicular nerves). It is fair to suggest that the prevertebral fascia provides a fixed basis upon which the pharynx and the larynx and oesophagus as well as the carotid sheaths can glide during movement of the neck as well as during swallowing.

The *pretracheal fascia* allows the pharynx, larynx and thyroid to glide forming a layer between sliding surfaces and lying deep to the infrahyoid muscles (the strap muscles which include the sternohyoid anteriorly, the flatter thinner sternothyroid deeply and laterally the superior belly of the omohyoid). The upward attachment of the pretracheal fascia is limited by the attachments onto the oblique line of the thyroid cartilage of these muscles as well as by the hyoid bone in the midline. This fascia splits around the thyroid gland where the isthmus connects the right and left lobes of the thyroid at the second–fourth tracheal rings. Laterally, the fascia fuses with the carotid sheath and is pierced by the inferior

---

[11] In tuberculosis of the spine, the commonest site is the thoracic spine, with the lumbar spine next and lastly the cervical spine. Sir Percival Pott (1714–1788) was a prominent English surgeon who established the field of orthopaedics.

thyroid artery as this vessel comes up from under the common carotid artery and leads into the lower thyroid pole. These landmarks are used during dissection of the thyroid gland at thyroidectomy. Inferiorly the fascia runs retrosternally into the anterior mediastinum by passing behind the distensible brachiocephalic veins and fusing with the fascia overlying the aortic root and with the fibrous pericardium.

The *Carotid Sheath* is more of a feltwork of areolar tissue rather than a distinct membrane which surrounds the common and internal carotid artery, the IJV and the Xth cranial nerve. It only thinly covers the IJV and runs from the base of the skull at the margins of the carotid canal (petrous temporal bone) and extends to the adventitia of the aorta and aortic arch. Where the carotid fascia runs under the sternomastoid it is adherent to the pretracheal fascia which blends with it. There is a loose areolar tissue lying behind the carotid sheath where the sympathetic trunk lies separately and in front of the prevertebral fascia. Typically in an extensive neck infection, purulent material can potentially track laterally from around the pharynx (for example if a fish bone or chop bone were to perforate the pharynx at this level) and pass behind the carotid sheath to point in the posterior triangle. Within the carotid sheath the common carotid artery (CCA) bifurcates at the level of the thyroid notch (the C3/4 vertebral junction) however, this bifurcation can be much higher and occur at the level of the greater horn of the hyoid bone (body of C3 vertebra). This is of clinical relevance during the operation of carotid endarterectomy where atheroma in the internal carotid artery (ICA) is removed for some patients presenting with a stroke or who are at high risk of a stroke. If the bifurcation is very high, there is limited space to place vascular clamps to control the vessels making access difficult.[12]

[12] In this circumstance, the posterior belly of the digastric muscle may need to be divided to provide a higher access to the ICA. Blind deep fracture of the styloid process will also provide better exposure. In extreme cases, subluxation of the mandible at the temporomandibular joint will expand necessary room.

The axial and sagittal views of these cardinal fasciae are shown in Diagram 2.6.

In addition to these four cardinal fasciae in the neck there are some subordinate fasciae that we need to consider. The fascia which runs between the carotids (the *alar* or *intercarotica* fascia) has a variable thickness and crosses the median plane between the carotid sheaths passing dorsally to the pharynx and fusing laterally with a separate fascia, the *buccopharyngeal fascia* lying behind the pharynx. The alar fascia is frequently separated from the visceral fascia and follows the course of the carotid arteries ventrally away from the visceral organs (the trachea and esophagus). This leaves a continuous retropharyngeal space lying dorsal to the intercarotid fascia, the so-called called "danger space" immediately in front of the prevertebral space between the alar and the prevertebral divisions of the deep layer of the deep cervical fascia that extends from the base of the skull through the posterior mediastinum and down to the level of the diaphragm. This danger space is so named because of its propensity to produce a descending necrotizing inflammatory mediastinitis first reported in 1938 by Pearse [13].[13]

Spread of infection from the neck to the mediastinum may therefore happen by: 1: spread along the pretracheal route to the anterior mediastinum (the same route a retrosternal goitre grows), 2: via the lateral pharyngeal route to the middle mediastinum and 3: via the retropharyngeal route and the so-called ***danger space*** (breaking through the alar fascia) into the posterior mediastinum. The nature of this infective mediastinitis as it is referred to has been graded into a Type 1, (localized to the upper mediastinum above the tracheal bifurcation), a Type 2A (extending to the lower anterior mediastinum) and Type 2B (extending to both the anterior and the posterior mediastinum) [14]. These fascial spaces are shown in axial and sagittal sections in Diagram 2.7a, b.

---

[13]Herman Pearse (1900–1983) was Professor of Surgery at Rochester New York and was a specialist hepatobiliary surgeon who worked with Robert Oppenheimer on the Manhattan Project. He researched the radiation burn effects of the atomic bomb.

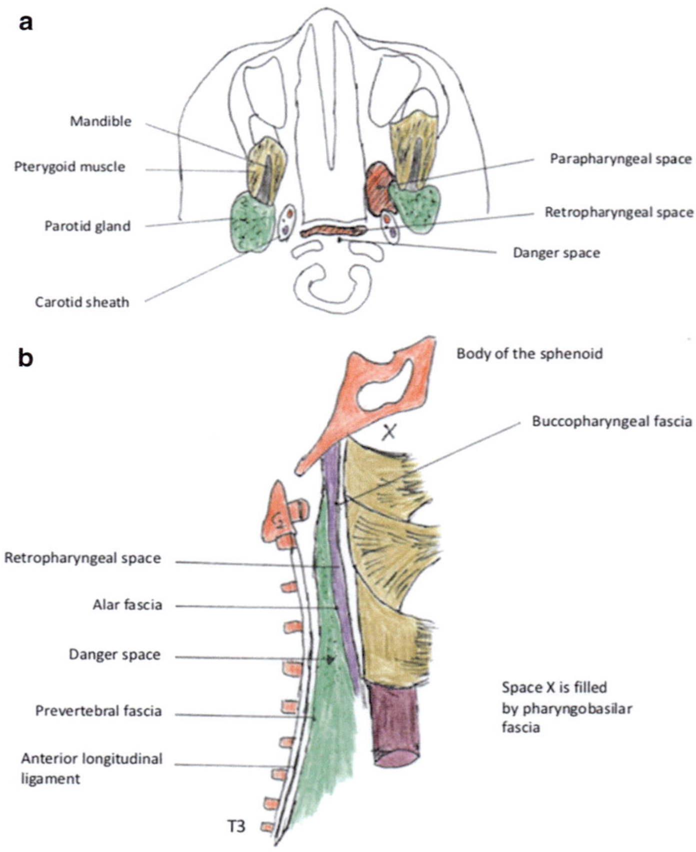

Diagram 2.7 Axial and sagittal views to demonstrate the deep fascial spaces that may transmit sepsis

(**a**) Axial view demonstrating the retropharyngeal space behind the alar fascia.

(**b**) Sagittal view. X is the space between the skull base and the origin of the superior constrictor filled in by pharyngobasilar fascia

There are two *other fasciae of relevance* in the Head and Neck which are often forgotten. The *first is the pharyngobasilar fascia* which fills the space between the base of the skull and the upper border of the pharynx (formed at this point by the superior constrictor muscle which hangs off the skull base like a hammock). This layer of fascia may be considered as a dense specialized thickening of the submucosa of the pharynx running on the inside of the musculature which can be traced down to the level of the soft palate. In effect, it is effectively the fourth layer stacked inside the three pharyngeal constrictors (inferior, middle and superior) which themselves are all stacked inside each other like a series of flowerpots. The fascia runs along all of the pharyngeal contours starting from the pharyngeal tubercle (the uppermost bony attachment point) in front of the foramen magnum to which the midline thickening of pharyngeal muscle fusion called the pharyngeal raphé is also attached. The fascia then passes over the top of the longus capitis muscle and the posterior margin of the foramen lacerum at the skull base up to the petrous part of the temporal bone just in front of the carotid canal. From there it is adherent to the cartilaginous portion of the auditory (pharyngotympanic or Eustachian) tube,[14] the sharp posterior border of the medial pterygoid plate and down on to the bulbous swelling at the bottom end of the plate (the pterygoid hamulus).

Similar to the superior constrictor, the pharyngobasilar fascia is suspended from the skull base but also from one medial pterygoid plate to the other where it is reinforced posteriorly by the pharyngeal raphé and designed to hold the nasopharynx permanently open for breathing. The lower edge of the fascia lies at the level recognized as Passavant's ridge which is conceptually level where the hard palate can abut against the pharyngeal wall. This ridge forms a functional muscular/fascial purse string that is designed to close off the nasopharynx during swallowing.

[14]The auditory tube equalizes the atmospheric pressure between the middle ear and the pharynx. It is discussed later in this volume. It was named after Bartolomeo Eustachi (1500?–74) an Italian surgeon and anatomist who described cardinal anatomy of the kidney, the hearing apparatus, the teeth and the circulation.

Clinical Relevance of This Area

The cartilaginous portion of the auditory tube entering the nasopharynx lies above the pharyngobasilar fascia but is adherent to it. There is a small triangular area (called the sinus of Morgagni) which forms above the hammock of the superior constrictor filled by the fascia and which also transmits the IXth cranial nerve (glossopharyngeal), the levator palati muscle, the ascending palatine artery and the palatine branch of the ascending pharyngeal artery.[15] The sinus of Morgagni is a lateral extension (or recess of the pharynx called the fossa of Rosenmüller) that extends across the base of the petrous temporal bone in front of the carotid canal. It gives origin to the levator palati muscle, making the muscle entirely intrapharyngeal.[16] A nasopharyngeal carcinoma located here can extend laterally to involve this sinus and also infiltrate the mandibular division of the trigeminal (Vth cranial) nerve running through the foramen ovale anteriorly causing Trotter's triad (conductive deafness from Eustachian tube obstruction, ipsilateral immobility of the soft palate (IX paralysis) and trigeminal neuralgia.[17]

The second other fascia of importance in the head and neck is the *buccopharyngeal fascia*. This fascia lies on the opposing surface of the pharyngeal constrictor to the pharyngobasilar fascia, forming a loose layer over the buccinator muscle and fusing with the periosteum on the posterior alveolar surface of the maxilla and the inner plate of the pterygoid process. The buccopharyngeal fascia is a connector between the superficial and deep fasciae and has

[15]Giovanni Battista Morgagni (1682–1771) was one of the most prominent eighteenth century anatomists whose book *De Sedibus et Causus Morborum per anatomem indigatis* (5 vols) established the discipline of anatomical (morbid) anatomy through the use of autopsy to define the organic effects of disease.

[16]Named after Johann Christian Rosenmuller (1771–1820) an Associate Professor of Anatomy and University Rector at Leipzig.

[17]Named after Sir Wilfred Louis Batten Trotter (1972–1939) Professor of Surgery at University College Hospital London. Trotter successfully performed a rib resection for empyema on King George V and was also consulted about the management of a recurrent oral cancer in Sigmund Freud.

connection to the tunica adventitia of the oesophagus. It forms part of the pterygomandibular raphe which runs down from the hamulus to the posterior edge of the mylohyoid line. Running forwards from this raphé is the buccinator muscle and backwards the superior constrictor [15].

To summarize:

The *investing layer*, *pretracheal* and *prevertebral* fasciae form components that are divisible into external, middle and deep layers. The middle layer (pretracheal) can also be divided into a muscular and a visceral layer. The deep fascia is superficial to the superficial cervical fascia which is an integral part of the subcutaneous tissue investing the platysma muscle. The attachment of the investing layer is to the ligamentum nuchae and vertebral spines and across the front to the hyoid bone coursing around the submandibular gland near the inferior surface of the mandible. In the suprahyoid area the layers invest the digastric and stylohyoid muscles with an extension coursing superiorly to envelop the parotid gland (as the parotid fascia or capsule) until it then extends from the mastoid process and on to the superior nuchal line.

The visceral division of the pretracheal fascia contains within it the thyroid and parathyroid glands and incorporates the trachea and the oesophagus. Superiorly this attaches to the thyroid cartilage with the posterior segment of this fascia extending between the carotid sheaths and running behind the oesophagus and the lateral lobes of the thyroid gland where it is referred to as the buccopharyngeal fascia because of its anatomic relationship to the pharynx and the buccinator muscle. Behind this fascia (and anterior to the alar fascia) is the retropharyngeal space which continues inferiorly as the covering of the trachea and the oesophagus. Posterior to the alar fascia (and anterior to the prevertebral fascia) lies the danger space. The buccopharyngeal and alar fasciae join one another inferiorly at the T1/T2 vertebral level [16]. Spaces can be considered as artificially divisible by the hyoid bone. There are spaces spanning the entire neck which include the retropharyngeal space, the danger space, the prevertebral space and the space within the carotid sheath. Those spaces bound inferiorly by the hyoid bone include the submandibular, pharyngomaxillary, masticator, parotid and peritonsillar spaces. Diagrams are attached to this section for the student to practice explaining the fasciae and neck spaces mentioned above that have clinical relevance in the spread of head and neck sepsis. Diagrams 2.6 and 2.7 show the axial and sagittal disposition of individual fasciae.

Q and A: Chap. 2 (Answers at the End of This Chapter)

1. The alar fascia of the neck:
   (a) Extends down to the diaphragm
   (b) Runs in front of the carotid sheath
   (c) Is retropharyngeal
   (d) Finishes at the level of the T3 thoracic vertebra at the insertion of the longus colli
2. The digastric triangle of the neck:
   (a) Has both of its borders formed by the digastric bellies
   (b) Has the hyoglossus muscle as its floor
   (c) Is solely innervated by the VII nerve
   (d) Arises from the third branchial arch
   (e) Is the point of commencement of Ludwig's angina
3. The carotid triangle:
   (a) Has as its floor the superior constrictor muscle
   (b) Lies above Chassaignac's tubercle
   (c) Has the bifurcation of the common carotid artery usually at the C4/5 junction
   (d) Is divisible into Farabeuf's triangle
   (e) Lies below the jugulodigastric lymph node
4. The investing layer of cervical fascia:
   (a) Is in continuity with the clavipectoral fascia
   (b) Is separable from the parotid fascia
   (c) Forms a sling around the omohyoid muscle
   (d) Covers the posterior triangle musculature which runs from the scalenus anterior, the levator scapulae, the splenius and the semispinalis
   (e) Is separable from the mandibulostylohyoid ligament

5. The pharyngobasilar fascia
   (a) Fills the space between the base of the skull and the upper pharyngeal musculature
   (b) Runs along the outside of the pharyngeal musculature
   (c) Attaches to the base of the skull behind the foramen lacerum and the behind the carotid canal
   (d) Leaves the origin of the levator palati muscle excluded from the pharynx
6. The digastric triangle of the neck:
   (a) Has both of its borders formed by the digastric bellies
   (b) Has the hyoglossus muscle as its floor
   (c) Is solely innervated by the VII nerve
   (d) Arises from the third branchial arch
   (e) Is the point of commencement of Ludwig's angina
7. The carotid triangle:
   (a) Has as its floor the thyrohyoid muscle
   (b) Lies above Chassaignac's tubercle
   (c) Has the bifurcation of the common carotid artery at the C4/5 junction
   (d) Is divisible into Farabeuf's triangle
   (e) Lies below the jugulodigastric lymph node
8. The investing layer of cervical fascia
   (a) Is in continuity with the clavipectoral fascia
   (b) Is separable from the parotid fascia
   (c) Forms a sling around the omohyoid muscle
   (d) Covers the posterior triangle musculature which runs from the scalenus anterior, the levator scapulae, the splenius and the semispinalis
   (e) Is separable from the mandibulostylohyoid ligament

Answers

1. a
2. a
3. d
4. a, c, e

5. a
6. b
7. d
8. a, c

References

1. Li J, Han Z. Sternocleidomastoid muscle flap used for repairing dead space after supraomohyoid neck dissection. Int. J Clin Exp Med. 2015;8(1):1296–300. PMID: 25785129 PMCID: PMC4358584. **This article suggests that transposing the sternocleidomastoid origin over the carotid vessels fills in the dead space of a Level II lymph node dissection below the lower pole of the parotid gland which can leak salivary fluid. Muscle transposition is associated with less superficial space infection whilst protecting the vasculature. Transposition relies on a fairly constant blood supply to the upper part via the occipital artery.**

References for Section "Triangles of the Neck"

2. Davies JC, Ravichandiran M, Agur AM, Fattah A. Evaluation of clinically relevant landmarks of the marginal mandibular branch of the facial nerve: a three-dimensional study with application to avoiding facial nerve palsy. Clin Anat. 2016;29:151–6.
3. See Tubbs RS, Rasmussen M, Loukas M, Shoja M, Mortazavi M, Cohen-Gadol AA. Use of the triangle of Farabeuf for neurovascular procedures of the neck. Biomed Int. 2011;2:39–42.
The Delphian node typically lies in the midline at cricothyroid level just above the thyroid isthmus. It is a metastatic node for a laryngeal squamous cell cancer or a thyroid cancer and is so called after the Oracle of Delphi who predicted ancient Greek prophesies. Clearance of this part of the muscular triangle is often not adequately performed in a radical neck dissection. [Oh E, Chung Y, Lee Y. Clinical significance of Delphian lymph node metastasis in papillary thyroid carcinoma. World J Surg. 2013;37(11):2594–9. https://doi.org/10.1007/s00268-013-2157-8].
4. In some textbooks the subclavian triangle is also the omoclavicular triangle.
5. See Cesmebasi A, Spinner RJ. An anatomic-based approach to the iatrogenic spinal accessory nerve injury in the posterior cervical triangle. How to avoid and treat it. Clin Anat 2015;28:761–6 and also Tubbs RS, Salter EG, Wellons JC 3rd., Blount JP, Oakes WJ. Superficial landmarks for the

spinal accessory nerve within the posterior cervical triangle. J Neurosurg Spine. 2005;3:375–8.
6. This point was described by Wilhelm Erb (1840–1921) using electrical stimulation experiments.
7. This area is discussed in detail in Volume 2 of this series on the Upper Limb.
8. Graves MJ, Henry BM, Hsieh WC, Sanna B, Pekala PA, Iwanaga J, Loukas M, Tomaszewski KA. Origin and prevalence of the accessory phrenic nerve: a meta-analysis and clinical appraisal. Clin Anat. 2017;30:1077–82.
9. Rusnak-Smith S, Moffat M, Rosen E. Anatomical variations of the scalene triangle: dissection of 10 cadavers. J Orthop Sports Phys Ther 2001; 31: 70–80 and also Klaasen Z, Sorensen E, Tubbs RS, Arya R, Meloy P, Shah R, Shirk S, Loukas M. Thoracic outlet syndrome: a neurologic and vascular disorder. Clin Anat 2014;27:724–32.
10. Kikuta S, Iwanaga J, Kusukawa J, Tubbs RS. Triangles of the neck: a review with clinical/surgical applications. Anat Cell Biol. 2019;52:120–7. **[This article provides a clinical overview of the importance of the neck triangles]**

References for Section "The Cervical Fasciae: The Fasciae of the Head and Neck"

11. Zhang M, Lee ASJ. The investing layer of the deep cervical fascia does not exist between the sternocleidomastoid and trapezius muscle. Otolaryngol Head Neck Surg. 2002;127:452–74.
12. Pearse HE. Mediastinitis following cervical suppuration. Ann Surg. 1938;108:588–611.
13. Pinto A, Scaglione M, Scuderi MG, Tortora G, Daniele S, Romano L. Infections of the neck leading to descending necrotizing mediastinitis: role of multi-detector row computed tomography. Eur J Radiol. 2008;65:389–94.
14. Feigl G, Hammer GP, Litz R, Kachlik D. The intercarotid or alar fascia, other cervical fascias and their adjacent spaces—a plea for clarification of cervical fascia and spaces terminology. J Anat. 2020;237:197–207.
15. Gavid M, Dumollard JM, Habougit C, Lelonge Y, Bergvandi F, Peoc'h M, Prades JM. Anatomical and histological study of the deep neck fasciae: does the alar fascia exist? Surg Radiol Anat. 2018;40:917–22.

The Neck Viscera: Thyroid, Parathyroids and Salivary Glands

3

Contents

The Infrahyoid Musculature: (The Strap Muscles)........ 35
The Thyroid Gland........ 39
Recurrent Laryngeal Nerve........ 46
Lymphatic Drainage........ 51
Nerve Supply........ 51
The Parathyroid Glands........ 51
Salivary Glands........ 53
Parotid Gland (See Diagram 3.5)........ 53
Submandibular Gland (Diagram 3.6)........ 62
Q and A: Chap. 3 (Answers at the End of This Chapter)........ 68
Answers........ 69
References........ 70

These glands, (thyroid and parathyroid), are located in the lower part of the anterior triangle of the neck encased by the infrahyoid muscles (sternohyoid and sternothyroid). The hyoid bone and its supra- and infrahyoid muscles are partially covered in this chapter but also in the chapters on the mouth and larynx.

One place to begin in this chapter is to consider how a knowledge of anatomy and the cervical fasciae (as discussed in Chap. 2) plays into the procedure of a thyroidectomy. Before we discuss the specific anatomy of the thyroid gland, we can recognize that the surgical approach is via a suprasternal incision (one finger breadth above the suprasternal notch) and proceeds through the subcutaneous tissue, the platysma and then the investing layer of

A. Zbar, *Anatomy--Head and Neck*,
https://doi.org/10.1007/978-3-031-69538-4_3

deep cervical fascia. Once in this plane under the investing layer of deep cervical fascia a top flap of all layers is lifted up as far as the level of the tracheal notch superiorly with the lower flap lifted downwards as far as the clavicles and the sternoclavicular joints inferiorly. The aim in this operation is then to find the midline between the two bellies of the sternohyoid muscles where there is only loose areolar tissue and no small bridging vessels. These sternohyoid muscles are then separated. Pulling off the much flatter and thinner strands of the sternothyroid muscle beneath which is usually moderately adherent to the gland. The gland lies in its pretracheal fascia and is made more clearly evident (i.e one enters the correct operative plane) as the veins on the surface of the thyroid enlarge and as the facia is peeled away.

For mobilization of the lateral aspect of the gland and so that it can be prolapsed and rotated into the wound, there is usually a short but relatively wide middle thyroid vein seen exiting the middle part of the lobe and running straight across to the internal jugular vein (IJV). This small vein needs to be formally ligated. After this, the finger can readily be passed around the thyroid lobe and it can usually be elevated. Any bleeding may occur in the lower end of the wound dependent upon the arrangement of the anterior jugular veins (AJV). These begin in the submental space and travel down in the investing layer of deep cervical fascia often with a small jugular venous arch connection in the suprasternal space before emptying into the external jugular vein (EJV) on both sides. These veins (and the thyroid isthmus between the lobes of the thyroid) have clinical significance as they may obstruct the view necessary (before their ligation) for the performance of an emergency or an elective tracheostomy. The AJV typically pierces the investing layer about the mid-level of the sternocleidomastoid (SCM) muscle and lies slightly behind it to join the EJV. There is variability as the AJV can on occasion replace the EJV (or rather there may be only one midline AJV and a composite relationship between the AJV and the EJV). In the circumstance where there is a median vein replacement this runs anterior to the SCM and there is no traditional EJV.

In this region from above downwards there are a few landmarks:

- The median thyrohyoid ligament: This is part of the thyroglossal apparatus connecting the inferior and posterior surfaces of the body of the hyoid bone to the upper edge of the thyroid cartilage. It is of importance in removal of a thyroglossal cyst and fistula (the Sistrunk's operation covered later in this chapter).

- The laryngeal prominence, notch, Adam's apple
- The cricothyroid ligament: along with the only extrinsic visible laryngeal muscle on the external surface of the larynx (the cricothyroid muscle).
- The isthmus of the thyroid gland: This is a constant but variable depth bridge of tissue joining the thyroid lobes over the second–fourth tracheal rings and which may need division during a tracheostomy. Note also that the left thyroid lobe (more commonly) is attached to a small extension of thyroid tissue (called the pyramidal lobe) that is adherent to the hyoid by a small muscle the *levator glandulae thyroidea* which is embryologically derived from the region of the foramen caecum (a developmental pit between the anterior 2/3 and the posterior 1/3 of the tongue).

The Infrahyoid Musculature: (The Strap Muscles)

These muscles are innervated via the cervical plexus through its ansa cervicalis (see Chap. 4). Nerve fibres from the C1 ventral root are transmitted along the hypoglossal nerve (Cranial XII) to innervate one of the suprahyoid muscles (geniohyoid) and one of the infrahyoid muscles (thyrohyoid). In the innervation of the infrahyoids, the nerves typically enter from the ansa cervicalis at a low level so that in very large thyroid masses where these muscles need to be divided in order to deliver the mass, they can be cut relatively high up in order to gain more room but resulting in less risk of their denervation. These infrahyoid muscles form from the prevertebral cervical myotomes and are normally supplied segmentally from above downwards with small tendinous intersections that are somewhat similar in appearance to the rectus abdominis. As these muscles are all in the same plane as other vertical strip muscles, they include those running from the chin—the suprahyoid muscles (the anterior and posterior bellies of the digastric, the stylohyoid, the mylohyoid and the geniohoid), the infrahyoid muscles (sternohyoid, sternothyroid, omohyoid and thyrohyoid). They would be embryologically continuous with the rectus abdominis and only interrupted by the thoracic cage forming a continuous sheet from the chin to the pubis innervated by C1-T12. In some patients (about 5% of dissected cadavers) this is completed by an anterior costal strip of similarly disposed muscle in the midline of the front of the chest called the rectus sternalis which when present fuses with the sternal tendon of the SCM). The muscle orientation is shown in Diagram 3.1.

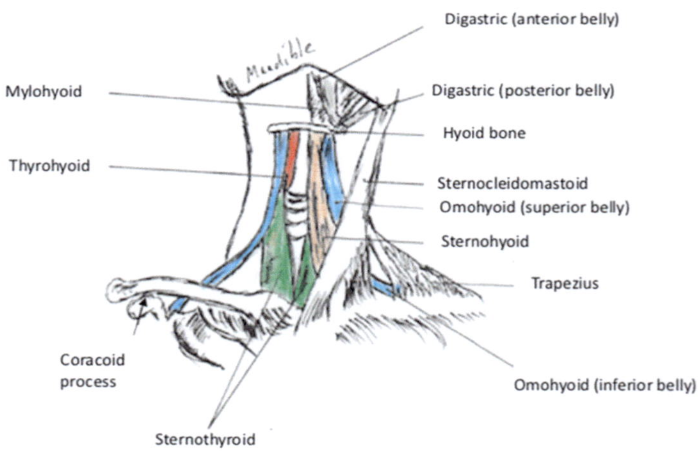

Diagram 3.1 The infrahyoid musculature. On the right the superficial muscles have been removed. Omohyoid (blue) is divided into a superior and an inferior belly (note the attachment to the upper margin of the scapula next to the suprascapular notch). Sternohyoid (brown), Sternothyroid (green), and thyrohyoid (red). The suprahyoid muscles include the mylohyoid (marked) and the anterior and posterior bellies of the digastric (grey)

Sternohyoid This muscle takes origin from the central aspect of the lower border of the hyoid bone and inserts into the bone at the back of the sternoclavicular joint (SCJ) and on to a variable part of the manubrium and even the clavicle. These two muscles which lie edge to edge at the hyoid diverge from one another and are rather rounded in cross section.

Omohyoid This muscle is more laterally located and arises from the lower border of the hyoid bone. The omohyoid is not usually exposed in a thyroidectomy. It passes laterally under the SCM and over the carotid sheath and the IJV where there is a central tendon (similar in appearance and glide to that which attaches the bellies of the digastric muscle). The inferior belly of the omohyoid then runs down and away from the central tendon crossing posteriorly in the supraclavicular triangle to attach to part of the transverse scapular ligament overlying the suprascapular notch. The intermediate tendon of the omohyoid has a double sleeve of investing cervical fascia and when cut as part of a neck dissection for cervical lymphadenectomy (in squamous oropharyngeal/laryngeal carcinoma or melanoma for example), the cut muscle retracts back towards the scapula. The omohyoid creates the lower divisions of the neck triangles (as discussed in Chap. 2) and is a useful landmark for the IJV and common carotid artery (CCA).

Thyrohyoid This is a shorter flatter muscle which is under cover of the sternohyoid muscle and also the omohyoid, The thyrohyoid arises from the lower margin of the greater horn (or cornua) of the hyoid bone to run down to the oblique lamina of the thyroid cartilage and which is end to end in its insertion with the origin of the sternothyroid. The thyrohyoid receives its nerve supply via Cranial XII but as described above by C1 fibres which hitchhike fibres in the superior root of the ansa cervicalis. The thyrohyoid covers the entry point of the internal laryngeal nerve (which provides sensation above the larynx and which travels through the thyrohyoid membrane with branches of the superior laryngeal artery. This artery (also called the infrahyoid artery) is a prominent branch of the superior thyroid artery. The internal laryngeal nerve is a branch of the superior laryngeal branch of the Vagus nerve (Cranial X).

Sternothyroid Although it is broader than the sternohyoid, the sternothyroid muscle is flatter and attaches at a lower level on the under surface of the manubrium well below the sternoclavicular joint (and without any clavicular attachment). The sternothyroid will also extend laterally from the manubrial body to the first costal cartilage which may have relevance in the extirpation of large retrosternal goitres. The upper origin of the muscle froms a line with the oblique line of the thyroid cartilage so that the two muscles can be thought of as lying in continuity. The sternothryoid neural supply is via C2/3 the lower root (*descendens hypoglossi*) of the ansa cervicalis. The attachment of the muscle on the thyroid cartilage is superficial to the pretracheal fascia and in front of the cricothyroid muscle with the sternothyroid lying anterior to the great vessels of the upper thorax and the root of the neck in front of the thyroid gland.

These infrahyoid muscles are all extrinsic laryngeal depressors with only the sternothyroid acting directly on the thyroid cartilage. Depression of the larynx increases the volume of resonation and is dynamically opposed by the laryngeal elevators (mylohyoid, palatopharyngeus, stylopharyngeus, salpingopharyngeus, inferior constrictor) each of which assists in preventing ascent of the hyoid bone during movement of the digastric. The latter muscle effectively fixes the base of the hyoid bone for the tongue. These depressors also help maintain the natural distance between the thyroid cartilage and the hyoid bone (where the larynx is drawn towards the hyoid via the thyrohyoid muscle in the early phase of swallowing) with depression of the larynx via the sternohyoid in the last phase of swallowing.

One final thing we can note when we remember the neck triangles formed is the presence of the anterior (so-called muscular triangle because of the infrahyoid musculature) that is bordered on each side by the SCM, laterally by the superior belly of the omohyoid and limited by the midline.

The Thyroid Gland

A pear-shaped lobe on each side is connected by an isthmus and spans the second–sixth tracheal rings extending as far as the oblique line of the thyroid cartilage. The gland is surrounded by the pretracheal fascia (attached to the arch of the cricoid cartilage) so that all thyroid masses move with swallowing. The thyroid gland is one of the largest endocrine glands with a neonatal weight of 2–3 g but an adult weight of 18–20 g and with approximate dimensions of $4 \times 5 \times 1$ cm. Beneath this pretracheal fascia there is a true thyroid capsule with the vessels extending between these fascial planes. The delicate lobes are moulded around the trachea with the superior thyroid artery accompanied by the external laryngeal nerve at the top and the inferior thyroid artery (ITA) accompanied by the recurrent laryngeal nerve (RLN) in the middle of the gland posteriorly.

The upper lobe lies in direct relationship to the inferior part of the inferior constrictor (also called the thyropharyngeus) and the cricothyroid. Posterior to the gland is the prevertebral fascia anterior to the longus colli muscle with some overlap to the medial part of the carotid sheath. This arrangement creates disposition of a triangular lobe lying on its side with a lateral medial and posterior surface. The lateral surface is tucked up against and beneath the upper end of the sternothyroid preventing any further upward expansion of a thyroid mass. The medial surface hugs the lateral side of the larynx and the trachea with the laryngopharynx and the upper oesophagus behind. At this point the oesophagus is flattened in the AP direction.

In brief, the gland develops as a caudal extension of the thyroglossal duct which arises from the foramen caecum (the junction point between the anterior 2/3 and the posterior 1/3 of the tongue). The thyroid is the first endocrine gland to develop as an outgrowth of the pharynx via the first and second pharyngeal pouches near the base of the tongue. The pharyngeal apparatus is formed by a combination of pharyngeal arches and pharyngeal pouches, pharyngeal grooves and pharyngeal clefts. These form the pharyngeal exterior whereas the pharyngeal interior is formed by the pharyngeal membranes. (An appreciation of these areas explains the development of the face which is covered in Chap. 13 of this volume). There are five pharyngeal (or branchial) arches (with rapid regression of the fifth arch) and four pharyngeal pouches, four pharyngeal grooves and four pharyngeal membranes. The mesoderm of each arch is covered externally by ectoderm and space between branchial arches is called the pharyngeal cleft (or groove). The arch is covered internally by endoderm and inside the space between two arches is called the pharyngeal pouch. This embryological development is shown simply in Diagram 3.2. Specifically, the thyroid develops from the endoderm at the junction of the foramen caecum and with growth progressively descends in front of the developing hyoid and laryngeal cartilages connected to the tongue via the thyroglossal duct. By week 7 of foetal development the gland solidifies and forms two lobes and an isthmus in the adult pattern with regression of the duct and persistence of the pyramidal lobe and attachment to the foramen caecum by the levator glandulae thyroidea smooth muscle. Estimates of the

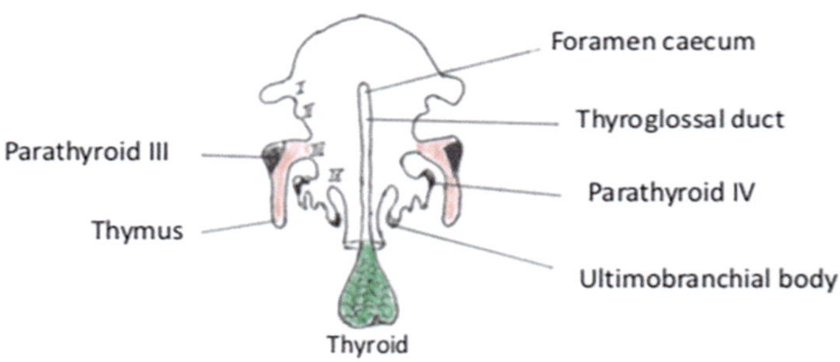

Diagram 3.2 Embryological development of the thyroid and parathyroid glands. The view is the anterior aspect of the pharynx at 4 weeks gestation. The top of the image is cranial towards the buccal cavity and the bottom is caudal towards the developing trachea and oesophagus. The thyroid originates from the foramen caecum and descends vertically forming the right and left lobes. The inferior parathyroids (III) form in the dorsal wing of the third pharyngeal pouch whereas the ventral wing forms the thymus (explaining why the inferior PT glands have the most variable positioning and can be mediastinal). Ectopia of the superior PT glands (IV) is over a smaller range in the neck

incidence of a pyramidal lobe (PL) vary with one 2015 paper in 166 patients finding a PL in 65.7% of cases, the PL being either isthmial or lobar in origin with a propensity to lie on the left-hand side. In this paper the PL was categorized as short (<15 mm), intermediate (15–30 mm) and long (>30 mm in length) [1].

Ectopic thyroid tissue is an anomaly of migration with the commonest type a failure of descent forming a suprahyoid mass. The so-called lingual (or high cervical) thyroid lies close to the tongue with excessive migration leading to mediastinal thyroid ectopia. Functioning thyroid tissue can aberrantly be found in the adrenal and pituitary glands, variably along the GI tract, in the female reproductive system and even in the iris of the eye. Based upon the anatomy of the thyroglossal tract and the levator glandulae thyroideae, most thyroglossal cysts are infrahyoid (25–65%) with about 20–25% suprahyoid masses. These masses typically move when the tongue is poked out (a manoeuvre irrelevant for other thyroid masses). The intimate embryological relationship between the tract and the front and under surface of the hyoid necessitates that the central body of the hyoid bone needs to be removed with the cyst and tract in such procedures. The distance between the foramen caecum and the hyoid is actually very short and during excision of a thyroglossal cyst or fistula, is assisted in the core out of the tract through some of the intrinsic muscle of the tongue by the anaesthetist placing a finger against the foramen caecum territory and pushing downwards. The procedure for *en bloc* removal of this tissue is called the Sistrunk's operation.[1]

Vascular supply of the thyroid gland: (Shown in Diagram 3.3).

- The **superior thyroid artery (STA)** is the first branch of the ECA and runs downward vertically from the CCA bifurcation piercing the pretracheal fascia at the apex of a lobe (with anterior and posterior branches forming a posterior anastomosis with the ITA).
- A separate branch from the left STA can supply the PL.
- The principal relationship of the STA is with the external laryngeal nerve (ELN).

[1] Named after the American surgeon Walter Ellis Sistrunk (1880–1933).

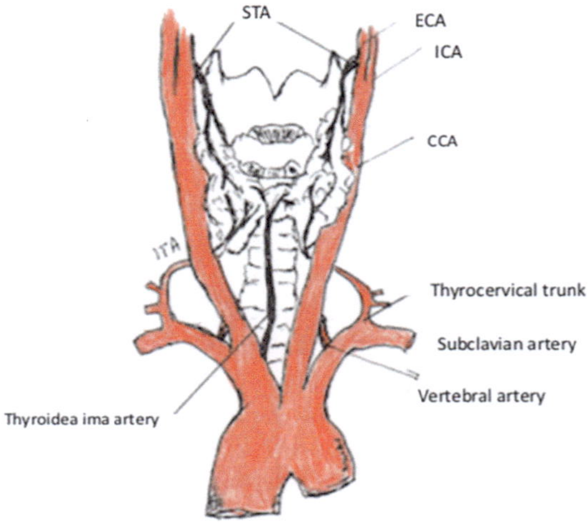

Diagram 3.3 The arterial blood supply of the thyroid gland. STA—Superior thyroid artery, ITA—Inferior thyroid artery. In this case the thyroidea ima artery originates from the brachiocephalic trunk
Legend: Superior thyroid artery (STA), ECA—External carotid artery, ICA—Internal carotid artery, Common carotid artery

- The STA has discrete branches including: the superior laryngeal artery (also called the infrahyoid artery) which is a robust vessel running into the substance of the thyrohyoid membrane with the internal laryngeal nerve. A separate branch is supplied to the lower edge of the SCM.[2]

[2]The arterial supply to the upper SCM is via the sternocleidomastoid branch of the occipital artery. This small vessel holds down Cranial XII as it crosses the CCA bifurcation. These small vessels are important if the SCM and a paddle of skin are ever rotated as a local myocutaneous flap. The SCM can be rotated based on this blood supply by detaching its clavicular origin and rotating the muscle across the front of the exposed carotid vessels and IJV to attach it to the under surface of the mandible. Such an approach may be used after a radical neck dissection where radiotherapy has been used and where there is a risk of wound breakdown and vascular exposure.

The ELN and its relationship to the upper thyroid lobe has been categorized in a number of classifications. In the past the superior pole of the thyroid was taken in a thyroidectomy by ligation of this bundle of tissue using a Kocher's enucleator (a scoop with a groove in it passed behind the bulk of the thyroid lobe where then an aneurysm needle passed a large silk suture to tie the upper lobe). It was realized that this bulk tie technique placed the ELN at risk for injury [2]. The ELN innervates the cricothyroid muscle (it is the only intrinsic muscle of the larynx not innervated by the RLN) and the task of the ELN is to stretch the vocal fold and to raise the pitch of the voice.[3]

The commonest classification of the STA/ELN relationship is the Cernea classification [3] emphasizing the closeness of the ELN to the thyroid lobe substance and to the STA such that:

Type 1	The ELN crosses the STA > 1 cm above upper pole of thyroid
Type 2a	The ELN crosses the STA < 1 cm above upper pole of thyroid
Type 2b	The ELN crosses the STA under cover of upper pole of thyroid

The Friedman classification [4] relates the ELN to the inferior constrictor such that:

Type 1:	The nerve runs superficial to the inferior constrictor muscle.
Type 2:	The nerve penetrates the lower part of the inferior constrictor muscle.
Type 3:	The nerve runs deep to the inferior constrictor muscle. (The Type 3 variant may account for the fact that the nerve is only variably identifiable).

[3]The effects of ELN damage can be quite subtle although a source of litigation in professional singers who may experience a moderately breathy voice, a loss of pitch and a particular inability to raise the pitch and maintain a good pitch range. The ELN has been called the nerve of Galli-Curci after the Milanese opera soprano Amelita Galli-Curci (1882–1963) in whom it was famously injured in 1935 in the USA during goitre surgery.

Another classification similar to the Cernea system is the Kierner classification [5] such that:

Type 1: The ELN crosses the STA > 1 cm above upper pole of thyroid
Type 2: The ELN crosses the STA < 1 cm above upper pole of thyroid
Type 3: The ELN crosses the STA under cover of upper pole of thyroid
Type 4: The ELN descends dorsal to the STA and crosses the STA branches immediately above upper pole of thyroid

In older textbooks the ELN passes superficial to the inferior constrictor muscle where it has been described as lying within Joll's (sternothyrolaryngeal) triangle which is formed laterally by the upper pole of the thyroid and the superior thyroid vessels, superiorly by the attachment of the strap muscles to the thyroid cartilage and medially by the midline. This is, however, a far less reliable landmark.[4]

- **The Inferior Thyroid Artery (ITA):** arises from the thyrocervical trunk from the first portion of the subclavian artery (before the subclavian artery runs behind the scalenus anterior muscle). The ITA approaches the thyroid from the lateral side of the neck by running under the CCA (an important operative landmark) and then it runs upwards to pierce the pretracheal fascia usually as a separate leash along the thyroid substance. The relationship of this artery to the RLN is of importance with the trend in years past to ligate the ITA in isolation during thyroid lobectomy as laterally as possible and distant to its entry into the gland in order to avoid RLN damage. With the increase in the use of total thyroidectomy (for both benign and malignant thyroid disease), it has become recognized that this approach leads to parathyroid ischaemia and insufficiency with troublesome postoperative hypocalcaemia so that the small ITA vessels are now ligated directly on the gland itself in an attempt to preserve parathyroid blood supply.

[4] Sir Cecil Joll (1885–1945) was an English thyroid surgeon (1885–1945).

- The ITA is the important developmental artery of the region, supplying the trachea-oesophageal anlage in the neck with oesophageal and inferior laryngeal branches before reaching the thyroid gland.

The remaining arterial supply of the thyroid is the variable **thyroidea ima artery** (TIA) evident in 3% of individuals[5] which is a persistent fetal vessel which can arise from the brachiocephalic trunk, (which is the most usual), the aortic arch directly, or even the left or right CCA and ascend on the anterior surface of the isthmus. It can rarely originate from the subclavian artery, the ITA, the pericardiophrenic artery, the suprascapular, the transverse cervical, the thyrocervical trunk or the internal thoracic artery [6]. On occasion when the TIA is present then the ITA is hypoplastic or absent. When rarely present, it is at risk of injury (with a superior mediastinal component of bleeding from its retracted components) during tracheostomy [7]. Vascular anastomosis in the thyroid of its arterial blood supply is usually in the posterior aspect of the lobes with some anterior anastomoses across the upper border of the isthmus.

- Venous drainage of the thyroid gland (Diagram 3.4): Three separate pairs of veins drain the thyroid; namely, a superior thyroid vein arising near the upper pole, the middle thyroid vein (previously mentioned) and typically a small leash of inferior thyroid veins. The superior thyroid vein when traced out commonly crosses the carotid bifurcation on its way to the IJV. In some cases, it may ascend towards the common facial vein. As stated, the short middle thyroid vein runs directly across to the IJV laterally preventing elevation of the thyroid lobe. The leash of inferior thyroid veins enters the left brachioceophalic vein inferiorly. This arrangement is part of the left brachiocephalic vein forming the anterior cardinal vein embryologically in a different manner than the right brachiocephalic vein. In utero a left superior vena cava (SVC) forms and regresses, coalescing into the left brachioce-

[5]First described in 1772 by Jonathan Neubauer. The thyroidea ima artery is also referred to as Neubauer's artery, or the accessory thyroid artery.

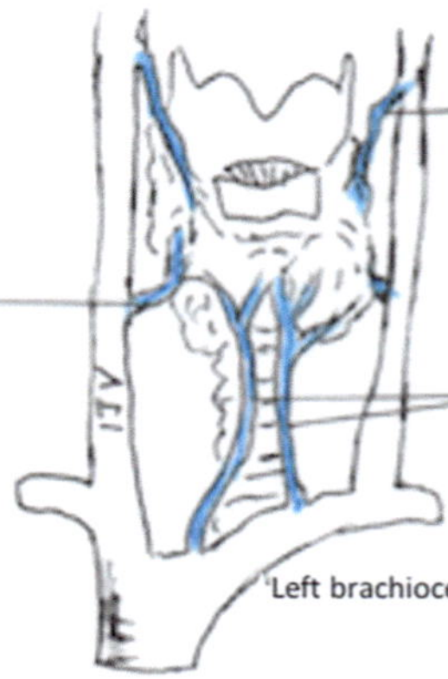

Diagram 3.4 The venous drainage of the thyroid gland. The leash of inferior thyroid veins drain into the left brachiocephalic vein with the middle thyroid vein a short tributary of the IJV that is initially ligated in order to mobilize the thyroid lobe
Legend: STV—Superior thyroid vein, SVC—Superior vena cava

phalic vein and also forming the variable accessory hemiazygos venous system. This means that the tributaries of the left brachiocephalic vein differ from those of the right brachiocephalic vein. These left brachiocephalic vein tributaries include the inferior thyroid veins, the thymic veins and the left superior intercostal vein. The latter runs behind the phrenic nerve in the mediastinum but in front of Cranial X and drains the first and second intercostal spaces. Its right-sided equivalent superior intercostal vein drains into the azygos. Thyroid veins may also receive tributaries from unnamed tracheal, laryngeal and oesophageal veins.

Recurrent Laryngeal Nerve

One of the principal considerations during thyroid surgery is identification (and variability) of the recurrent laryngeal nerve (RLN). Of importance, the course of the last 2 cm of the RLN is critical to the suspensory ligament of Berry which itself is divisible into a superficial (vascular) fascial layer and a deeper (fibrous) layer with the RLN typically moving between both layers. Within the superficial layer the RLN lies closely to the terminal branches of the ITA, the organ of Zuckerkandl and the superior parathyroid (PT) gland. The risk of a permanent RLN injury with thyroidectomy varies between 0.27% and 0.75% overall and is dependent upon the mechanism of injury. There is a worse prognosis with electrical (diathermy) injury, ischaemia, inadvertent ligation or crushing as opposed to the better outcome with a stretch neurapraxia. It should also be pointed out that the technique of mobilization of the thyroid lobe alters the anatomical position of the RLN from its normal *in situ* place where rotation of the lobe tends to stretch it vertically.

Firstly, there is a variable relationship between the RLN and the ITA. More commonly the RLN lies behind the ITA, however, it can on occasion pass between the branches of the ITA. On occasion a minute vessel is visible on the nerve directly. At the upper border of the thyroid isthmus it is not uncommon for the RLN to divide into two branches with typically the larger anterior branch being the motor laryngeal branch and the posterior one sensory only [8]. The RLN inside the larynx communicates with the internal branch of the superior laryngeal nerve and supplies the mucous membrane below the vocal folds as well as all of the intrinsic muscles of the larynx (except the cricothryoroid). The RLN also gives off cardiac branches close to its origin which supply the trachea, oesophagus and the inferior part of the pharynx. The RLN will always be located behind the pretracheal fascia and the fascial membranous connection which attaches to the cricoid cartilage (the so-called suspensory ligament of Berry). This 'ligament' is a condensed part of the pre-tracheal fascia attaching the thyroid gland to the crico-tracheal anlage and was first reported by Berry as an anatomical landmark in 1888.[6]

[6]Sir James Berry (1860–1946) Canadian born British surgeon.

This relationship has important clinical significance in some cases. As the position of the RLN in relation to the ligament of Berry is shifted by lobe rotation (from its *in situ* position), there is the formation of a genu (bend) in the extra-laryngeal part of the nerve with a greater risk of traction to the anterior (motor) branch as it takes off from the main RLN trunk. It is at this point that the RLN may be vulnerable and also where there can be troublesome bleeding, particularly when the ligament is dense or when there is excessive nerve branching [9]. One further landmark (which is considered in the surgical but not the anatomical literature) is the organ of Zuckerkandl.[7] This is embryologically the most posterior aspect of the thyroid lobe near the ligament of Berry and has a close relationship to the superior PT gland. This area of tissue forms from the lateral thyroid anlage as a fusion of the regressive fifth and the ventral portion of the fourth pharyngeal pouches such that this landmark is considered like an arrow that points to the RLN location. This region represents the ultimobranchial bodies (which form the C (parafollicular) calcitonin-producing cells of the thyroid) and also the superior parathyroid glands. As these areas fuse at this point with the thyroid gland this accounts for the relatively close association between the organ and the superior parathyroid gland. There is a Pelizzo grading based on the size of the organ (ranging from miniscule to up to 1 cm in diameter) [10–12].

Debate has centred around the technique of direct exposure of the course of the nerve where particular attention is paid to its relationship to the landmarks already described from a lateral approach as the nerve runs upwards in the trachea-oesophageal groove and into the larynx. In some difficult cases after ligation of the superior pole a superior (top down) approach can be used to isolate the RLN at the ligament of Berry at the lower end of the inferior constrictor muscle. An inferior (bottom up) approach is less advisable lifting the thyroid up against the tra-

[7]This 'organ' was first described in 1867 by Otto Wilhelm Madelung (1846–1926) who referred to it as the posterior horn of the thyroid (or in 1902 by Emil Zuckerkandl (1849–1910) as the "processus posterior glandulae thyroideae").

chea as this requires a longer RLN dissection and a greater risk of neurapraxia.[8]

Another area of anatomical (and embryological) interest is the so called non-recurrent nerve (NRLN). At the point where the RLN enters the larynx it is more appropriate to refer to it as the inferior laryngeal nerve in order to distinguish it from the superior laryngeal nerve. One nerve innervates the region below the vocal cords whilst the other supplies sensation to the area above the rima glottidis (the laryngeal opening). There is a chance that the RLN on the right side may be non-recurrent (hence the term non-recurrent inferior laryngeal nerve).

An appreciation of the anatomy can be obtained by understanding the vascular anomaly typically associated with a NRLN. In development, the RLN nerve arises from the Cranial X developing with the sixth branchial arch. The fourth arch is the only arch to remain with the fifth and sixth resorbing and with the RLN running up under the fourth arch which on the right side forms the right subclavian artery (RSA). The normal anatomy is then for the right-hand side RLN to run around the RSA and to ascend into the neck lying in the trachea-oesophageal groove. On the left side, the sixth branchial arch forms the ductus arteriosus (connecting the aorta and the pulmonary artery) with the normal left-hand side arrangement of the RLN running around the arch of the aorta to get to the trachea-oesophageal groove. A NRLN relies on abnormal embryological formation of the aortic arch where a right SCA forms beyond the take-off of the left SCA distal to the ductus arteriosus. This occurs either without an innominate (brachiocephalic) artery or as a variant (a right aortic arch where the pulmonary artery is located on the right side but with the vessels disposed in a similar manner). The prevalence of this NRLN anomaly is about 0.5–1% overall and is as a result of the abnormal absorption of the fourth right branchial arch so that in a left-sided aortic arch the right SCA aberrantly runs behind the oesophagus

[8] Similar lateral, superior and inferior mobilizations have been described with the more novel transaxillary, retroauricular and minimally invasive thyroidectomy (MIVAT) approaches.

in order to reach the right arm. For these reasons the NRLN is an entirely right-sided phenomenon.[9]

The position adopted by the vocal cords after an RLN palsy.

The motor function of the RLN is critical, innervating all intrinsic muscles of the larynx except the cricothyroid muscle. The anatomy of the larynx is covered in Chap. 15 of this book. The single muscle abducting the cords and opening the airway (rima) is the posterior cricoarytenoid muscle, meaning that in an RLN injury at thyroidectomy, the vocal cord on the palsied side is unable to abduct and is joined by the contralateral healthy vocal cord which prolapses across the midline, resulting in a tiring or weakened, hoarse voice. This is the basis of Teflon injection of the cord to assist this position. The patient with bilateral RLN palsy often requires a tracheostomy. Given the principle that more total thyroidectomies are being performed for benign thyroid disease such as multinodular goitre (along with for thyroid carcinomas) there has been the theoretical risk of a higher number of bilateral RLN injury (although this remains extremely small in experienced hands). By contrast, the cadaveric position of the vocal cord lies half-way between the abducted and the adducted position since there is no abduction/adduction intrinsic muscle activity.

One final point of interest has been the argument proffered by the biologist Professor Richard Dawkins that the presence of the RLN is a marker for evolution and against the notion of intelligent design. This argument follows the dissection of the RLN in a giraffe (which may be viewed on social media platforms) suggesting that the nerve is an evolutionary hangover from fish although the counter argument is that the task of the RLN in the thorax is rather to supply branches to the oesophageal and cardiac plexi

[9]The vascular anomaly was described by Aaron Arkin in 1936 and referred to as *arteria lusoria* (meaning 'quirky' artery) although dysphagia associated with the vascular anomaly (referred to as *dysphagia lusoria*) which may occur in 10% of cases of arteria lusoria was actually described by Bayford in 1789. Some cases of NRLN have been associated with an aplasia of the intracranial circulation, the Circle of Willis. There is a classification of NRLN which is dependent upon the point at which it arises directly from the Cranial X. An NRLN may be found proximally (near the cricoarytenoid joint entry) or distally (in the trachea-oesophageal groove at the lower pole of the thyroid gland).

branches as it progressively develops and that there is a failure of regression of supplying components. For Dawkins, the intelligent designer would just redesign such an arrangement whereas in evolution such a 'mistake' cannot be amended.

Lymphatic Drainage

The lymphatics of the thyroid follow the arteries, entering upwards the anterosuperior group of deep cervical nodes and downwards behind the origin of the ITA into a posteroinferior group. Some pass downwards with the pretracheal nodes in the midline to a particular node (called the Delphian node) which is located in the midline at the upper isthmus where it is found in about 20% of central neck dissections. On occasion, the commonest thyroid cancer, (papillary thyroid cancer) may present as an isthmial nodal mass with an occult microscopic tumour located in one (or both) thyroid lobe (s) correlating with primary tumour size, the presence of lymphovascular invasion and multicentricity.

Nerve Supply

The middle cervical sympathetic ganglion supplies this area with sympathetic fibres entering the gland travelling along branches of the ITA. Some sympathetic fibres run with the STA from the superior cervical ganglion as well as others derived from cardiac and laryngeal branches. The gland has vagal (Cranial X) fibres but their function is unknown.

The Parathyroid Glands

These two pairs of small tan-coloured glands (approximately 6 × 3 × 2 mm) are typically embedded in the posterior part of the thyroid but with importantly variable position. Locating an abnormal parathyroid (PT) gland (or glands) becomes critical in the management of hyperparathyroidism either in parathyroid adenoma or in PT hyperplasia. Normal PT glands are typically between 30 and 60 mg in weight. In 90% of cases there are four PT glands, however, they can be supernumerary and with a total weight not exceeding 200 mg. Because of the embryology alluded to, the superior PT is more constant in its position, usually lying below the STA near the posterior surface of the thyroid lobe and level with the first tracheal ring. The inferior PT is much more variable and may lie at the lower pole of the thyroid but much lower either in the upper thymus, the mediastinum or in the so-called thyrothymic ligament, (a collection of loose areolar tissue in the lower thyroid that can be pulled up and resected from the neck incision). The inferior PT is usually lateral to the RLN. These glands may be identified at surgery by having a small petechial blood blush as they are manipulated and occasionally small vessels can be seen running on them.

Several take away points are:

- The older technique of lateral isolated ITA ligation (in order to avoid RLN injury) during thyroidectomy has largely been abandoned because this disrupts the PT blood supply and leads to a higher incidence of perioperative hypocalcaemia.
- Ectopic (or aberrant locations) of the superior PT can include those found within the carotid sheath necessitating formal examination of this region ipsilaterally if a PT adenoma has not been found. The superior (IV) PT glands are uncommonly ectopic in location because they develop with the thyroid from the fourth branchial pouch and with the C-cell complex. They rarely can migrate to the trachea-oesophageal groove or be retrotracheal or retropharyngeal (very rare).
- Ectopic inferior PT gland sites can include those embedded within the thyroid lobe, thyrothymic examples and mediastinal locations. Remnants of thyroid tissue are found in about half the cases in this thyrothymic area and in half of cases these cell rests are bilateral [13]. These III PT glands may be found along the line of descent into the superior border of the pericardium.
- Mirror image symmetry usually occurs for both the superior and inferior PT glands [14].
- Intraoperative anatomic localization has been improved recently with a range of techniques including: preoperative neck US and Tc sestamibi SPECT scanning. Alternatives

include Tc-Thallium subtraction scanning. Intraoperative localization has been aided by rapid on-table PTH assay and near infrared autofluorescence (NIRAF).

Salivary Glands

Discussion of the anatomy of the salivary glands has overlap with the anatomy of the face, the layout of the autonomic nervous system of the head and neck, the suprahyoid region and the temporal and infratemporal fossae. All of these areas are considered elsewhere in this volume and should be cross-checked across chapters. The principal glands of study here are the parotid and submandibular glands with the sublingual gland considered in the discussion of the oral cavity (Chap. 13). In addition to the major salivary glands there are on microscopy grid count an estimated 750–1000 minor salivary glands (based upon mucosal strips and geometry) which are located principally in the palate but also along the oral cavity in the buccal, labial and lingual submucosa and the floor of the mouth. These glands are the sites of stones (sialolithiasis), chronic inflammation (sialadenitis and von Mikulicz syndrome/Sjogren's syndrome) and of tumours. For interest the clinical correlates of anatomy of these glands shows that nearly 80% of neoplastic lesions are located in the parotid (about 15% of which are locally aggressive or frankly malignant), 15% in the submandibular gland (of which nearly half can be malignant) and 5% in the minor salivary glands (nearly 90% of which are malignant).

Parotid Gland (*See* Diagram 3.5)

The area below the zygomatic arch houses the parotid gland and the masseter muscle as well as the insertion into the mandibular coronoid process of the temporalis muscle. The parotid is a watershed area where the investing layer of deep cervical fascia splits around the gland filling the complex space located between the mastoid process and the angle of the mandible. For the purposes of anatomic definition (and for the classification of types of parotidectomy) the gland is somewhat artificially divided into a super-

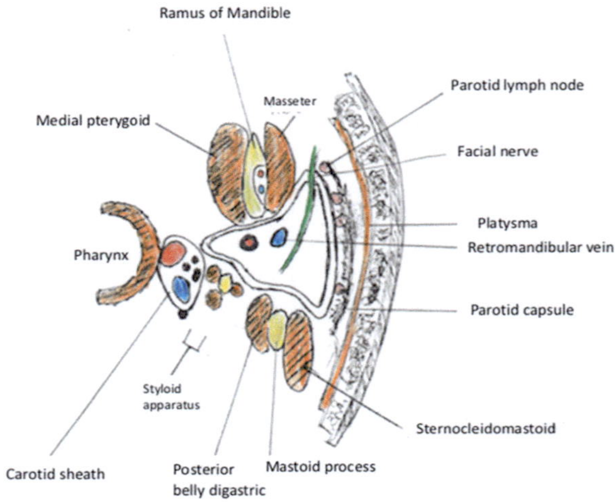
Ramus of Mandible
Masseter
Medial pterygoid
Parotid lymph node
Facial nerve
Platysma
Retromandibular vein
Pharynx
Parotid capsule
Styloid apparatus
Sternocleidomastoid
Carotid sheath
Posterior belly digastric
Mastoid process

ficial and a deep parotid lobe which are separated by the so-called faciovenous plane which includes the facial nerve (Cranial VII). Those excisions superficial to the Cranial VII are considered as conservative (or superficial) parotidectomies. With 10% of parotid tumours occurring in the 'deep' lobe, these are removed by a total parotidectomy taking out the deep lobe piecemeal and increasing the likelihood of partial or total facial nerve paralysis. The relation of the deep surface of the parotid gland is the side of the pharynx and the termination of the external carotid artery (ECA) into the superficial temporal and maxillary arteries.

Diagram 3.5 *Top image.* The relationships of the parotid gland. In the superficial lobe of the parotid is the faciovenous plane with the VII in front of the retromandibular vein. The ECA divides in the substance of the gland into the superficial temporal artery and the maxillary artery. Deep to the gland is the carotid sheath (containing the CCA, the IJV and Cranial nerves IX, X, XI and XII) as well as the styloid apparatus (with its muscles the styloglossus, the stylopharyngeus and the stylohyoid). These muscles represent separate compartmental nerves of the branchial arches; namely, the second (VII-stylohyoid), the third (IX -stylopharyngeus).

Ramus of mandible, Masseter, Parotid lymph node, Facial nerve (VII), Platysma, Retromandibular vein, Parotid capsule fascia, Sternocleidomastoid, Mastoid process, Posterior belly digastric, Styloid apparatus, Carotid sheath (Internal carotid artery ICA, Cranial IX, X, XI), Cranial XII lies in front outside the sheath. Pharynx, Medial pterygoid

Middle Image: Orientated relations of the parotid. The nerves of the muscles of facial expression include: temporal, zygomatic, buccal, mandibular and cervical. The green area above the parotid duct is an accessory lobe of parotid called the socia parotidis

Lower Image: Variations of the Cranial VII. Type 1 is separated into a temporofacial and cervicofacial branch. Type 2 has a temporal communication. Type 3 connects between the two main branches. Type 4 has complex neural anastomoses

The shape of the parotid gland is like an inverted triangle filling in the space deeply as far as the styloid process. This orientation effectively creates separate lateral, anterior and deep surfaces and is surrounded on all of its surfaces by a thickened specialized part of the fascia (the parotid fascia) which limits the spread of infection (such as in Mumps parotitis). The upper pole is in front of the cartilaginous part of the external auditory meatus (EAM) and the lower pole extends below the angle of the mandible overlapping part of the posterior belly of the digastric muscle. This means that a parotid tumour may present as a high neck mass. At the upper end of the gland is the parotid duct (of Stensen) and commonly an aggregate of parotid tissue which sits above the duct called the *socia parotidis.*[10] The depth of the gland embraces the masseter muscle on its outer surface and the medial pterygoid muscle on its inner surface. At this point, a thickening, the stylomandibular ligament separates the inner surface of the gland from the medial pterygoid sending a fascial extension to separate off the submandibular gland. On the deep surface at the anterior border of the parotid, the duct emerges with the delicate branches of Cranial VII. The deep part of the gland is indented by the mastoid process lying against the styloid apparatus (stylohyoid, styloglossus and stylopharyngeus) with this area representing the embryological guy ropes of the different cranial nerves that compartmentally supply individual branchial arches. The Cranial VII innervates the second branchial arch), the Cranial IX (Glossopharyngeal) the third pharyngeal arch and the Cranial XII (Hypoglossal) the innervation of the styloglossus. This area deeply relates to two ligaments, the stylohyoid and stylomandibular. Deeply the styloid process separates the deep part of the gland from the ICA, the side of the pharynx (mainly the superior constrictor muscle) and the IJV.

The principal association (and anatomical importance) of the gland is its association with Cranial VII. The basis of the conservative superficial parotidectomy exposing the VII arose because of the surgical procedure of enucleation of apparently encapsu-

[10]Named after the Dutch anatomist Nicolas Steno (1638–1686).

lated tumours (the commonest the mixed salivary or pleomorphic adenoma) which was followed by a very high rate of locoregional recurrence of this benign tumour since the capsules were invariably microscopically infiltrated. This high local recurrence rate was obviated by a reappraisal of the anatomy of the gland where the VII separated the superficial and deep lobes and where there was a standardization of operative location and identification of the main VII to preserve its function. The relationships of the gland are shown in Diagram 3.5. Embedded within the gland (from superficial to deep) are VII, the retromandibular vein and the ECA. Parotid (preauricular) lymph nodes are embedded under the parotid capsule. The parasympathetic nervous system (PSNS) secretomotor (also called sudomotor) supply for salivation are distributed to the gland via the auriculotemporal branch of the mandibular division of Cranial V (Trigeminal), the branch referred to as V_3. These deliver postganglionic PSNS fibres which have synapsed in the otic ganglion at the skull base and which hitch-hike along V_3 to get to their destination at the side of the face. The parotid duct courses across the front of the masseter and pierces the buccinator muscle opening onto the mucosa as a visible papilla opposite the second upper molar tooth. It has a surface landmark from the front of the tragus of the ear to the lateral junction point of the upper and lower lips (the cheilion).

The main concern during parotidectomy (as already mentioned) is detection of the main VII. Several points are worth noting. The filaments of VII at the front of the parotid gland are extremely delicate and typically are subdivided (although with considerable variation and overlap) into a zygomaticofacial and cervicofacial branch (Diagram 3.6). The typical branches to the muscles of facial expression are: temporal, zygomatic (to the orbicularis oculi), buccal, marginal mandibular (to the depressor anguli oris and the depressor labii inferioris muscles) and cervical (to the platysma). These branches are remembered by placing a hand along the side of the face with its five splayed fingers. Argument has been made over the most crucial branch with some suggesting the zygomatic branch (if injured requiring liquid tears and partial lid closure as a lateral tarsorrhaphy procedure) or the

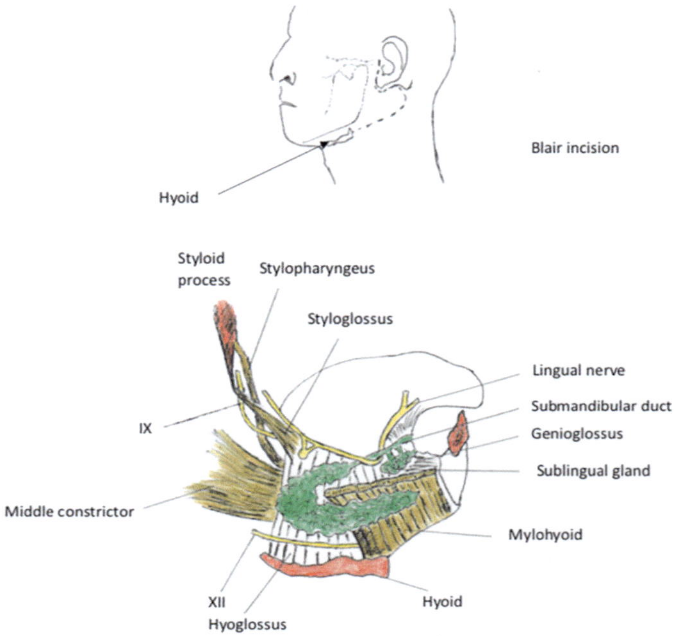

Diagram 3.6 Dissection of the submandibular gland. The *top image* shows the Blair incision for a parotid gland excision (*dashed line*). The *image below* shows the superficial and deep lobes of the gland which embrace the free posterior edge of the mylohyoid muscle (shown cut across). The submandibular and sublingual glands are shown in *green*. Under the mylohyoid is the hyoglossus on which runs the lingual nerve (with its submandibular ganglion) and the hypoglossal nerve. The glossopharyngeal nerve wraps deeply around the stylopharyngeus (the only muscle it innervates) above the middle constrictor and deep to the hyoglossus. The lingual nerve swerves around the submandibular duct and runs on its medial side into the tongue to supply the sensation and transmit PSNS secretomotor fibres to the sublingual and minor salivary glands

buccal branch which results in drooling. Bell's palsy[11] is a lower motor neurone paralysis of these muscles of facial expression and is distinct from an upper motor neurone (supranuclear) VII palsy where the brow muscle (the frontalis) which is bilaterally represented in the cerebral cortex has preserved function.

The VII emanates from the skull via the stylomastoid foramen and enters the substance of the parotid gland in an almost vertical disposition (coming up towards the surgeon) where it is found by performance of a Blair incision.[12] This incision runs from the zygomatic arch just in front of the tragus and across to the tip of the mastoid process in a gentle curve, then proceeding down two fingerbreadths below the angle of the mandible (so as not to injure the marginal mandibular VII) and as far as the palpable greater horn of the hyoid bone. The flap is dissected off the cartilaginous portion of the EAM as far as the junction of its cartilaginous and bony portions. Just below this junction is a small palpable tubercle with the Cranial VII lying immediately beneath this spur. The cartilaginous portion of the EAM is part of the extension of the conchal cartilage and the bony portion is part of the tympanic part of the squamous temporal bone. Another anatomical landmark is to place the eponychial fold of the thumbnail on the tip of the mastoid process and the Cranial VII will lie in that block of tissue as far forward and as far deep as the end of the thumb. The point here is that the main VII lies deeper than one would think. Other ways of finding the main VII can be used usually as part of a reoperation where fibrosis obscures the normal landmarks. One way is to find the delicate buccal branch near Stensen's duct (which is palpable). Another method is to find the marginal mandibular branch and trace this backwards. Both methods have the risk of injury or neurapraxia [15].

The facial nerve has a number of anatomical variations in its terminal connexions: (Diagram 3.5). These include:

---

[11] Named after the nineteenth century English anatomist Sir Charles Bell (1774–1842)

[12] Vilray P Blair (1871–1955) was an American head and neck and plastic reconstructive surgeon.

Type 1 (where there are two main separations—the temporal and cervicofacial—and where there is little terminal connection).
Type 2 where distal anastomoses only occur within the temporofacial component.
Type 3 where there is an isolated connection between the two main branches.
Type 4 (and others) where there are combinations of differing complexity.

According to a paper by Gataa et al. [16] Type 1 is noted in 16%, Type 2 in 23%, Type 3 in 30%, Type 4 in 19% and others in 10% of dissections.

Behind the VII is the retromandibular vein which is an anterior confluence of the superficial temporal vein along with a middle temporal vein, stout maxillary veins and a transverse facial vein. The retromandibular vein divides into an anterior and a posterior division at the lower end of the gland. The anterior branch typically joins the facial vein and empties forward into the IJV. The posterior branch runs backwards piercing the investing layer of deep cervical fascia and is joined by the posterior auricular vein to form the EJV. The EJV runs down on the sternocleidomastoid piercing the fascia to empty via a valve into the subclavian vein about 1 cm above the clavicle. The posterior auricular vein may be joined by a mastoid emissary vein which connects it directly to the sigmoid sinus (allowing mastoiditis to lead to sigmoid sinus thrombophlebitis). The superficial lymph nodes embedded in the parotid gland drain the auricle, the anterior scalp and the upper face with deeper nodes receiving lymph from the EAM, the middle ear, the auditory tube, nose, palate and the deep cheek. Enlarged lymph nodes in the parotid may represent metastatic sites from any of these primary sites mentioned above.

The secretomotor function of the parotid gland is part of the parasympathetic autonomic nerve supply of the head and neck (explained in Chap. 5). In this system, the chain of command comes from a nucleus and then runs as a preganglionic pathway to a ganglion. From there is a postganglionic pathway to the target tissue. In this case, the inferior salivatory nucleus (lying within the midbrain) leads to the otic ganglion via Cranial IX (the glossopharyngeal nerve) via the lesser petrosal nerve which runs in the middle cranial fossa. Following synapse in the otic ganglion (which lies just below the skull base below the foramen ovale), connection continues as postganglionic secretomotor fibres which use the local Cranial V to hitchhike to get to the parotid gland. The local nerve here to use is the auriculotemporal nerve (part of V_3) splitting around the origin of the middle meningeal artery and running along the side of the temple and parotid region. Sympathetic fibres for the parotid travel along the middle meningeal artery and control the precapillary sphincters over the gland. The skin over the angle of the mandible and the parotid capsule is innervated via the great auricular nerve (C2,3) a branch of the cervical plexus (See Chap. 4). The great auricular nerve is large and supplies part of the ear lobe but may be sacrificed with minimal morbidity and used as a cable graft should the Cranial VII need to be sacrificed in a parotidectomy for malignant disease. The disruption of the SNS and PSNS within the auriculotemporal nerve after dissection leads to Frey's syndrome (a syndrome of gustatory sweating) with salivation. In this circumstance where the auriculotemporal nerve is damaged sympathetic fibres grow into parasympathetic axons. This syndrome named after a patient Lucille Frey and leads to sweating and redness over the side of the face on salivation. These days the better treatment is by injection under the skin of the area with methylene blue but in the past an anatomical approach was taken to the pathology with a range of options. These included auriculotemporal nerve injection and ablation, phenol injection of the otic ganglion and sectioning of the lesser petrosal nerve in the middle cranial fossa.[13]

The remaining structure in the region is the masseter muscle (which can be considered in association with the muscles of mastication and those of the temporal and infratemporal fossae). The muscles of mastication are branchial muscles which are innervated by the motor nucleus of Cranial V (located in the midbrain).

[13]The nerve is also referred to as the lesser superficial petrosal nerve, the tympanic nerve or Jacobson's nerve. The nerve runs in the middle ear at the inferior tympanic canaliculus providing the principal sensory innervation to the auditory tube and the mastoid air cells. It can be the site of a glomus paraganglionoma which can present with deafness and tinnitus.

The muscle has a tricipital origin from the zygomatic arch inserting into the broad plate of the ramus of the mandible. This quadrate-shaped muscle covers the coronoid process of the mandible (the insertion point of the temporalis) and has an external insertion that somewhat mirrors the insertion of the medial pterygoid on the inner surface of the mandibular ramus. The masseteric nerve runs between the deep, intermediate and the superficial parts of the muscle. The nerve supply is from the motor (anterior) division of V_3 running in front of the temporomandibular joint (TMJ) via the mandibular notch. There is a sensory (proprioceptive) part of Cranial V which relays in the midbrain via the mesencephalic nucleus creating a local reflex arc. Here afferent neural stimuli defining the position of the jaw in space synapse with the motor aspect of the arc (through the motor nucleus of Cranial V) ensuring that there is not an excessive bite. The action of the masseter is to close the jaw and to draw the mandible forwards as well as to slew the mandible from side to side during chewing.

Submandibular Gland (Diagram 3.6)

The submandibular region (aka the suprahyoid region) lies between the body of the mandible and the hyoid bone and incorporates the submental and digastric triangles. The deep part includes the floor of the mouth and the root of the tongue. The muscles of the area are the digastric (s), stylohyoid, mylohyoid, hyoglossus, styloglossus, genioglossus and geniohyoid. In front running vertically is the anterior belly of the digastric sitting on the mylohyoid (running to the internal mylohyoid line from the body of the hyoid) which then sits on the hyoglossus running perpendicularly to the mylohyoid. Deep to the hyoglossus is the bulk of the tongue formed by the spreading fibres of the genioglossus. The lingual nerve, the submandibular ganglion and much lower down Cranial XII all lie under the free edge of the mylohyoid and sit on the surface of the hyoglossus. Deep to the hyoglossus is the lingual artery and the deep lingual vein.

The occipital artery runs superiorly from the posterior margin of the ECA along the lower edge of the posterior belly of the digastric with the posterior auricular artery running in the same direction but along the upper border of the muscle. The anterior belly of the digastric is innervated by the nerve to mylohyoid, the only motor branch of the larger (largely sensory) V_3 mandibular nerve. By comparison, the one sensory part attached to the small motor root of V_3 is the buccal nerve (not to be confused with the buccal branch of VII).

The submandibular area houses the submandibular gland, the submandibular ganglion and the submandibular (Wharton's) duct.[14] The fascia overlying attaches to the mylohyoid line splitting around the mylohyoid and the submandibular gland. This important space under the mylohyoid can fill during sepsis of the floor of the mouth (known as Ludwig's angina) which can be life threatening through airway obstruction and which can originate from dental or tonsillar sepsis.[15] The anterior belly of the digastric arises near the symphysis menti. The posterior belly of the digastric comes from the pit of the mastoid process with the two having an intermediate synovial tendon which is bound to the greater horn and body of the hyoid bone. The muscle acts to raise the hyoid bone and assist in swallowing, synergizing with the infrahyoid muscles by stabilizing the hyoid bone in such a way that it can act as a stable platform for tongue movement.

The anterior belly is innervated by the *nerve to mylohyoid* (on which it sits). This nerve arises from the inferior alveolar nerve (V_3) at the point of the mandibular foramen just above the mylohyoid line. The *nerve to mylohyoid* pierces the sphenomandibular ligament which is a fascial extension from the spine of the sphenoid just in front of the medial pterygoid muscle in the ridge of bone above the mandibular foramen called the lingula. This ligament is part of the remnant of the first branchial arch cartilage (whose compartmental nerve is the V_3 mandibular nerve). The upper part of this cartilage gives rise to the malleus (of the middle ear) and the lower part is fused to the medial aspect of the devel-

[14]Named after Thomas Wharton (1614–1673) a British scientist who described various body glands.

[15]Named after the German surgeon Wilhelm Friedrich von Ludwig (1790–1865) who described Ludwig's angina in 1836.

oping mandible. By contrast, the posterior belly of the digastric is innervated by Cranial VII and is accompanied by a small submental artery which supplies part of the floor of the mouth and the sublingual gland. The region is **bilaterally** drained by lymphatics running from the floor of the mouth and the tip of the tongue to submental lymph nodes. The posterior belly of the digastric passes deep to the lower pole of the parotid gland and is a landmark for the carotid bifurcation and an approach to the ICA during a carotid endarterectomy operation. The posterior belly of the digastric muscle is crossed by the facial vein and the submandibular gland with the neurovascular bundle, (the IJV, the carotid bifurcation and XII) underneath.

Stylohyoid Muscle This muscle is a small slip arising from the styloid process and passing alongside the upper border of the posterior belly of the digastric. The muscle splits around this posterior digastric to insert into the body and greater horn of the hyoid bone. It is innervated by VII and pulls the hyoid bone upwards and backwards during swallowing. It is a landmark muscle in neck dissection.

The submandibular gland appears in the region like a small walnut located under the mandible against the mylohyoid muscle. The normal weight of the gland is approx. 15 g which is divided into a superficial and a deep lobe orientated like a 'U' lying on its side and wrapping around the free posterior border of the mylohyoid muscle (Diagram 3.6). The mylohyoid is seen running medially and forwards to a central fibromuscular raphe which runs between the mandibular symphysis and the central body of the hyoid bone. The submandibular duct comes from the deep part of the gland. An appreciation of this anatomy is critical in submandibular gland excision. The gland is removed by a curvilinear incision over the gland 2 fingerbreadths below the angle of the mandible (so as to avoid injury to the marginal mandibular VII). This nerve is also protected by extending the incision down to the deep fascia (capsule) of the gland reflecting the upper flap so that the nerve is safeguarded. The posterior aspect of the gland is grooved very closely by the facial artery which needs to be formally ligated. The upper part of the gland just under the mandible directly against the medial pterygoid muscle also has a close association with the facial artery as it runs forwards on to the mandible and this needs a second formal ligation. These double ligations free up the back and the top of the gland.

If the free border of the mylohyoid is retracted, the deep part of the gland comes into view revealing the hyoglossus running at right angles to the mylohyoid underneath. On the top of loose fascia lies the lingual nerve (which at this level is quite large) and which is held down by a double attachment of the small submandibular ganglion (one of the four parasympathetic ganglia of the head and neck). Lower down lying on the hyoglossus (although not usually seen during a submandibular gland excision) is the Cranial XII. The submandibular duct lies directly against the mucosa and against the mylohyoid muscle. The duct runs medially between the sublingual gland and the geniohyoid to open alongside the frenulum at the sublingual papilla inside the mouth. The duct has a particularly special relationship with the lingual nerve which hooks superficially around the duct and which then runs deep to it on its medial side. In cases of a submandibular stone which is palpable in the mouth, these can be retrieved intraorally but a suture should be placed around the duct between the mucosa of the gum and the mandible and held up to prevent the stone falling back into the gland. An incision can then be made directly over the stone to release it and leave a small intraoral fistula which does not require suture. There is always the possibility that this blind suture holding the duct can injure the lingual nerve which is superficial and submucosal at this point and which descends between the ramus of the mandible and the medial pterygoid muscle.

The lingual nerve passes below the attachment of the superior constrictor muscle (and below where the superior constrictor is attached at the pterygomandibular raphe) and runs between the mucosa and the mandible just behind and below the last (third) molar tooth where it is accessible for anaesthetic injection. The lingual nerve has a large gingival branch which supplies all of the mucous membrane of the lingual sulcus up to the midline and continues on to supply the mucous membrane of the side of the anterior 2/3 of the tongue. More details of this nerve are considered in Chap. 13 on the mouth and palate.

The lingual nerve then lies close to the side of the tongue crossing the styloglossus and the upper hyoglossus (Diagram 3.6) in its swerve around the submandibular duct. The parasympathetic nervous system (PSNS) supply of the submandibular (and sublingual) glands follows the typical PSNS pattern.

- The nucleus for these glands is the superior salivatory nucleus in the pons.
- The preganglionic pathway is via the chorda tympani (nervus intermedius of VII).
- This nerve synapses in the submandibular ganglion.
- The postganglionic pathway hitchhikes along the available lingual nerve (V_3)
- On its way to the targets—the submandibular and sublingual glands.

In brief, the sublingual gland of Nuhn[16] lies on the mylohyoid between the mandible and the genioglossus, forming the sublingual mucosal fold. It joins its fellow on the other side in the median plane at the origin of the genioglossus muscle. There is a leash of 8–20 small ducts which open into the mouth on the summit of the sublingual fold and the gland is supplied by the sublingual branch of the lingual artery and by the lingual nerve. The PSNS supply is supported by sympathetic fibres from plexi formed on the facial and lingual arteries.

There are several muscles in this region yet to consider as well as structural orientations in the floor of the mouth. Beneath the mylohyoid is the *hyoglossus*, a quadrate muscle running in the opposite direction from the bulk of the body and the greater horn of the hyoid bone into the side of the substance of the tongue. The hyoglossus interdigitates at its upper outer end with the styloglossus muscle. As an extrinsic muscle of the tongue the nerve supply to hyoglossus and styloglossus is Cranial XII. The hyoglossus depresses the side of the tongue and assists genioglossus in enlarging the oral cavity.

[16]Named after Anton Nuhn (1814–1889) a German anatomist.

Styloglossus lies at the upper outer end arising from the tip of the styloid process and part of the stylohyoid ligament. The styloglossus passes into the side of the tongue below the superior constrictor muscle with Cranial IX curving parallel and deeply to its lower border (Diagram 3.6). The muscle pulls the tongue upwards and laterally.

Geniohyoid lies inferiorly and anteriorly on the side of the lower tongue taking origin from the mandibular mental spine and attaching to the hyoid bone. It lies directly alongside its contralateral fellow horizontally and on top of the mylohyoid and it pulls the hyoid bone forward effectively increasing the volume of the front of the oral cavity to receive a food bolus. Geniohyoid is innervated by the C1 nerve root that is transmitted via Cranial XII through the superior root of the ansa cervicalis (cervical plexus). The anatomy of the cervical plexus is covered in Chap. 4.

Genioglossus forms a fan-like muscle that is the bulk of the side of the tongue and which extends from the tongue tip to the hyoid bone. Genioglossus joins its fellow on the opposite side in a similar way to geniohyoid. The posterior and inferior fibres of genioglossus when acting together, protrude the tongue as well as depress its central part as occurs in sucking motions designed to increase the volume of the oral cavity. The anterior fibres of genioglossus retract the tongue tip and this is the muscle which when paralyzed, moves the tongue when it is protruded towards the affected side.

- All of these extrinsic muscles of the tongue (muscles with -*glossus* in their name; hyoglossus, styloglossus, genioglossus) except for one muscle (palatoglossus) are innervated by Cranial XII. (This point is expanded with explanation in Chap. 13).
- Geniohyoid and Thyrohyoid are innervated by C1 roots hitchhiking along Cranial XII as part of the superior root of the ansa cervicalis
- The hyoglossus is an important landmark for the deep structures in the tongue. The lingual artery passes deep to the styloglossus with the IX nerve passing in the same plane but somewhat higher up. This nerve is particularly delicate and innervates the mucous membrane of the posterior third of the tongue from the vallate papillae.

- The angle between the stylohyoid ligament and the greater horn of the hyoid bone houses the middle constrictor fibres which fan out behind the posterior border of the hyoglossus to join their fellow muscle in a midline pharyngeal raphé.

Q and A: Chap. 3 (Answers at the End of This Chapter)

1. The parotid fascia is innervated by:
   (a) The transverse cervical nerve
   (b) The great auricular nerve
   (c) The auriculotemporal nerve
   (d) The zygomaticofacial nerve
2. The non-recurrent inferior laryngeal nerve
   (a) May be bilateral
   (b) Is associated with a distal right subclavian vessel take off distal to the left subclavian artery
   (c) Runs in the tracheo-oesophageal groove
   (d) Runs a retro-oesophageal course
3. The digastric triangle of the neck:
   (a) Has both of its borders formed by the digastric bellies
   (b) Has the hyoglossus muscle as its floor
   (c) Is solely innervated by the VII nerve
   (d) Arises from the third branchial arch
   (e) Is the point of commencement of Ludwig's angina
4. In a submandibular gland excision:
   (a) The deep and superficial parts of the gland wrap around the hyoglossus muscle
   (b) The facial artery needs to be ligated both superiorly and posteriorly
   (c) Has the marginal mandibular division of the VII deep to the capsule
   (d) The duct lies deep to the lingual nerve
   (e) The submandibular ganglion is routinely excised
5. In a thyroidectomy
   (a) The external laryngeal nerve can be injured during ligation of the inferior thyroid artery
   (b) The inferior thyroid artery is ligated close to the gland

   (c) the organ of Zuckerkandl relates to the superior parathyroid gland
   (d) May result is excessive traction of the anterior motor branch of the RLN during lobe rotation
6. Regarding the parotid gland:
   (a) It is split into a superficial and a deep lobe by the VII nerve
   (b) Has a socia parotidis attached to the parotid duct of Stensen
   (c) The maxillary artery divides deep to the gland
   (d) Has a parasympathetic innervation from the pterygopalatine ganglion
7. The infrahyoid musculature is
   (a) Innervated by the hypoglossal nerve
   (b) Innervated in part by the C1 ramus
   (c) Innervated high in its segmentation
   (d) Innervated by the ansa cervicalis except for the omohyoid
8. The external laryngeal nerve
   (a) Is a direct branch of the recurrent laryngeal nerve
   (b) Innervates the cricothryoid muscle and the thryopharyngeus
   (c) Has no relationship to the superior thyroid artery
   (d) Perforates the thyrohyoid membrane with the superior laryngeal vessels

Answers

1. b
2. b, d
3. a
4. b, e
5. b, c, d
6. a, b, c
7. b
8. b

References

1. Gurleyik E, Gurleyik G, Dogan S, Cobek U, Cetin F, Onsal U. Pyramidal lobe of the thyroid gland: surgical anatomy in patients undergoing total thyroidectomy. Anat Res Int. 2015;2015:384148.
2. Patnaik U, Nilakantan A. Identification of external branch of the superior laryngeal nerve in thyroid surgery: is it always possible? J Thyroid Disorders Ther. 2013;2(2):1000127. https://doi.org/10.4172/2167-7948.1000127.
3. Cernea CR, Nishio S, Hojaij FC. Identification of the external branch of the superior laryngeal nerve (EBSLN) in large goiters. Am J Otolaryngol. 1995;16(5):307–11.
4. Friedman M, Lo Savio P, Ibrahim H. Superior laryngeal nerve identification and preservation in thyroidectomy. Arch Otolaryngol Head Neck Surg. 2002;128:296–303.
5. Kierner AC, Aigner M, Burian M. The external branch of the superior laryngeal nerve: its topographical anatomy as related to surgery of the neck. Arch Otolaryngol Head Neck Surg. 1998;124:301–3.
6. Singh R. Study of Thyroidea Ima artery: narrative review of its prevalence and clinical significance. Basic Sci Med. 2022;11(1):1–4.
7. Kamparoudi P, Paliouras D, Gogakos AS, Rallis T, Schizas NC, Lazopoulos A, Chatzinikolaou F, Sarafis P, Serchan P, Katsikogiannis N, Sarika E, Zarogoulidis P, Karapantzos I, Barbetakis N. Percutaneous tracheostomy—beware of the thyroidea-ima artery. Ann Trans Med. 2016;4:449.
8. Sritharan N, Paddle PM, Snyder SK, Serpell JW. The ligament of Berry. In: Randolph GW, editor. The recurrent and superior laryngeal nerves. Cham: Springer; 2016. p. 103–13. https://doi.org/10.1007/978-3-319-27727-1_10.
9. Sasou S, Nakamura S-I, Kurihara HS. Suspensory ligament of Berry: its relationship to recurrent laryngeal nerve and anatomic examination of 24 autopsies. Head Neck. 1998;20(8):695–8.
10. Pelizzo MR, Toniato A, Gemo G. Zuckerkandl's tuberculum: an arrow pointing to the recurrent laryngeal nerve (constant anatomical landmark). J Am Coll Surg. 1998;187:333–6.
11. Bomeli SR, Wojtczak B, Abdullah H, Kania RE, Terris RE. The recurrent laryngeal nerve and the tubercle of Zuckerkandl. In: Randolph GW, editor. The recurrent and superior laryngeal nerves. Cham: Springer; 2016. p. 95–101. https://doi.org/10.1007/978-3-319-27727-1, XVII, 313, ISBN 978-3-319-27725-7.
12. Kandil E, Singer M, Deniwar A, Randolph GW. Surgical approaches to the recurrent laryngeal nerve. In: Randolph GW, editor. The recurrent and superior laryngeal nerve. Cham: Springer; 2016. p. 139–44.
13. Sackett WR, Reeve TS, Barraclough B, Delbridge LW. Thyrothymic thyroid rests: incidence and relationship to the thyroid gland. J Am Chem Soc. 2002;195:635–40.

14. Scharpf J, Kyriazidis N, Kamani D, Randolph G. Anatomy and embryology of the parathyroid glands. Oper Tech Otoloaryngol. 2016;27:117–21.
15. Martinez Pascual P, Maranillo E, Vazquez E, Simon de Blas C, Lasso JM, Sanudo JR. Extracranial course of the facial nerve revisited. Anat Rec. 2019;302:599–608.
16. Gataa IS, Faris BJM. Patterns and surgical significance of facial nerve within the parotid gland in 43 patients. Oral Maxillofac Surg. 2017;20:161–5.

The Prevertebral Muscles and the Cervical Plexus

4

Contents

Platysma 73
Sternocleidomastoid (SCM) 74
Trapezius 75
XI: The Spinal Accessory Nerve 76
The Cervical Plexus 82
Q and A: Chap. 4 (Answers at the End of This Chapter) 88
Answers 90
References 90

The platysma, sternocleidomastoid, trapezius, scaleni and prevertebral musculature are outlined in this chapter, along with the anatomy of the cervical plexus.

Platysma

The first layer exposed in any neck dissection is the platysma, a thin sheet of muscle in the superficial fascia which lies in front of the cutaneous branches of the cervical plexus. This muscle spreads from the chin onto the front of the chest and somewhat into the superior part of the posterior triangle of the neck being attached to the lower mandible and running over the pectoralis major and the deltoid muscle laterally. Superiorly the muscle fibres extend beyond the chin and mingle with the muscles of the lips and the

A. Zbar, *Anatomy--Head and Neck*,
https://doi.org/10.1007/978-3-031-69538-4_4

lower face where they form part of the risorius muscle [1, 2]. A superficial musculoaponeurotic system (SMAS) in the face has been anatomically proposed which defines the fibro-adipose mesh network connecting the muscles of facial expression to the skin creases. There is some anatomical variability of the platysma which can extend as far as the orbicularis oculi with both the platysma and the cervical skin having the same embryological myoblast origin. The muscle is innervated on its under surface by the cervical branch of VII and it forms part of the *panniculus carnosus* of lower animals which includes subcutaneous muscle in other sites such as that the palmaris brevis in the hand, and the dartos in the scrotum. These act as fright muscles and in cattle as flinching muscles designed to remove pests and perching birds. In the Australian *Tachyglossus echidna* it covers most of the body and allows the animal to change its shape into a ball as protection.

Sternocleidomastoid (SCM)

This muscle has a thicker tendinous sternal head arising from the upper anterior manubrium and a more fleshy and thinner, strip-like clavicular head which originates from the upper surface of the medial one third of the clavicle. The two heads fuse about half-way up the neck with a thick anterior border inserted into the anterior surface of the mastoid process and thence on to the lateral half of the superior nuchal line. The space between the sternal and the clavicular heads is a landmark site for a percutaneous IJV approach in the insertion of a central venous line catheter. Separate parts of the muscle are recognized as the sterno- and cleido-occiopitalis. Deep to its upper part lies the cervical plexus whereas deep to its lower part are the contents of the carotid sheath.

The blood supply of the SCM is both proximal (via the sterno-mastoid branch of the occipital artery) and distal (via the sterno-mastoid branch of the superior thyroid artery). The Cranial XI (spinal accessory nerve) innervates the muscle deeply, running through it at the junction of its upper and lower two-thirds. There are additional proprioceptive branches to the SCM which arise from the C2,3 parts of the cervical plexus. Acting alone, the SCM tilts the head ipsilaterally (to its own side) with a rotation of the face such that the face is turned to the opposite side. If both muscles act together, the neck is flexed. The SCM also acts as an accessory muscle of inspiration.

The SCM is innervated by the anterior horn cells of their own side only, whereas the trapezius has bilateral innervation so that the head can be coordinated to turn to the side in order to see what is happening. (As an example the right SCM turning the head to the left side has the right cerebral cortex controlling all these muscles). The movement of the head into the wry neck position allows the ear to approach the shoulder (an action opposed by splenius capitis on the contralateral side). The SCM also, however, functions as a rotator of the atlanto-axial joint. In this sense the actions of the SCM are a little more complex as it is a muscle that seldom contracts in isolation. Its precise actions are therefore dependent upon the activity of other prevertebral muscle groups, for example when the face is protracted forward on the neck.

Trapezius

The trapezius arises from the external occipital protuberance of the skull and the medial one third of the superior nuchal line down to the spinous processes of all the cervical vertebrae along with attachment to the ligamentum nuchae and extending its origin along the spinous processes of all of the 12 thoracic vertebrae (and their interspinous ligaments). At the thoracic spine level the muscle is aponeurotic and in the shape of a diamond with the opposite side. The occipital fibres are inserted into the lateral one third of the clavicle posteriorly and then progressively into the medial border of the acromion and as this carries on to the superior lip of the crest of the scapular spine. The lower part of the muscle is inserted into the medial root of the scapula spine more as a recurved or rolled tendon often in this area with an intervening bursa. The muscle belies its origin with the occipital myotomes and is innervated by the spinal XI as well as by proprioceptive fibres (C3,4) from the cervical plexus. The size of the muscle creates a complex action. It retracts the scapula, with the upper and the lower fibres important in scapular rotation behaving alternately like a wingnut. Some can elevate or depress the acromion and spine of the scapula, with upper fibres shrugging the shoulder. Assisting in shoulder abduction and acting together, the trapezius muscles extend the neck. Accessory nerve injury prevents typical shrugging of the shoulder.

XI: The Spinal Accessory Nerve

This nerve passes out of the posterior end of the SCM and lies on the levator scapulae embedded in the investing layer of deep cervical fascia in the roof of the posterior triangle. The fibres for this nerve arise in the spinal nucleus of the XI and the cervical (spinal) part of the medulla destined for the upper 5–6 spinal segments near the anterior grey column. This nerve then re-enters the skull via the foramen magnum joining fibres arising from the medulla oblongata (the cranial portion of XI which arises from the caudal pole of the nucleus ambiguus and near the dorsal X nucleus). The spinal XI re-exits via the jugular foramen with the IX and X nerves. The spinal XI separates and passes posteriorly and inferiorly across the transverse process of the atlas on its way to the SCM. One may consider the cranial XI (which supplies innervation to the soft palate, pharynx and larynx) as more appropriately part of the Cranial X. [3]

Levator Scapulae This thin muscle arises from the transverse processes of the upper four cervical vertebrae and descends down in the posterior triangle to be inserted into the medial border of the scapula from the upper angle to the area opposite the scapular spine. The levator scapulae is part of the developing upper limb bud and as a consequence its nerve supply reflects this origin being supplied by the dorsal scapular nerve principally via C5. Levator scapulae is an elevator of the shoulder as its name implies. Diagram 4.1 shows the muscles visible in the posterior triangle which include: Scalenus anterior, Scalenus medius, Scalenus posterior, Levator scapulae, Splenius capitis and Semispinalis capitis as one progressively moves backwards and upwards.

The Scaleni (Diagram 4.2) The muscles are so named, the scaleni (*Gk uneven*) as they are all of different lengths. These are a

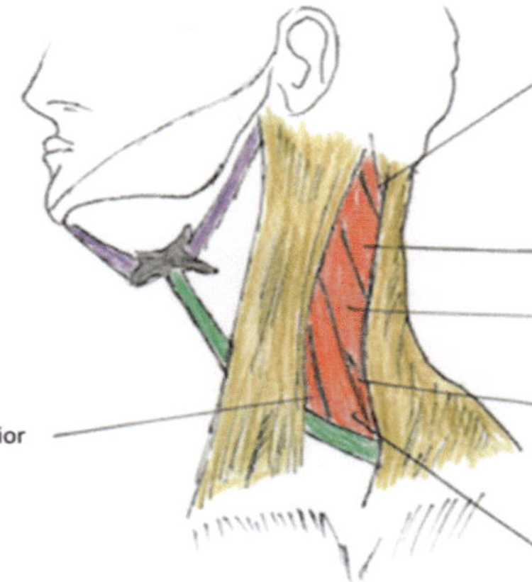

Diagram 4.1 Muscles of the posterior triangle of the neck. *Blue* attaches the anterior and posterior belly of the digastric to the hyoid bone (*black*)

relatively thick mass of muscles lying within the prevertebral fascia which run from the transverse processes of the first four cervical vertebrae to the upper two ribs. Their task is to elevate the ribs as accessory muscles of inspiration and to laterally flex the neck. The arrangement is similar in embryological structure to that of the intercostal muscles and the abdominal muscles. In the chest and the abdomen the intercostal or thoracoabdominal neurovascular bundles respectively, lie between the innermost and the internal muscular layer. In the chest this is between the innermost and internal intercostals and in the abdominal wall between the transversus abdominis nuscle and the internal oblique muscle. In this circumstance in the head and neck, the brachial plexus lies between the scalenus medius (the equivalent inner muscle) and the scalenus anterior (the equivalent innermost muscle). These arrangements are therefore the same except that in the neck it is rotated 90° to the vertical).

The nerve supply to the scaleni is via twigs from the lower 5 or 6 ventral rami which are locally distributed.

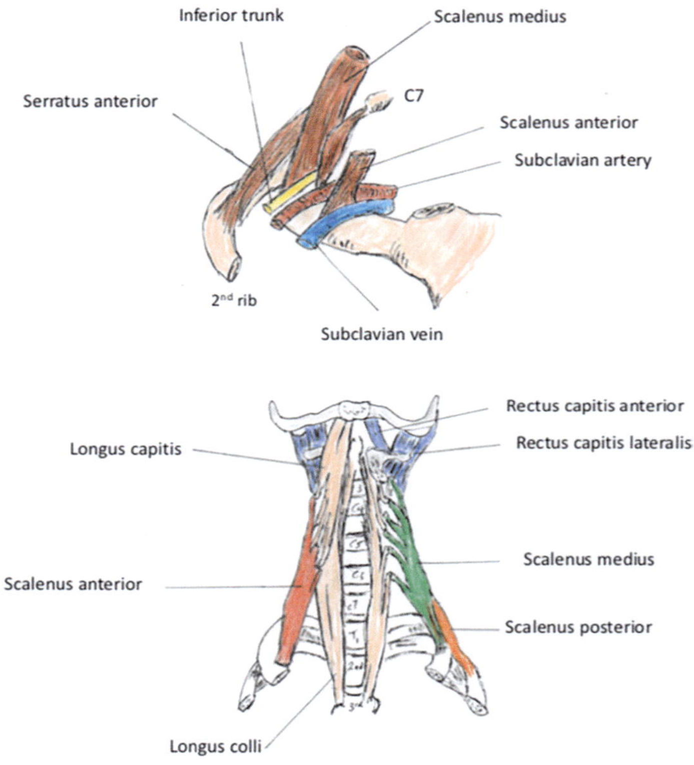

Diagram 4.2 *Top image:* The insertion of the scalenus anterior divides the subclavian artery and separates it from the subclavian vein. The thin muscle in front of the lower trunk of the brachial plexus is the scalenus minimus (originating from the anterior tubercle of the transverse process of C7)
Notations: Scalenus medius, C7, Scalenus anterior, Subclavian artery, Subclavian vein, second rib, Scalenus anterior, Inferior trunk
Bottom image: Scalenus anterior (C3–C6 anterior tubercles)—interdigitates with the longus capitis (anterior tubercles of the transverse processes of C3–C5)
Scalenus medius (posterior tubercles of the transverse processes of C2–C7) interdigitates with the medial fibres of the longus colli. The bottom end of T3 represents the inferior limit of the prevertebral fascia
Scalenus posterior is shown originating from the posterior tubercles of C5–7

The scalenus anterior is an important anatomical landmark in the root of the neck.

- The scalenus anterior arises from the anterior tubercles of the third–sixth cervical vertebra and attaches to the scalene tubercle on the first rib (Diagram 4.2). These slips of muscle are separate and they lie in their origin end to end with slips of the muscle above, the longus capitis. The subclavian vein lies in front, with the subclavian artery behind. The subclavian artery is divided on the basis of its relationship to the scalenus anterior (first part above the muscle, second part behind the muscle and third part beyond the muscle).
- The phrenic nerve runs behind the prevertebral fascia on top of the muscle and runs obliquely from the lateral to the medial muscle border. The nerve then enters the chest at the superior thoracic aperture behind the subclavian vein but in front of the subclavian artery passing medial to the apex of the lung on the suprapleural membrane (Sibson's fascia) and in front of Cranial X. Running medially is the ascending cervical artery (when present) which is a branch of the thyrocervical trunk. In front of all of this are the transverse cervical vessels and suprascapular vessels. It is at this level on the right side that the RLN is given off of Cranial X. Just above this level is a lymph node lying on the inferior belly of the omohyoid (the jugulo-omohyoid lymph node) which drains the side of the tongue (and may be enlarged as a presentation of cancer of the tongue).
- In the root of the neck, the IJV runs in front as does the inferior belly of the omohyoid muscle and the transverse cervical and suprascapular vessels.
- The thyrocervical trunk is medial to the muscle along with Sibson's fascia with the pleura and the vertebral artery lying supero-medially.[1]
- The longus colli muscle lies medially creating a small pyramidal space with the medial edge of the scalenus anterior where the base is the subclavian artery, and the neck of the first rib

[1]Named after the British anatomist Francis Sibson—1814–1876.

with Sibson's fascia. The apex of this space is Chassaignac's tubercle of C6 and is the point where the CCA can be directly palpated or compressed. This space also contains the stellate ganglion, the vertebral artery and the vertebral vein. The inferior thyroid artery (ITA) arches across this space medially as does the thoracic duct low down on the left side with the right lymphatic duct similarly on the right side arching medially over the lung apex to enter the IJV/Subclavian vein confluence.

- The vertebral artery (a branch of the first part of the subclavian) heads above this pyramidal space to reach the foramen transversarium in the C6 vertebral transverse process. Here the vertebral artery has a sympathetic plexus lying over it (the vertebral plexus) with the tiny middle cervical ganglion. From medial to lateral lying at the back of the neck of the first rib is the vein, artery and stellate ganglion with a connecting loop between the middle and the inferior cervical ganglia called the *ansa subclavia.*
- The next lateral branch of the subclavian artery is the thyrocervical trunk which divides into transverse cervical, suprascapular and ITA branches. From the lower surface of the convexity of the vessel is the origin of the internal thoracic artery. Anteriorly and inferiorly the vertebral vein runs forward to empty into the brachiocephalic vein, however, it can occasionally travel through the empty foramen transversarium of C7.
- From behind the scalenus anterior is the second part of the subclavian artery from which arises the costocervical trunk and which passes backwards over the lung apex to the neck of the first rib dividing into the superior intercostal artery and an ascending deep cervical artery running upwards to anastomose with the occipital artery.
- Laterally, are the trunks of the brachial plexus and the third portion of the subclavian artery. There is a variably described dorsal scapular artery which can arise here running laterally through the brachial plexus and passing deep to levator scapulae. This vessel forms part of the scapular anastomosis (a natural connexion of collaterals between this third part of the subclavian artery and the circumflex scapular vessels which arise from the third part of the axillary artery). This native col-

lateral circulation opens when there is an occlusion between the third parts of the subclavian and axillary arteries.

Behind the scalenus anterior lies the scalenus medius.

The **scalenus medius** is a larger muscle but is less regarded in anatomy teaching. It arises from the posterior tubercles of all the cervical transverse processes and is inserted into a rough oval shaped region on the superior surface of the first rib behind the depression left for the subclavian artery. The scalenus medius is directly pierced by the dorsal scapular nerve and by the upper segmental two roots of the long thoracic nerve (nerve to serratus anterior). The serratus anterior muscle is attached posteriorly just at this point to the back of the first rib with the cervical pleura lying just below here. Scalenus medius is typically innervated by the anterior rami of the lower cervical nerves (C3–8). On occasion a fourth muscle the **scalenus minimus** (the so-called Sibson's muscle) can lie below the lower edge of the scalenus anterior.

The **scalenus posterior** is a small muscle lying behind, deep to the first interdigitation of serratus anterior and inserted along the outer border of the second rib. Scalenus posterior is innervated by the anterior rami of C6–8.

- The other prevertebral muscles include: the longus colli, the longus capitis and higher up the rectus capitis anterior and lateralis muscles.
- Longus colli is so named because it is the longest of the muscle slips extending from the anterior tubercle of the atlas down to T3 (also attaching to the transverse processes of the C3–6). It is the muscle that holds in the prevertebral abscesses derived from Pott's disease (thoracic Tuberculosis) and is the inferior limit of the prevertebral fascia.
- Laterally (and more superiorly) is the longus capitis passing from the anterior tubercles of C3–6 to the base of the skull in front of the rectus capitis anterior and in front and to the side of the foramen magnum.
- The rectus capitis anterior arises from the anterior surface of the lateral mass of the atlas up to the base of the skull just anterior to the occipital condyle and adjacent to the hypoglossal canal.

- The rectus capitis lateralis arises from the transverse process of the atlas and passes to the jugular process of the occipital bone. It is separated from the attachment of the rectus capitis anterior by the ventral ramus of the first cervical nerve which supplies both muscles.

The origins and disposition of the scaleni and rectus capitis muscles are shown in Diagram 4.2.

Another relevant landmark muscle of the region is the **subclavius**. This muscle arises from the costochondral junction of the first rib and is inserted into the subclavian groove on the inferior surface of the clavicle. It is enclosed by the upper attachment of the clavipectoral fascia and holds the clavicle down to the first rib. It may possibly prevent shards of a clavicle fracture injuring the subclavian vein. Subclavius is innervated by the nerve to the subclavius (C5, 6) which is a rootlet branch of the brachial plexus. This nerve may importantly contribute to the formation of an accessory phrenic nerve and can be damaged in brachial plexus injuries where it can be a sign of a root or trunk nerve avulsion injury that renders this injury irreparable (This clinical point is considered in greater detail in Chap. 4 Upper Limb of Volume 2 in this book series).

The Cervical Plexus

The cervical plexus forms the sensory coverage to the neck and part of the side of the face and ear and the motor roots to the diaphragm and infrahyoid musculature. This plexus forms from simple loops of the upper four cervical nerve ventral primary rami after each has already received a grey ramus communicans from the superior cervical ganglion. It lies in effect in series with the brachial plexus on the scalenus medius and is held down behind the tough prevertebral fascia.

Diagram 4.3 is a progressive schematic which allows the reader to develop the structure of the cervical plexus for themselves.

Sensory Branches: include

- The cutaneous branches of the cervical plexus supply the front and the sides of the neck.
- The first branch of C2 is the lesser occipital nerve which is quite slender and which runs up along the posterior border of the SCM to supply the posterior part of the neck up to the nuchal line and the postauricular area.
- The great auricular nerve (C2, 3) is a large nerve running vertically upwards on the SCM to supply the skin over the angle of the mandible as well as the parotid fascia. It extends to supply the cranial surface of the auricle and the lateral lobar surface below the EAM, as well as the skin over the mastoid region. It passes partially within the parotid gland supplying the deep layer of parotid fascia. It is a useful cable graft should any part of Cranial VII need to be sacrificed in parotid surgery.[2]
- The transverse cervical nerve of the neck (previously known as the anterior cutaneous nerve of the neck) is derived from C2 and C3 and emerges as a single trunk behind the mid-border of the SCM to be distributed from the chin to the suprasternal space in the midline
- From C3 and C4 there is a large supraclavicular nerve passing inferiorly which divides into a medial, intermediate and lateral component and which covers the skin sensation over the cape area of the shoulder and extending as far as the second intercostal space. The medial branch extends to the sternal angle and the sternoclavicular joint, the intermediate branch passing as far down as the anterior axillary line and the lateral branch passing across the acromion to half way down over the deltoid

[2]The great auricular nerve is a particular site attacked in leprosy.

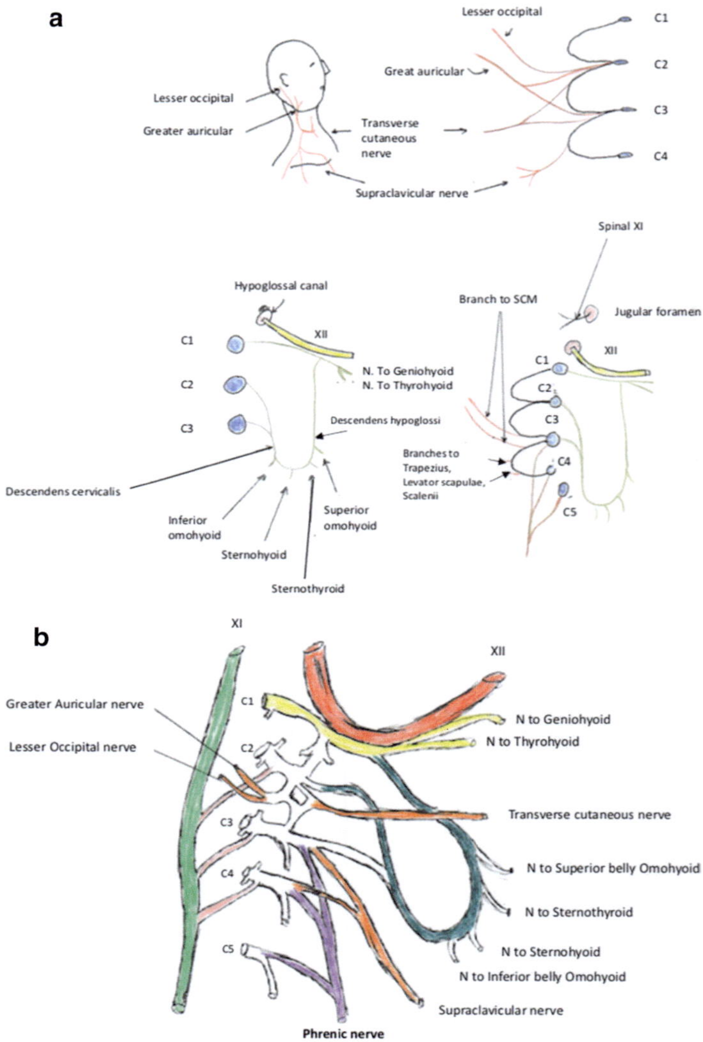
a
Lesser occipital
C1
C2
Great auricular
Lesser occipital
Greater auricular
C3
Transverse
cutaneous
nerve
C4
Supraclavicular nerve
Spinal XI
Hypoglossal canal
Branch to SCM
Jugular foramen
XII
C1
N. To Geniohyoid
N. To Thyrohyoid
C2
C3
Descendens hypoglossi
Branches to
Trapezius,
Levator scapulae,
Scalenii
C4
C5
Descendens cervicalis
Inferior
omohyoid
Sternohyoid
Superior
omohyoid
Sternothyroid
b
XI
XII
Greater Auricular nerve
Lesser Occipital nerve
N to Geniohyoid
N to Thyrohyoid
Transverse cutaneous nerve
N to Superior belly Omohyoid
N to Sternothyroid
N to Sternohyoid
N to Inferior belly Omohyoid
Supraclavicular nerve
Phrenic nerve

Diagram 4.3 The cervical plexus
(**a**) The *top left* schematic images shows the radiation of the cutaneous elements (lesser occipital, greater auricular, transverse cervical and supraclavicular)
Notations: Transverse cutaneous nerve, Supraclavicular nerve, Greater auricular nerve, Lesser occipital nerve
The *top right image* shows the origins of the cutaneous elements from the cervical roots
The *bottom left image* shows the innervation of the infrahyoid muscles via the *ansa cervicalis* (lower root as the *descendens hypoglossi* to sternothyroid, sternohyoid and omohyoid). Geniohyoid and thyrohyoid are innervated by C1 roots traveling with the Cranial XII
The b*ottom right image s*hows the motor elements of the plexus including the phrenic nerve and segmental proprioceptive branches to the sternocleidomastoid and trapezius and motor to the levator scapulae (C3, 4), scaleni and other prevertebral muscles (C1,2 to rectus capitis; C1–3 to Longus capitis, C2–4 to Longus colli and intertransversarii). The spinal XI is formed from the upper C1–C4 roots which enter the skull via the foramen magnum and which split off through the jugular foramen to innervate the SCM and the trapezius muscles
(**b**) Combined sensory and motor elements of the cervical plexus

muscle and posteriorly over the shoulder as far as the spine of the scapula (posterior axial line).

- The supraclavicular nerve is one point where part of the cutaneous supply of the upper limb (namely the shoulder) is not supplied by branches of the brachial plexus (the other area being the inner aspect of the upper arm which is sensorily innervated by the intercostobrachial nerve—the collateral branch of the second intercostal nerve). One can imagine that in the formation of the cutaneous nerve supply of the upper limb that this area over the shoulder cape region has been dragged down with development of the upper limb bud.

Muscular Branches: include

- Additional segmental branches to other prevertebral muscles (the longus capitis, the longus colli and the scaleni).
- Formation of a unique loop with C1 that transmits along Cranial XII. There is a meningeal branch returning around the hypoglossal canal (and innervating part of dural sensation over the posterior cranial fossa) and a specific branch to the superior root of the *ansa cervicalis* loop (also called the *descendens hypoglossi*). These C1 fibres are destined for motor innervation to the higher hyoid-related musculature—the geniohyoid and the thyrohyoid. The Cranial XII fibres only innervate the tongue musculature with their cell bodies located in the hypoglossal nucleus of the medulla. These tongue muscles have formed from occipital myotomes which drag the XII nerve with them by passing between the ICA and the ECA (as do only a few other structures including Cranial IX and the pharyngeal branch of Cranial X). As Cranial XII has no sensory component, it resembles Cranials III, IV, VI and XI.
- The superior root of the ansa cervicalis lies over the front of the carotid sheath innervating the infrahyoid musculature (sternohyoid, sternothyroid and omohyoid). Further proprioceptive branches come from C2 and C3 (to the sternocleidomastoid) and from C3 and C4 (to the trapezius).
- The inferior root of the ansa cervicalis (the *descendens cervicalis*) loops around from C2 and C3 to complete the circle on the lateral side of the IJV.
- The principal motor supply of the cervical plexus is the **phrenic nerve** the sole motor innervation of the diaphragm which is principally C4 (with some contributions from C3 and also C5). Below the subclavian vein it can be joined by an **accessory phrenic nerve** derived from the nerve to subclavius which can descend in front of the subclavian vein. The accessory phrenic nerve (when present) can also arise directly from the ansa cer-

vicalis or even the nerve to stylohyoid. (The phrenic nerve is considered in greater detail in Volume 3, Chap. 3 of this book series). In brief, it is a mixed nerve which is also sensory to large parts of the parietal pleura, pericardium and upper peritoneum [4].

- The dermatomes of the neck in addition to the cutaneous branches of the Cervical plexus supplying the anterior and lateral part of the neck include the greater occipital and third occipital nerves from the posterior rami of C2 and C3 respectively for the back of the neck. It should be noted that C1 does not supply any skin at all. C2 supplies most of the posterior aspect of the neck up to the occiput and the auricle as well as the face over the angle of the mandible with C3 providing a cylindrical area of the neck and with C4 extending over the clavicles and shoulder down to the scapular spine.
- Connections between the C4 and C5 roots are large if the brachial plexus is prefixed (meaning that it has a higher root take off with more C4 and less T1 contribution).

Try and build Diagram 4.3 from scratch to form the sensory and motor components of the cervical plexus.

1. Begin by drawing the five cervical foraminae and above this the hypoglossal canal and the jugular foramen.
2. On the sensory side join C2 and C3 to form posteriorly the lesser occipital and great auricular nerves and anteriorly the transverse cutaneous nerve of the neck. The C2,3,4 fibres drop down to form the supraclavicular nerve.
3. On the motor side there are segmental branches to the prevertebral muscles. Draw a straight line from Cranial XII. Join a branch to XII from C1. This innervates the upper hyoid muscles geniohyoid and thyrohyoid.
4. Loop branches of C2 and C3 with this C1 link to form the *ansa cervicalis* (which innervates the infrahyoid muscles—sternohyoid, sternothyroid and omohyoid).
5. Below link C3 and C4 to form the phrenic nerve (occasionally replaced by a C5 branch—the accessory phrenic nerve from the nerve to the subclavius).

When the phrenic nerve is replaced, a brachial plexus injury where the rootlets are avulsed can paralyze the hemi-diaphragm. This may also occur if the brachial plexus is prefixed.

6. Additional positional proprioceptive fibres are derived from C2,3 to innervate the SCM and from C3,4 to innervate the trapezius forming a local reflex arc.
7. In clinical practice an ultrasound-guided cervical plexus block can be used for carotid endarterectomy and a deep block can be useful for vocal cord surgery, dental abscesses in patients with difficult airways, lymph node resections and some plastic surgical repairs.

Q and A: Chap. 4 (Answers at the End of This Chapter)

1. The sternocleidomastoid:
   (a) Has a dual blood supply
   (b) Is solely innervated by the spinal XI
   (c) Has bilateral central innervation
   (d) Tilts the head ipsilaterally turning the face to the other side
2. Regarding the scalenus anterior muscle:
   (a) It lies in series with the longus capitis
   (b) Lies behind the subclavian vessels
   (c) Has the phrenic nerve running on its surface from medial to the lateral border of the muscle
   (d) Is crossed by the inferior belly of the omohyoid
   (e) The inferior thyroid artery and Sibson's fascia are inferiorly located
   (f) Chassaignac's tubercle lies laterally
3. The subclavius muscle:
   (a) Is enclosed by the clavipectoral fascia
   (b) Has a direct innervation from the segmental spinal nerves
   (c) Can incorporate the accessory phrenic nerve
   (d) Protects the subclavian vein

4. Regarding the Cervical Plexus
   (a) The descendens hypoglossi supplies the infrahyoid muscles
   (b) Proprioceptive branches supply the sternocleidomastoid and trapezius separately
   (c) The phrenic nerve is purely motor
   (d) C1 provides hitchhiking branches to all the infrahyoid muscles
   (e) The medial supraclavicular nerve extends to the sternal angle
5. The infrahyoid musculature is:
   (a) Innervated by the hypoglossal nerve
   (b) Innervated in part by the C1 ramus
   (c) Innervated high in its segmentation
   (d) Innervated by the ansa cervicalis except for the omohyoid
6. The accessory nerve
   (a) Has a cranial segment which supports the Vagus and provides pharyngeal and palatal innervation
   (b) Has spinal segments which arise below the medulla
   (c) Runs between the scalenus anterior and the scalenus medius
   (d) Exits the skull via the foramen magnum
7. The accessory phrenic nerve
   (a) Arises from the upper trunk of the brachial plexus
   (b) May pass in front of the subclavian vein
   (c) Cannot be injured in a brachial plexus injury
   (d) Is found in less than 10% of dissections
8. The cervical plexus
   (a) Forms from the upper 3 cervical nerves uniting to form loops
   (b) Usually forms 2 loops (C1–2 and C2–3)
   (c) Never connects to the brachial plexus
   (d) Has an anterior primary ramus which is entirely motor
   (e) Forms a loop with the ascending branch of C2 below the transverse process of the atlas
   (f) Has each root receiving a grey ramus communicans from the superior cervical ganglion

Answers

1. a, d
2. a, d
3. a, c, d
4. a, b, e
5. b
6. a
7. a, b
8. d, f

References

1. Sandulescu T, Stoltenberg F, Buechner H, Schmidt-Park H, Linnerz F, Jast J, Franzmann M, Blaurock-Sandulescu T, Naumova EA, Arnold WH. Platysma and the cervical superficial musculoaponeurotic system—comparative analysis of facial crease and platysmal band development. Ann Anat. 2020;227:151414.
2. Hwang K, Kim J-Y, Lim JH. Anatomy of the platysma muscle. J Craniofac Surg. 2017;28:539–42.
3. Rezigallah AA, et al. The accessory nerve. Sudan J Med Sci. 2012;7:125–9.
4. Loukas M. Surgical anatomy of the accessory phrenic nerve. Ann Thorac Surg. 2006;82:1870–5.

The Autonomic Nervous System of the Head and Neck

5

Contents

Sympathetic Nervous System (SNS) of the Head and Neck 92
SNS Fibres Hitchhike Along the Relevant Arteries 95
Parasympathetic Nervous System (PSNS) of the Head and Neck 97
Ciliary Ganglion: Diagram 5.3a 100
Submandibular Ganglion: Diagram 5.3b 104
Pterygopalatine Ganglion: Diagram 5.3c 105
Otic Ganglion: Diagram 5.3d 106
Q and A: Chap. 5 (Answers at the End of This Chapter) 107
Answers 109
Reference 109

In the somatic nervous system, the motor supply to somatic muscle has its cell bodies located in the motor nuclei of cranial nerves or in the anterior horn cells of the spinal cord, with the nerves entering the motor end plates directly. By contrast, in the autonomic nervous system (ANS) as a whole, the motor part concerned with the innervation of cardiac and smooth muscle and the bodily glands comprises a pathway from the CNS to the target organ interrupted by a synapse within an intervening ganglion.

This very basic difference effectively divides the ANS into a preganglionic and a postganglionic pathway with the preganglionic cell bodies part of the CNS itself. If these are part of the sympathetic nervous system (SNS) these cells are located in the thoracolumbar outflow part of the spinal cord. These cells lie in

A. Zbar, *Anatomy--Head and Neck*,
https://doi.org/10.1007/978-3-031-69538-4_5

the lateral horn (called the intermediolateral cell column). If they are part of the parasympathetic nervous system (PSNS) these occur in certain cranial nerve nuclei and in the lateral horn cells of the sacral segments S2, 3, and 4 (the craniosacral outflow).

The postganglionic cell bodies go from the ganglia into the peripheral nervous system. If these are sympathetic, the ganglia are either in the sympathetic trunk itself (the paravertebral ganglia) or lie in other ganglia which are variably called the collateral ganglia. If this is part of the PSNS, the ganglia are collectively referred to as terminal ganglia as they are typically located within the walls of the viscus or tissue target. With the PSNS there are also certain discrete named mixed head and neck ganglia, four of which are the:

- ciliary
- submandibular
- pterygopalatine and
- otic

Sympathetic Nervous System (SNS) of the Head and Neck

The function of the SNS in the head and neck is largely to control precapillary sphincters (vasomotor), as well as pilo-erector function and in the sudomotor (secretomotor) control of the sweat glands. The SNS system is distributed via the paravertebral ganglia and specifically as part of the sympathetic chain via the superior, middle and inferior cervical ganglia. Sympathetic activity is derived specifically from the thoracolumbar outflow arising in the segments T1-L2 in the intermediolateral cell column which is a group of cells located between the sensory and motor horns of the spinal cord as shown in Diagram 5.1.

To explain the SNS in the body simply, in brief in a cross section of the spinal cord the intermediolateral cell column contributes fibres into the ventral spinal nerve which then typically leave

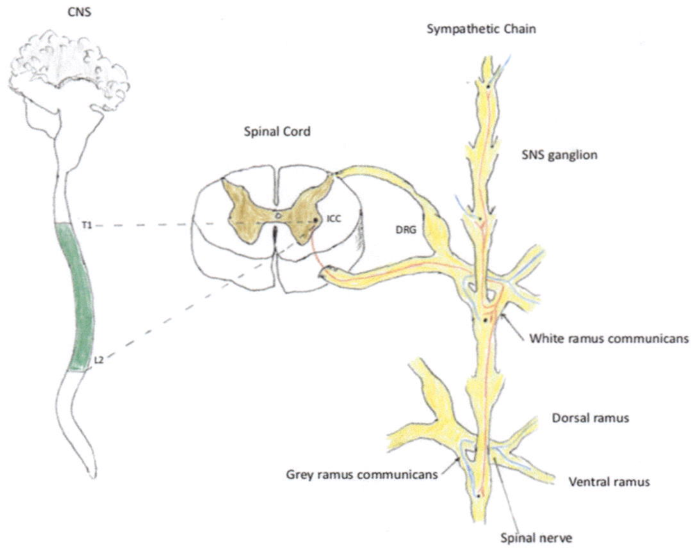

Diagram 5.1 The sympathetic nervous system: Basic structure. Cells for the thoracolumbar SNS outflow (T1–L2) reside in the intermediate cell column (ICC) in the spinal cord. Myelinated preganglionic fibres (*white rami communicantes*) may synapse locally or head up and down the sympathetic chain before synapsing. Postganglionic unmyelinated fibres (*grey rami communicantes*) deliver fibres to viscera and tissues principally controlling precapillary sphincters but in the head and neck also innervating sweat glands, hair follicles and the dilator pupillae muscle (pupillary dilatation)

the nerve to enter one of the paravertebral ganglia. These fibres are myelinated preganglionic fibres which because of their myelination are referred to as the *white rami communicans*. They may or may not necessarily synapse in the ganglion at that level but they can just as equally use the ganglion as a relay station without synapsing. Once however they do synapse these postganglionic SNS fibres are no longer myelinated and are known as *grey rami communicans*. The possibility is of course that these fibres can ultimately move lower down or higher up depending upon their target tissue where they can ultimately synapse. In the rest of the body they may of course also pass for long distances as preganglionic fibres to perhaps get to the preaortic ganglia (like the coeliac or the aorticorenal ganglia) before synapsing. In other circumstances they may directly synapse in the adrenal medulla (which effectively behaves like a giant ganglion) where epinephrine or norepinephrine is directly released.

In the normal circumstance the preganglionic fibre of the PSNS system is typically long with a short postganglionic fibre (often known as an intramural fibre) within the substance of the viscus or target tissue. That is to say that the postganglionic PSNS system is typically short.

The reverse is the case with the SNS where the preganglionic fibre is long and this long preganglionic fibre is referred to as a *splanchnic nerve*. Examples of these splanchnic nerves exist in the thorax as the greater (typically T5–9), the lesser (T10, 11) and the least (T12) splanchnic nerves which then synapse in the coeliac and aorticorenal preaortic ganglia respectively.

So in summary there are only several options for the SNS fibres here after having reached a sympathetic trunk ganglion:

1. Synapse with cell bodies in a trunk ganglion (either in the one entered or by running up or down to an adjacent trunk ganglion);
2. Leaving the trunk ganglion without synapsing only to synapse in a collateral ganglion;
3. Passing to the suprarenal medulla and synapse there with the medulla functioning as a specialized ganglion.

As there is no SNS in the cervical region or for that matter from the lower lumbar and sacral parts of the cord outflow, those preganglionic fibres destined to run with cervical nerves must ascend in the SNS trunk to cervical ganglia. (In the lower lumbar and sacral regions these fibres descend to lower lumbar and sacral ganglia).

The SNS trunk extends alongside the vertebral column from the base of the skull to the coccyx with (in theory at least) one ganglion per level for each spinal nerve where the upper 4 unite to form the superior cervical ganglion, 5 and 6 unite as the middle ganglion and 7 and 8 fuse with the T1 ganglion as the cervicothoracic (or stellate) ganglion. Elsewhere there is therefore one ganglion less than the number of spinal nerves such that there are 11 thoracic, 4 lumbar and 4 sacral ganglia. Every spinal nerve receives a grey ramus but the cervical lower lumbar and sacral nerves do not have white rami because there is no SNS outflow in these segments.

SNS Fibres Hitchhike Along the Relevant Arteries

In the neck, the preganglionic sympathetic fibres ascend and descend as a discrete trunk from the upper thoracic ventral rami (as already stated) towards the cervical ganglia. This trunk runs vertically anterior to the longus colli and the longus capitis muscles behind the carotid sheath on the ends of the transverse processes of the vertebrae. Inferiorly, the SNS chain lies medial to the vertebral artery and on the left it is crossed anteriorly by the thoracic duct and on the right by the arching inferior thyroid artery (ITA). Although superiorly the trunk effectively ends in the superior cervical ganglion, it is continued on the surface of the ICA as what is called the internal carotid nerve.

The *superior cervical ganglion* is a large (2.5 cm) ganglion lying on the longus capitis typically opposite the second or the third cervical vertebra. It has a number of communicating branches including:

- communicators to the IX, X and XII cranial nerves
- grey rami communicantes to the upper four cervical ventral rami
- the internal carotid nerve
- laryngopharyngeal branches which contribute to the pharyngeal plexus
- the external carotid nerves (running on the ECA and its branches).

- contributors to the superior cervical cardiac plexi on the left this is part of the superficial cardiac plexus, on the right it descends into the chest (either in front of or behind the subclavian artery) to be part of the deep cardiac plexus at the bifurcation of the trachea.

The *middle cervical ganglion* is very small lying on the ITA at about the level of the cricoid cartilage. It has several branches:

- grey rami communicantes passing to the fifth and sixth cervical ventral rami
- thyroid branches forming an ITA plexus (communicating with the RLN and the external laryngeal nerve -ELN)
- middle cervical cardiac nerve which is a slender branch to the deep cardiac plexus which on the right-hand side accompanies the superior cervical cardiac nerve
- ansa subclavia (a slender branch which loops around the subclavian artery to join the stellate ganglion. The ansa subclavia supplies the subclavian artery sending branches across to the phrenic nerve.

The cervicothoracic ganglion may exist as either one or two parts. It can represent the fused inferior cervical and T1 (and/or) T2 ganglia. If separate the inferior cervical ganglion is small lying behind the CCA and the vertebral artery anterior to the eighth cervical ventral ramus. If combined as a *stellate ganglion* it lies at the neck of the first rib receiving a white ramus communicans from the first thoracic ventral ramus. The branches (whether a fused ganglion or not) include:

- gray rami communicantes from the seventh and eighth cervical ventral rami
- ansa subclavia connexions
- communications with the vertebral plexus on the vertebral artery
- inferior cervical cardiac nerve which joins the deep cardiac plexus.
- SNS outflow for the head and neck (which is concerned with pupillary dilatation)
- Forms the deep petrosal nerve which combines with PSNS nerve fibres running in the greater petrosal nerve to form an input nerve to the pterygopalatine ganglion (the nerve to the pterygoid canal

also called the Vidian nerve).[1] What is unusual in this ganglion is that the preganglionic PSNS and the SNS actually combine as separate branches in the pterygopalatine fossa where the PSNS fibres are the only ones which synapse and where the pterygopalatine ganglion is a relay station for autonomic (PSNS and SNS) activity for the glands and sinuses of the middle third of the face (*see below*).

Parasympathetic Nervous System (PSNS) of the Head and Neck

The **Parasympathetic (PSNS) system** in the head and neck is part of the craniosacral outflow which includes centres coalesced around:

- III cranial nerve (in the midbrain)
- VII nerve nuclei
- IX nerve and
- Cranial X.

There are several structural points regarding the PSNS:

1. The PSNS is visceral and is not distributed to the trunk, limbs, suprarenal or gonads.
2. Preganglionic fibres of cranial origin originate in the Edinger-Westphal oculomotor (III) nucleus, the superior and inferior salivatory nuclei and the dorsal motor nucleus of the X.
3. The postganglionic vagal fibres are located in the viscera (heart lungs and gut) and the postganglionic cells for the EW nucleus, the salivatory nuclei end on the four head and neck PSNS ganglia respectively.

---

[1] Named in honour of the Italian surgeon Guido Guidi (1509–1569) who was locally known as Vidus Vidius. He was the personal physician to King Francis I of France and then to Cosimo di Medici. Guidi was the grandson of the great artist Domenico Ghiralndaio and also a personal friend of the artist and ceramicist Benvenuto Cellini (1500–1571).

4. For completeness, the preganglionic fibres of sacral origin arise from the lateral horn cells of S2,3 and 4 constituting the pelvic splanchnic nerves entering the inferior hypogastric plexus and run up from the pelvic origins to the level of the splenic flexure.
5. The four head and neck ganglia (ciliary, submandibular, pterygopalatine and otic) are specifically distributed via local Cranial V fibres that sensorily serve glands of the orbit, nose and nasal pharynx and mouth as well distributing PSNS function to the sphincter pupillae and the ciliary muscle of the eye.
6. Postganglionic fibres of the SNS and fibres of Cranial V run through these ganglia which act as a relay station **but do not synapse there**.
7. The ganglia are each similar in structural plan possessing a PSNS, SNS and a sensory root. Specifically, the PSNS root carries the preganglionic fibres from the nucleus and represents the essential ganglionic function which is glandular secretomotor (sudomotor). In some textbooks the PSNS root is referred to as the motor root. The SNS root contains postganglionic fibres from the superior cervical ganglion whose preganglionic fibres lie in the lateral horn of T1–T3. The sensory root contains the cell bodies of the Trigeminal (V) ganglion.

Diagram 5.2 shows the basic structure of PSNS stimulation of head and neck glands (mucous and salivary).

The easiest way to understand this is by starting with the target tissues for secretion.

- These include the pupil (and the ciliary body), the submandibular (and sublingual) glands, the lacrimal gland and the parotid gland (*Bottom of* Diagram 5.2).
- Each target tissue has its own ganglion: the eye (ciliary), the submandibular and sublingual glands (submandibular), lacrimal apparatus (pterygopalatine) and the parotid gland (otic).
- For each ganglion there is a nucleus: for the oculomotor, the nearby EW nucleus; for the submandibular and the lacrimal

glands, the superior salivatory nucleus and for the parotid gland, the inferior salivatory nucleus (*Top of* Diagram 5.2).

- Each nucleus conveys to its individual ganglion via a **preganglionic CNS pathway** (directed by a specific cranial nerve or part of a cranial nerve) **with each postganglionic pathway distributed to its relevant target by hitchhiking along the nearest available branch of V.**

(*Second Line* Diagram 5.2)

The preganglionic pathway of the ciliary ganglion is distributed via III.
That of the submandibular ganglion is brought in via the chorda tympani branch of VII.
That for the lacrimal gland is brought in by the greater petrosal branch of Cranial VII.
That for the parotid gland is brought by the lesser petrosal branch of Cranial IX.

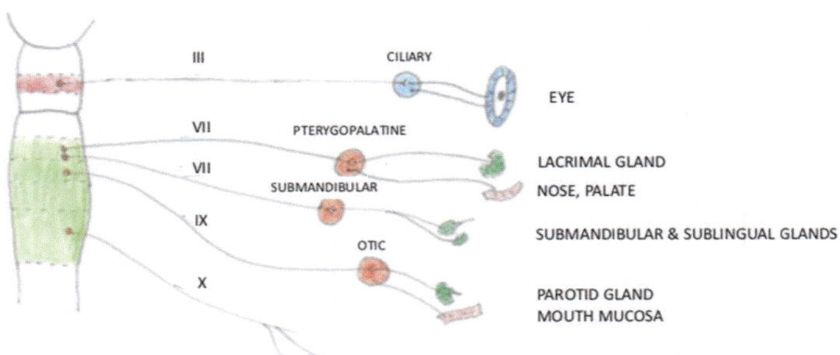

Diagram 5.2 Basic structure of the parasympathetic nervous system (PSNS) for the head and neck. Central nuclei travel to the four ganglia and link as postganglionic fibres to local branches of Cranial V to lead to salivation and lacrimation. The III nuclei are located in the midbrain and the remainder of the relevant nuclei are pontine. Vagal fibres are distributed to the rest of the body

(*Third Line* Diagram 5.2)

The postganglionic pathway for the ciliary ganglion is via the short ciliary nerves to the sphincter pupillae and the ciliary body of the iris. The effect here is pupillo-constriction and ciliary muscle accommodation.

The pathway for the postganglionic fibres of the submandibular and sublingual glands is brought by the lingual nerve (V_3).

The postganglinonic fibres for the lacrimal gland arrive via the zygomaticofacial nerve (V_2) after synapse in the pterygopalatine ganglion which **in the inner orbit then jump across** to get to the lacrimal gland as part of V_1 via the lacrimal nerve (which has most laterally made its way through the superior orbital fissure. The role of the superior orbital fissure is to transmit nerves and vessels from the middle cranial fossa to the orbit.

The postganglionic pathway to the parotid gland is also via V_3 through the distribution along the parotid and the side of the face in the auriculotemporal nerve.

It should be noted that the embryological development of the face is such that the orbit and vertex is sensorily innervated by V_1, the middle third of the face by V_2 and the side of the chin and the neck are pulled up against the temple as V_3 so that the parotid territory and the submandibular territories are both V_3 innervations.

Each of these ganglia has some unique features.

Ciliary Ganglion: Diagram 5.3a

The ciliary ganglion is about the size of pinhead lying between the optic nerve and the lateral rectus muscle. There is a long slender filament from cell bodies in the Cranial V ganglion (V_1) via the nasociliary nerve with the fibres extending to the eyeball. The SNS root of the ciliary ganglion comes from the superior cervical ganglion via branches of the internal carotid nerve entering the ophthalmic nerve from the internal carotid plexus to supply the dilator pupillae and the blood vessels in the outer coat of the eye. These relay straight through the ganglion without synapse in the short ciliary nerves. Cranial III has a short stout branch coming from the nerve to the inferior oblique muscle and entering the ganglion with its PSNS pre-ganglionic fibres from III for synapse within the ganglion. This nerve is part of the inferior division of III traveling through the superior orbital fissure. These nerves enter from lateral to medial in accordance with a mnemonic as **L**azy **F**rench **T**erriers **S**it **N**earby **I**n **A**nticipation; (i.e. **L**acrimal, **F**rontal, **T**rochlear, **S**uperior division of III, **N**asociliary, **I**nferior division of III and **A**bducent). In this schema, the most medial structure VI travels the most lateral and circuitous course and is subject in a non-specific way to the effects of raised intracranial pressure. The effect is for a lateral rectus palsy to function as a non-localizing (or so-called non-lateralizing) sign when the intracranial pressure rises.

Postganglionic cells from the ciliary ganglion pass with the short ciliary nerves to the eyeball and innervate the sphincter pupillae muscle and also the ciliary muscle. The ciliary muscle reduces the tension in the suspensory ligament of the lens to make the lens fatter and able to accommodate to focus closer objects.

The EW nucleus is effectively two basic structures in the midbrain and is a part of the III complex (preganglionic PSNS motor neurons). The other part controls a range of stress-related peptidergic functions.

The Pupillary Reflex (Diagram 5.4) is a reflex which involves adaptation to vision at various levels of illumination, with constriction of the pupil (miosis) directly and consensually. The physiology and anatomy of this reflex is complex. The pupillary light reflex neural pathway has an afferent limb and two efferent limbs. The afferent has nerve fibres in Cranial II (optic) with efferent fibres running along Cranial III (oculomotor). The afferent limb runs along II and synapses in the pretectal nucleus in the midbrain at the level of the superior colliculus. The efferent limb is the pupillary motor output from the pretectal nucleus to the ciliary sphincter muscle of the iris. The pretectal nucleus projects both crossed and uncrossed fibres to both the ipsilateral and the contralateral EW nuclei located nearby. Each of these EW nuclei then has its preganglionic PSNS fibres exiting via III in the ciliary ganglion. The contralateral efferent limb results in the consensual reaction [1].

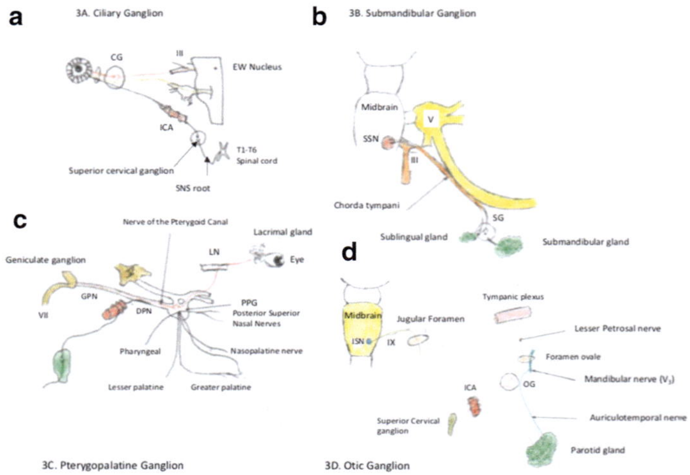

Diagram 5.3 The structure of the four PSNS ganglia
(**a**) Ciliary ganglion (CG). The CG has a sensory root (via the nasociliary branch of the ophthalmic division of Cranial V), a sympathetic root (arriving along the internal carotid artery as the carotid nerve) and a PSNS root (derived from the Edinger-Westphal nucleus located in the mid-brain) that is distributed through the inferior branch of Cranial III. The motor nuclei of Cranial III lie alongside the EW nucleus in the midbrain. Postganglionic PSNS fibres innervate the sphincter pupillae (causing pupillary constriction) and the ciliary body (altering the zonula fibres that change lens shape and lead to accommodation)
The sympathetic root is derived from T1–T6
Legend: EW Edinger-Westphal nucleus
ICA Internal carotid artery
(**b**) The Submandibular ganglion (SG) has the chorda tympani (derived from Cranial VII) which runs along with the lingual nerve (V3). Postganglionic PSNS fibres are distributed to the submandibular and sublingual glands
Legend: SG—Submandibular ganglion
SSN—Superior salivatory nucleus

(**c**) Pterygopalatine ganglion (PG). The ganglion is mixed with only the PSNS fibres synapsing. There are SNS fibres derived from the superior cervical ganglion running along the internal carotid artery as the carotid nerve. The autonomic branches to the PG include the sympathetic (SNS) element called the deep petrosal nerve and the PSNS element via the greater petrosal branch of Cranial VII after it has left the geniculate ganglion. The SNS and PSNS nerves combine to form the nerve to the pterygoid canal (Vidian nerve) which enters the pterygopalatine fossa through its roof. Postganglionic fibres from the PG go to the nose, pharynx, hard and soft palate and the infraorbital skin, mucous glands, sinuses and soft tissues of the middle 1/3 of the face. The PG acts as a relay station with canalicular and foraminal connections to the nasal, pharyngeal, infraorbital and palatal regions merging the distribution of blood vessels, sympathetics, sensory afferents and secretomotor parasympathetics. Postganglionic fibres for lacrimation travel along V2 in the zygomaticofacial nerve which then jumps across to the lacrimal nerve (V1) to travel to the lacrimal gland promoting tear production.
Legend: PPG—Pterygopalatine ganglion
LN Lacrimal nerve
DPN Deep petrosal nerve
GPN Greater petrosal nerve
NPC Nerve of the pterygoid canal (Vidian nerve)
(**d**) Otic ganglion (OG). Preganglionic PSNS fibres originate from the inferior salivatory nucleus in the midbrain and travel through the tympanic canaliculus as a branch of Cranial IX, the lesser petrosal nerve. These are joined with SNS fibres from the superior cervical ganglion traversing through the OG. The postganglionic sudomotor fibres travel to the parotid gland via the auriculotemporal branch of the mandibular nerve (V3) to the side of the face
Legend:
OG Otic ganglion
ICA Internal carotid artery
ISN Inferior salivatory nucleus

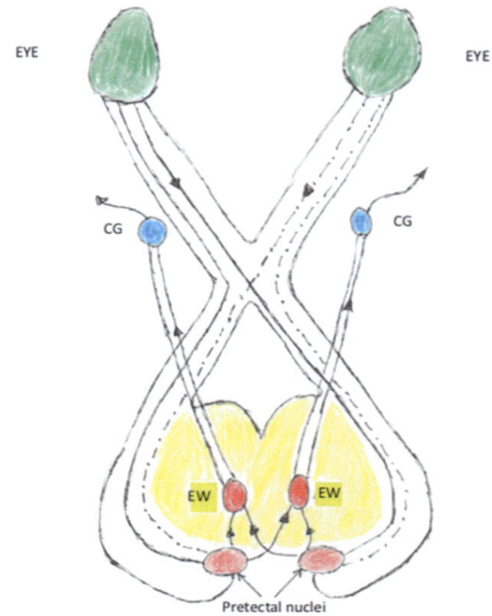

Diagram 5.4 The pupillary reflex. Afferents run in the optic nerve and relay in the pretectal nucleus. There is bilateral connection to the Edinger-Westphal nuclei (EWN) and hence bilaterally to the ciliary ganglion for ipsilateral and consensual pupillary constriction
Notations: CG Ciliary ganglion
EW Edinger-Westphal nucleus

Submandibular Ganglion: Diagram 5.3b

This small ganglion lies on the hyoglossus muscle suspended by two attachments to the lingual nerve. The posteriorly located attachment carries the preganglionic chorda tympani fibres and the anterior branch carries the postganglionic axons for distribution via the lingual nerve. These are secretory to the submandibular and the sublingual glands as well as to numerous unnamed glands in the anterior 2/3 of the tongue and the mucous membrane of the mouth. The ganglion is also a relay station for postganglionic SNS fibres which run along the facial and the lingual arteries and which arise from the superior cervical ganglion. The central nucleus of this ganglion is the superior salivatory nucleus in the midbrain (Diagram 5.2). The sensory root cell bodies lie in the Cranial V ganglion.

Pterygopalatine Ganglion: Diagram 5.3c

This small pyramidal ganglion lies within the pterygopalatine fossa (which is a deep extension of the pterygomaxillary fissure running in the depth of the face between the lateral pterygoid plate and the maxillary tuberosity). This fossa lies inside the infratemporal fossa and is a relay station for blood vessels, somatic sensory nerves and the autonomic nervous system (both SNS and PSNS). This fossa is discussed in Chap. 8. In brief the fossa connects to the middle 1/3 of the face, the nose, the palate and the pharynx distributing SNS fibres, sensory (V_2) fibres, postganglionic secretomotor fibres to the glands of the region and the sinuses with terminal branches of the maxillary artery and concomitant draining maxillary veins.

The pterygopalatine ganglion lies near the sphenopalatine foramen leading to the nose and is surrounded by small branches of the maxillary artery. It is suspended from the inferior aspect of the maxillary nerve (V_2) as it runs in the roof of the pterygopalatine fossa leading forward from the foramen rotundum in the middle cranial fossa. The unusual feature of this ganglion is that the autonomic nerve supply is not mixed but rather is separately divided as a sympathetic root (part of the internal carotid nerve) which is called the **deep petrosal nerve** and the PSNS preganglionic nerve, the **greater petrosal nerve** which has been derived from Cranial VII before it enters the internal acoustic meatus. These two petrosal nerves form a combined nerve which runs across the roof of the pterygopalatine fossa entering via a small foramen called the pterygoid (Vidian) canal. The combined nerve (SNS + PSNS) is called the **nerve to the pterygoid canal (Vidian's nerve)**.[1]

To recall, postganglionic fibres supply not only the lacrimal gland (V_2 and then a jump across to V_1 via the lacrimal nerve) but also glands that relay into the nose (via the sphenopalatine foramen), the palate via the descending palatal canal (moving forwards to the hard palate as the greater palatine nerves or backwards to the soft palate as the lesser palatine nerves) and to the pharynx backwards via a small **palatovaginal canal** in the sphenoid. The termination is in the middle third of the face as the infraorbital nerve. A few of the fibres included are taste fibres from the palate which run in the greater petrosal nerve with their pseudounipolar cell bodies in the geniculate ganglion of Cranial VII as it turns in the middle ear. These relay centrally in the gustatory nucleus in the midbrain.

The pterygopalatine ganglion has branches which include orbital branches as 2–3 filaments which enter the orbit via the inferior orbital fissure and which are sensory to the orbital periosteum. The important component of the ganglion are the postganglionic secretory fibres the lacrimal gland. There are also the nasopalatine nerve and the posterior nasal nerves (lateral superior posterior nasal) which pass through the sphenopalatine foramen to the mucous membrane of the nose. The pharyngeal branch passes posteriorly through the palatovaginal canal to the mucous membrane of the sphenoid sinus and to the roof of the pharynx. The small terminal branches of the maxillary artery at this level follow the components of the pterygopalatine ganglion as infraorbital, posterior superior alveolar, greater (and lesser) palatine, nasopalatine and pharyngeal branches as well as the artery of the pterygoid canal. Greater palatine arteries and nerves run forwards to supply the hard palate whereas those branches running backwards to the soft palate are called lesser palatine nerves and arteries. The canals located in the sphenoid bone (pterygoid and palatovaginal) are discussed in more detail in Chap. 6.

Otic Ganglion: Diagram 5.3d

This small ganglion is located just below the skull base lying between the mandibular nerve (V_3) as it exits the *foramen ovale* and the origins of the tensor palati muscle (which arises from a small area at the root of the medial pterygoid lamina called the scaphoid area). The otic ganglion is adjacent to the nerve to the medial pterygoid muscle. Similar to the other ganglia, a number of fibres relay through, however, the only synapse point is for preganglionic PSNS fibres which reach the ganglion via the lesser petrosal nerve (Cranial IX). The postganglionic pathway is via the auriculotemporal nerve (V_3), a branch of the mandibular trigeminal. Other nerve fibres traversing the ganglion include motor fibres to both tensors (the tensor palati and the tensor tympani) which are derived from the nerve to the medial pterygoid muscle. SNS fibres also traverse the ganglion running through from the plexus on the middle meningeal artery which exits the foramen spinosum lying right against the foramen ovale. These foraminae are discussed in greater detail in Chap. 6. The cell nucleus of the otic ganglion is the inferior salivatory nucleus lying near to Cranial IX and its tympanic branch to the tympanic plexus.

The unique features of each ganglion to remember are:

- In the ciliary ganglion there is a separate sensory, sympathetic and parasympathetic root, the latter distributed via the inferior division of Cranial III.
- In the pterygopalatine ganglion the autonomic root (nerve to the pterygoid canal) is formally created by fusion of the SNS element (deep petrosal nerve) and the PSNS element (greater petrosal nerve).
- In the otic ganglion, a unique feature is its somatic motor root from the nerve to medial pterygoid.

Central brain stem connections of these nerves involved in salivation and lacrimation are discussed in Chap. 7.

Q and A: Chap. 5 (Answers at the End of This Chapter)

1. The nerve of the pterygoid canal (Vidian nerve)
   (a) forms from the greater and lesser petrosal nerves
   (b) has preganglionic Cranial VII fibres
   (c) can be a conduit for intracranial spread of a parotid tumour
   (d) travels between the greater wing of the sphenoid and the lateral pterygoid plate
2. The otic ganglion is a station for:
   (a) Sensory synapse of the mandibular nerve
   (b) Passage of a motor root for the lateral pterygoid muscle

   (c) Parasympathetic synapse of the lesser petrosal nerve
   (d) Parasympathetic synapse of the greater petrosal nerve
   (e) Is the smallest of the PSNS head and neck ganglia
3. The pupillary reflex
   (a) Is afferent to the pretectal nucleus
   (b) Disappears on the efferent limb of the contralateral side with an oculomotor nerve palsy
   (c) Has only ipsilateral connection for the Edinger-Westphal nucleus
   (d) Relies on the ciliary ganglion for pupillary dilatation
4. The autonomic ganglia of the head and neck
   (a) Each have a sensory root
   (b) Is a relay synapse station for sympathetic and parasympathetic preganglionic fibres
   (c) Have sympathetic plexi which align with the arterial circulation
   (d) Connect to their nuclei via postganglionic pathways leading from cranial nerves III, VII and IX
5. Sphlanchnic nerves
   (a) Convey visceral efferents only
   (b) Greater, lesser and least synapse in the preaortic ganglia
   (c) Include preganglionic lumbar and sacral segments
   (d) Do not include postganglionic fibres
6. Concerning the Pterygopalatine ganglion:
   (a) Preganglionic fibres arising from the superior salivatory nucleus travel via the nervus intermedius
   (b) Preganglionic fibres synapse in the geniculate ganglion
   (c) Postganglionic fibres travel in the lesser and greater palatine nerves
   (d) Is typically the largest of the PSNS head and neck ganglia
   (e) Connects to the nose via the sphenopalatine formane located just above the middle concha
   (f) Has no orbital branches
   (g) Cannot be anaesthetically blocked via the nasal cavity

Answers

1. b, c
2. c, e
3. a
4. a, c
5. b, c
6. a, c, d, e

Reference

1. Kozicz T. The Edinger-Westphal nucleus: a historical structural and functional perspective on a dichotomous terminology. J Comp Neurol. 2011;519:1413–34.

The Skull and Its Foraminae

6

Contents

The Cranial Fossae ... 114
Ossification of the Skull ... 121
Sphenoid (Diagram 6.4) ... 122
Temporal Bone (Diagram 6.6) ... 126
SCALP ... 129
Temporal Fossa and the Zygomatic Arch ... 132
Temporalis ... 132
Q and A: Chap. 6 (Answers at the End of This Chapter) ... 133
Answers ... 135
References ... 135

Firstly, some remarks on general skull and cranial topography. If possible go over and confirm some of these general points with a skull handy.

The component parts of the skull are the cranium and the facial skeleton with the main facial elements including the orbit, the maxillae, zygomatic (triradiate malar) and the mandible. With the zygomatic bone there is a zygomaticofrontal suture, a zygomaticomaxillary suture and a completing zygomatic arch which covers both the temporal and infratemporal fossae. The zygomatic bone meets the lateral wall of the orbit against the greater wing of the sphenoid. On the medial side the orbit is formed by the process of the frontal bone, the orbital lamina of the ethmoid bone and the lacrimal bone where these separate off the upper part of the nasal cavity.

A. Zbar, *Anatomy--Head and Neck*,
https://doi.org/10.1007/978-3-031-69538-4_6

If you have access to a skull turn it to one side and note the slit between the tuberosity of the maxilla (its rounded most posterior part) and the lateral pterygoid plate. This is the pterygomaxillary fissure which is the entry and exit point to the infratemporal fossa (and ultimately more deeply to the pterygopalatine fossa) where the maxillary artery runs into the depth of the face and where the maxillary veins drain out. Further forwards, we note the inferior orbital fissure which forms the inferolateral floor of the orbit. The arrangement of these maxillary buttresses (or rather the cranial attachment to the maxilla) forms the basis of the middle third of the face, fractures of which affect the zygomatic bone and arch, the frontal processes of the maxilla and the pterygoid laminae. An understanding of this 3-dimensional anatomy demonstrates how a cheek fracture fragment separates at three points and can be displaced in any direction or involve the orbital floor.

The maxillae join in the midline and are articulated by their palatine processes posteriorly with the palatine bone, an L-shaped plate the horizontal lamina of which forms the posterior one third of the hard palate and the perpendicular lamina of which forms with the maxilla the lateral wall of the nasal cavity. In this arrangement the maxilla lies in front and the medial pterygoid plate sits behind. Appreciating this point can aid in understanding that there is a small area of separation between the pterygomaxillary fissure, its medial extension (the pterygopalatine fossa) and the nasal cavity. Separate individual assessment of the palatine bone shows that there is a notch in the upper margin of the perpendicular lamina which creates a sphenopalatine foramen transmitting the sphenopalatine branch of the maxillary artery and the nasopalatine nerve (emanating from the pterygopalatine ganglion). If one imagines the pterygopalatine fossa as a corridor with sides, a roof and a floor (as well as with entry and exit doors) one of these exits is via this sphenopalatine foramen into the nose. In fact it is how all of the assembled fibres of the pterygopalatine ganglion and the vessels which may run through it or alongside it (sensory, SNS, PSNS, arterial and venous) are all distributed (in this case) to the nose. Even though the only thing to synapse in the ganglion is the PSNS pathway, it acts as a relay station for neurovascular organizational distribution.

It is possible to equate the formation of the elements of the cranium to those of the developing vertebrae. In the adult, the solid part of the skull fuses the occipital and sphenoid bones. The solid, medial and inferior part of the cranium is thus the fusion of the occipital and the sphenoid bones with the foraminae of the middle cranial fossa being essentially like the intervertebral foraminae. Carrying this analogy further, the cranial vault would find homology with the vertebral arches (the pedicles and the laminae) so that only the occipital bone forms a complete arch to surround the foramen magnum. The inferior margin displays a facet (the occipital condyle) which then articulates with the superior articular facets of the atlas. Laterally, the occipital bone projects out to form the jugular process which lies just behind the jugular foramen, in effect a homologue with the vertebral transverse process. In this case the ventral ramus of C1 is separated here from the cranial nerves traversing the jugular foramen (IX, X and XI) with Cranial XII traversing its own canal above the occipital condyles.

Diagram 6.1 Sutures and points.

Examine a skull and note that on its lateral aspect is the pterion where the coronal suture and the frontal bone articulate with the greater wing of the sphenoid and with the inferior angle of the parietal bone. The **pterion**, rather than a discrete single point is more of an H-shaped area or pattern of sutures between the frontal, parietal, temporal and sphenoid bones with the squamous part of the temporal bone articulating with the greater wing of the sphenoid and overlapping to the parietal bone. Inferiorly, the mastoid part of the temporal bone continues as a suture with the parietal bone meeting the occiput at the **asterion**.

The occipital plate moves up *between the posterior edges of the two parietal bones joining these at the lambdoid suture*. In some cases there are collection of smaller bones here called the Wormian bones. These parietal bones form the greatest part of the dome of the skull. The *sagittal suture* is a median suture separating the parietal bones with the *coronal suture* separating the frontal bone articulation anteriorly. In some cases, the two halves of the frontal bone fail to fuse leaving a *metopic suture*. The midline meeting place of the bones is called the **bregma** which in the neonate and infant is the site of the anterior fontanelle.

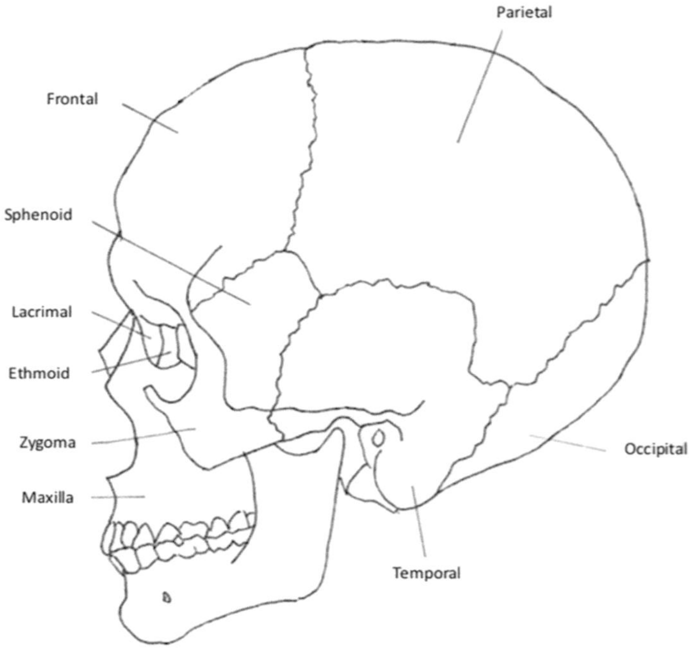

Diagram 6.1 Lateral view of the intact skull. The *pterion* overlying the middle meningeal artery is a neurosurgical landmark for a burr-hole craniotomy in extradural haematoma at the junction of the frontal, sphenoid, parietal and squamous temporal bones. The *bregma* is the junction point between the coronal and sagittal sutures (anterior fontanelle)
Notations: Parietal, Occipital, Temporal, Maxilla, Zygoma, Ethmoid, Lacrimal, Sphenoid, Frontal

The Cranial Fossae

Examination of the inner surface of the skull cap (*calvarium*) shows a deep midline groove which widens as it is traced backwards for the superior sagittal sinus. Pits laterally are for the arachnoid granulations (protrusions of the arachnoid mater) which sit either in the sinus or outside in the lateral blood lakes. Grooves for both the anterior and posterior meningeal branches are evident laterally behind the coronal suture and at roughly the level of the precentral gyrus.[1]

The internal part of the base of the skull is divided into three layers (Diagram 6.2) like the steps of a staircase: anterior, middle and posterior cranial fossae.

The **anterior cranial fossa** is level with the mid-orbit, the middle fossa with the zygomatic arch and the posterior fossa lying just above the superior nuchal line. The anterior fossa houses the frontal lobe, the middle the temporal lobes and the posterior the tentorium cerebelli and the cerebellum and brain stem. The posterior margin of the anterior fossa is the sharp concavity of the free edge of the lesser wing of the sphenoid with the medial end of this lesser wing projected backwards as the anterior clinoid process. The base of the lesser wing is perforated by the optic canal. The anterior fossa shows ridged undulations of the orbital plate of the frontal bone with a spur, the *crista galli* in the midline projecting for attachment of the *falx cerebri* separating the two cerebral hemispheres and on either side the thin multiply perforated cribriform plate of the ethmoid transmitting the olfactory filaments.[2] There is a small foramen caecum in front of this area for the transmission of an emissary vein.

The **middle cranial fossa** is deeper than the anterior cranial fossa and is an H-shaped or butterfly zone formed largely by the greater wing of the sphenoid which extends laterally to the squamous temporal bone and backwards is limited by the thick cortical petrous temporal bone. The body of the sphenoid forms the *sella turcica* (Turkish saddle) holding in life the hypophysis (pituitary gland) with an anterior hump the *tuberculum sellae* and the back of the sella forming the steep dorsum sellae extending to the posterior clinoid processes. Dura mater forms a sleeve over this area as the *diapragma sellae* and extends along the sides of the region to close off the cavernous sinus. The dorsum sellae is pierced by the pituitary stalk with the ICA grooving its medial and

[1] The calvarium is named after Calvary, a skull-shaped hill outside Jerusalem where Jesus Christ was crucified. The site outside Jerusalem's walls was also called Golgotha (Hebrew skull 'Galgola'—גולגולת).

[2] Cribriform meaning 'sieve-like'.

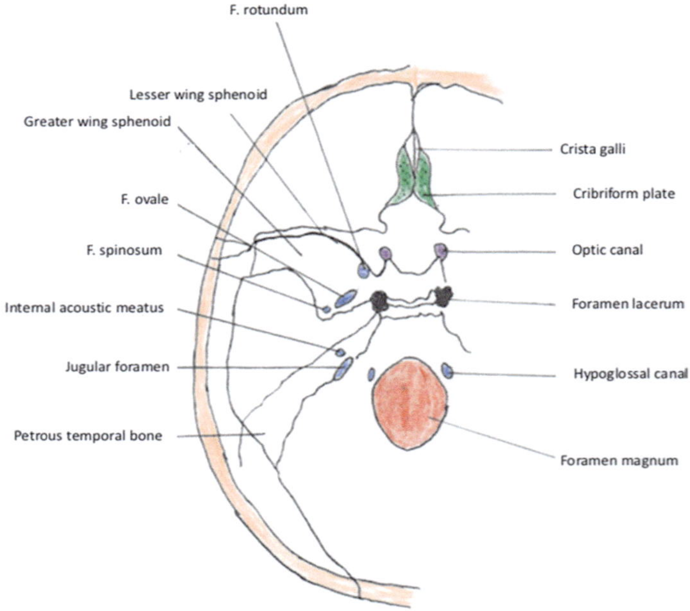

Diagram 6.2 Internal view of the skull—the cranial fossae. The anterior cranial fossa is limited posteriorly by the free edge of the lesser wing of the sphenoid. The middle cranial fossa has the greater wing of the sphenoid anteriorly and is limited posteriorly by the petrous temporal bone. Behind this point lies the posterior cranial fossa

bottom edge. A small middle clinoid process is evident at the lateral end of the tuberculum sellae compartmentalizing the dura and separating the cavernous sinus from the pituitary fossa. Near the attachment of the dura to the optic canal is the optic chiasm and above this the anterior communicating artery and the rostrum of the corpus callosum. The sella houses the hypophysis (the pituitary fossa) below which lies the sphenoid sinus. This anatomy is the basis of a trans-nasal trans-sphenoidal microscopic hypophysectomy for a microadenoma of the pituitary gland.

The part between the ICA and the *foramen lacerum* carries the greater petrosal nerve. The trigeminal (V) ganglion lies alongside the cavernous sinus occupying a dural space called Meckel's cave (*Cavum trigeminale, cisterna trigeminalis*).[3] The Cranial VI travels along the apex of the petrous temporal bone near a small bony spike attaching the petroclinoid ligament which extends half way up the dorsum sellae and which lies against the large sensory root of V_3 (the smaller motor root lies more deeply). Above this ligament is the superior petrosal sinus and laterally is a small groove visible for the lesser petrosal nerve before it exits the skull via the foramen ovale.

The middle cranial fossa houses multiple important foraminae to observe. These should be identified both inside the cranial vault and outside the skull for complete orientation.

Start with the foramen ovale which perforates the greater wing of the sphenoid and which lies behind the more medial foramen rotundum. It leads downwards into the infratemporal fossa transmitting the mandibular nerve (sensory and motor roots), the lesser petrosal nerve and an emissary vein running between the cavernous sinus to the pterygoid venous plexus. There may also be an accessory meningeal branch of the first portion of the maxillary artery which supplies the trigeminal ganglion. There can also be an accompanying meningeal branch of the mandibular nerve (V_3) the nervus spinosus which innervates the mastoid antrum and mastoid air cells.

In front of this is the **foramen rotundum** which pierces the greater wing of the sphenoid just below the superior orbital fissure. It leads into the pterygopalatine fossa and transmits the maxillary nerve (V_2).

The **superior orbital fissure** is seen from behind (but better from in front of the skull at the back of the orbit). It is a retort-shaped space that is wider at its medial end with a long axis that is directed upwards lying between the lesser and the greater wings

[3]Johann Friedrich Meckel (1781–1833) was a Professor of anatomy, pathology and zoology at Halle Germany.

of the sphenoid bone and designed to transmit structures leaving the middle cranial fossa and entering the orbit. There is an order of these structures which has been described before from lateral to medial. In brief as a reminder it transmits the ophthalmic veins, the ophthalmic nerve (V_1) and the Cranials III, (superior and inferior divisions), IV and VI.

Behind the foramen ovale is the small **foramen spinosum** transmitting the middle meningeal artery which runs from the infratemporal fossa away from the first (mandibular) section of the maxillary artery. The anterior branch of this artery proceeds across the pterion to the parietal bone and the posterior branch passes to the squamous temporal bone. The pterion is the site of a burr-hole craniotomy in those patients who present with a potentially life-threatening extradural haematoma.

In some cases there is an additional foramen between the ovale and spinosum called the **foramen of Vesalius** that transmits a sphenoidal emissary vein.[4] Posteromedial to the foramen ovale is the very irregular **foramen lacerum** bound by the apex of the petrous temporal and medially by the sphenoid body. It is not a strict foramen but rather a point of ossification fusion. It has the ICA running over it but little apart from small veins runs "through" it.

Between the anterior and the middle cranial fossa at the end of the free edge of the lesser wing of the sphenoid is the sphenoparietal venous sinus which empties into the cavernous sinus. The superior ophthalmic veins enter the medial end of the superior orbital fissure to also drain into the cavernous sinus. This sphenoparietal sinus is of relevance in the sphenoparietal neurosurgical approach to a posterior communicating artery aneurysm. Bridging Sylvian veins between the brain and the dura can be displaced to avoid venous injury and widen this operative space peeling the dura away from the inner aspect of the superior orbital fissure [1].

The **posterior cranial fossa** is the largest and the deepest of the three cranial fossae. It is deeply concave where posteriorly

[4]Named after Andreas Vesalius (1514–1564) a Belgian anatomist who was Professor of Anatomy at the University of Padua and who published the Fabrica humani corporis in 1543 one of the first illustrated dissection manuals.

and in its interior it is grooved by the transverse sinus at the internal occipital protuberance. The sagittal sinus usually turns right along the transverse groove at this point. The other transverse groove at the inflow of the straight sinus is usually narrower and turns leftwards. Evident in the posterior cranial fossa is the **jugular foramen** which is formed by the jugular notch of the petrous temporal bone and the shallower jugular notch of the occipital bone. The jugular foraminae are asymmetric with the larger jugular vein receiving the sigmoid and the sagittal/transverse sinuses (usually the right). The groove of the sigmoid sinus is also referred to in some textbooks as the sigmoid sulcus. Posteriorly a large mastoid emissary vein enters the sinus directly and is a portal for the transmission of mastoid sepsis. The jugular foramen separates the petrous temporal from the condylar occipital bones. The back end of this foramen transmits the sigmoid sinus for formation of the IJV **below** the skull base which is formed by the drainage of the **inferior petrosal sinus**. The jugular foramen from behind forwards transmits Cranials XI, X and IX.

The posterior cranial fossa is bounded in front by the dorsum sellae and the steep vertically disposed clivus (as part of the sphenoid) and a fusion point of the basi-occiput. The clivus is related to the basilar venous plexus which is the proximal extension of the internal vertebral venous plexus. Laterally is the petrous temporal bone with the **internal acoustic meatus** (transmitting Cranials VII and VIII). Beyond and above is the facial canal conducting the Cranial VII between the petrous temporal bone and the stylomastoid foramen where the VII leaves the skull. The remainder completing this region is the mastoid part of the temporal bone and the condylar part of the occipital bone. There is in addition for completion a small posteroinferior piece of the parietal bone. The foramen magnum transmits the medulla oblongata and is made up of the basilar part of the occipital bone anteriorly and laterally by the condylar section (plus a small amount of the squamous temporal).

Take the opportunity of locating the foraminae and listing their contents on both the side of the cranial fossae and on the under surface of the skull (Diagram 6.3).

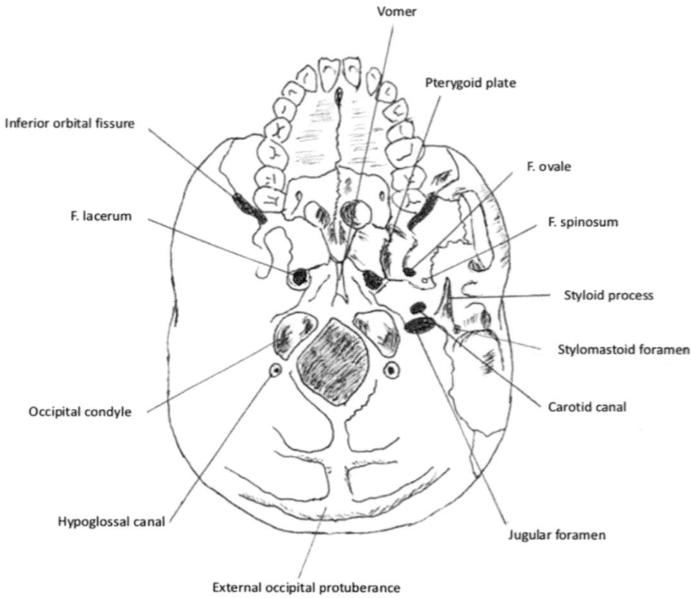

Diagram 6.3 The inferior view of the intact skull. By passing pipe cleaners through the foraminae, note the location of those that can be seen from the inferior skull view and which can be traced to the internal cranial fossa view (*foramen ovale*, *foramen spinosum*, *jugular foramen*, *foramen lacerum* and the *foramen magnum*). The inferior view shows the position of the *carotid canal*, the *stylomastoid foramen* and the *hypoglossal canal*

Ossification of the Skull

In the anterior cranial fossa the ethmoid is the only part to ossify in cartilage (endochondral ossification). The rest of the skull ossifies in membrane (intramembranous ossification). Division is into the neurocranium (protecting the brain) and the viscerocranium (forming the facial skeleton). The neurocranium is divisible into the chondrocranium (forming the skull base) and the membranous part (forming the calvarium). There are recognizable phases of development including the embryonic phase (first 8 weeks) and the foetal phase (up until birth) forming the cranial sutures. The neural crest is responsible for formation of the viscerocranium (frontal, sphenoid, squamous temporal) and facial bones whereas the somites of the paraxial mesoderm are involved in formation of the cribriform plate, sphenoid, parietal, petrous temporal, clivus and occipital bones.

The neonatal skull is of disproportionate size between the large cranial vault with respect to the small face (One-eighth of the cranial bulk versus one-half in adults). In adults there is growth of the maxillary sinuses and the dentition so that there is a normal vertical height of the orbit when compared with either the maxillary or the mandibular height. The bones of the vault and the face are all formed at birth but they are all mobile on one other. The occipital, temporal, sphenoid, frontal and mandible are in more than one piece at birth. The two frontal bones unite by the second year closing the anterior fontanelle (at the junction of the frontal, sagittal and coronal sutures) and which is rarely palpable after 18 months. The posterior fontanelle lies between the parietal and the squamous occipital a (at the junction of the sagittal and lambdoid sutures). The smallness of the face in infants is a result of the small mandible and maxilla, the non-eruption of teeth and the small size of the maxillary sinuses and nasal cavities. The posterior fontanelle closes by the end of the first year. Overall growth occurs at the skull base with requisite remodeling [2]. Growth occurs in length at the coronal suture, in breadth at the sagittal sutures and in height at the parietotemporal suture.

The following is a brief description of the individual skull bones and where appropriate their anatomical and clinical relevance.

Two of the bones which are separately studied by neurosurgical and ENT trainees are the *sphenoid bone* and the *temporal bone*, both of which are considered here in more detail.

Sphenoid (Diagram 6.4)

This bone may be available to you separated in your anatomy lab for more concentrated study. It should be examined now.

Orientate the isolated bone identifying its components. It is squeezed at the base of the skull between the temporal bone and the basi-occiput. It looks like a bat's wing with its central body block, its lesser wing on top and its greater wing broader underneath along with the two pterygoid processes. The anterior part articulates with the cribriform plate and this smooth area is called the *jugum sphenoidale* which leads posteriorly to the part of the bone forming the optic canals. As you move more posteriorly is the elevated *tuberculum sellae* and behind this the *sella turcica* which holds the hypophysis (pituitary gland). At the back is the *dorsum sellae* leading down to the clivus which supports the cerebral pons.

To recap:

The bulk of the greater wing projects over the front of the middle cranial fossa with the *foramen rotundum* medially to transmit the maxillary nerve (V_2). Behind and laterally lies the *foramen ovale* transmitting the mandibular nerve and the accessory meningeal artery and often the lesser petrosal nerve. Behind lies the *foramen spinosum* transmitting the middle meningeal artery and in 40% of cases medial to the foramen ovale is the emissary sphenoidal foramen (*foramen Vesalii*) transmitting an emissary vein running from the cavernous sinus to the pterygoid venous plexus.

Laterally the greater wing has a temporal component which forms part of the boundary of the infratemporal fossa (see Chap. 8) and an infratemporal part which forms behind the tuberosity (posterior limit) of the maxilla a space with the lateral pterygoid plate. This area is noted in the lateral aspect of an articulated skull and is called the *pterygomaxillary fissure* (the point where the maxillary artery enters the depth of the face and where maxillary veins drain outwards). Deep to this pterygomaxillary fissure lies the *pterygopalatine fossa* (see Chap. 8).

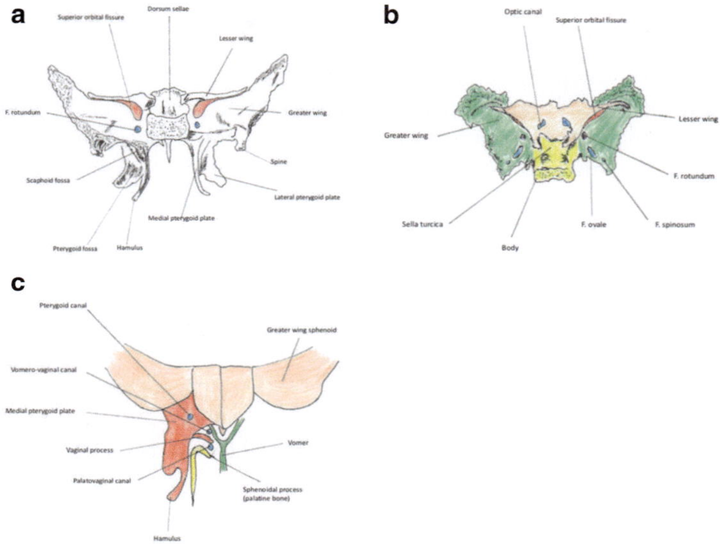

Diagram 6.4 Sphenoid bone
(**a**) Posterior view of the isolated bone
(**b**) Superior view of the isolated bone
(**c**) Simplified schematic view of the articulation between the greater wing and the vaginal process of its pterygoid plate with the palatine bone (*palato-vaginal foramen*) and with the rostrum and the vomer. Between the vomer and the vaginal process lies the *vomerovaginal canal* which transmits the sphenopalatine vessels. This canal lies medial to the palatovaginal canal and above the sphenoidal process of the palatine bone

Anteriorly the sphenoid contributes to part of the formation of the inferior orbital fissure with the gap between the lesser and the greater wings forming the superior orbital fissure where contents of the middle cranial fossa are trans mitted to the orbit. This is schematically shown in Diagram 6.5. The pterygoid plates slope downwards from where the greater wing and the body join. The pterygoid fossa between the lateral and medial plates contains the medial pterygoid muscle and the tensor palati (tensor veli palatini; *Lt. veli = curtain*). Above the pterygoid fossa is a small oval shaped scaphoid fossa for attachment of the tensor palati muscle. This anterior part of the pterygoid process holding both plates is the posterior wall of the pterygopalatine fossa and is pierced by the pterygoid canal. One may consider the pterygopalatine fossa like a room with exit and entry widows where one of the entry windows at the back is the pterygoid canal transmitting the nerve of the pterygoid canal (combined SNS deep petrosal nerve and PSNS greater petrosal nerve). This entrance is the manner in which the autonomic nervous system is distributed through the pterygopalatine fossa to the middle one-third of the face, the palate, the pharynx and the nasal cavity/sinuses.

The entire lateral surface of the lateral pterygoid plate gives origin to the lower head of the lateral pterygoid, but its inner sur-

Diagram 6.5 The superior orbital fissure
(**a**) The fissure is retort-shaped with some structures arising within the tendinous ring (coloured red) giving origin to the rectus muscles. These *intraconal* structures include the inferior and superior divisions of Cranial III, the nasociliary nerve and Cranial VI. The remainder (superior and inferior ophthalmic veins, Cranial IV, lacrimal and frontal nerves) are *extraconal*. The Cranial II and its accompanying ophthalmic artery run separately through the optic canal (**b**) Front view of the bones making up the orbit. The optic canal and superior and inferior orbital fissures are visible. The bones include the frontal, zygomatic, maxillary, sphenoid, ethmoid, lacrimal and palatine

a

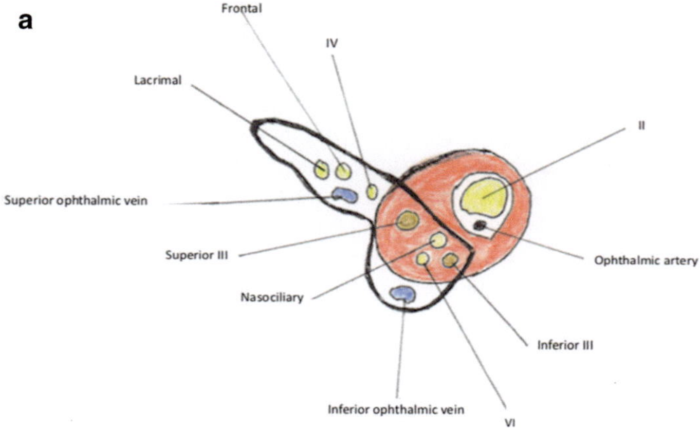
Frontal
IV
Lacrimal
II
Superior ophthalmic vein
Superior III
Ophthalmic artery
Nasociliary
Inferior III
Inferior ophthalmic vein
VI

b

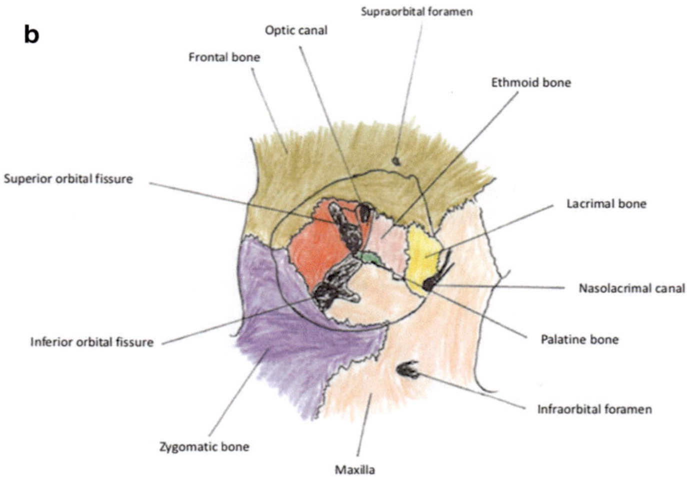
Supraorbital foramen
Optic canal
Frontal bone
Ethmoid bone
Superior orbital fissure
Lacrimal bone
Nasolacrimal canal
Palatine bone
Inferior orbital fissure
Infraorbital foramen
Zygomatic bone
Maxilla

face gives origin to the upper head of the medial pterygoid. Note the bottom end of the medial pterygoid plate. It is narrower and longer than its lateral fellow and is rounded off into a *hamulus* (*Lt. = hook*). The tensor palati (tensor veli palatini) curls around this hamulus and it attaches the *pterygomandibular raphe* which gives origin to the superior constrictor muscle of the pharynx (running posteriorly) and the buccinator muscle (running anteriorly). Superiorly the medial pterygoid plate is prolonged under the body of the sphenoid as a vaginal process which articulates anteriorly with a sphenoidal process of the palatine bone and medially with the vomer (Diagram 6.4c). These two articulating bones convert this connexion into a small canal the *palatovaginal canal* transmitting the pharyngeal branch of the maxillary artery and the pharyngeal nerve from the pterygopalatine ganglion. The posterior smooth margin of the medial pterygoid plate attaches the pharyngobasilar fascia and part of the superior constrictor muscle.

The central part of the sphenoid is called the rostrum which articulates with the perpendicular plate of the ethmoid at the upper nasal septum between the two sphenoidal air sinuses. The body of the sphenoid articulates with the nasal septum in the midline, and with the ethmoid anteriorly and the vomer inferiorly.

Temporal Bone (Diagram 6.6)

One of the bones studied in isolation by otolaryngologists is the temporal bone which fills the space between the occipital and sphenoids and the squamous (flat) part of the parietal bone. The posterior inferior part of the temporal bone is the petrous temporal, a dense cortical bone shelf with this part not quite reaching the sphenoid but leaving only the area of the *foramen lacerum* between them. The apex of the petrous temporal bone is squeezed between the basiocciput and the greater wing of the sphenoid as far as this foramen. The very irregularly edged 'foramen' is poorly named since little traverses it and it is more strictly a point of ossific fusion giving the impression of a foramen. This point can be noted on examination of the skull looking for the petroclival (petro-occipital) suture, the spheno-petrosal suture

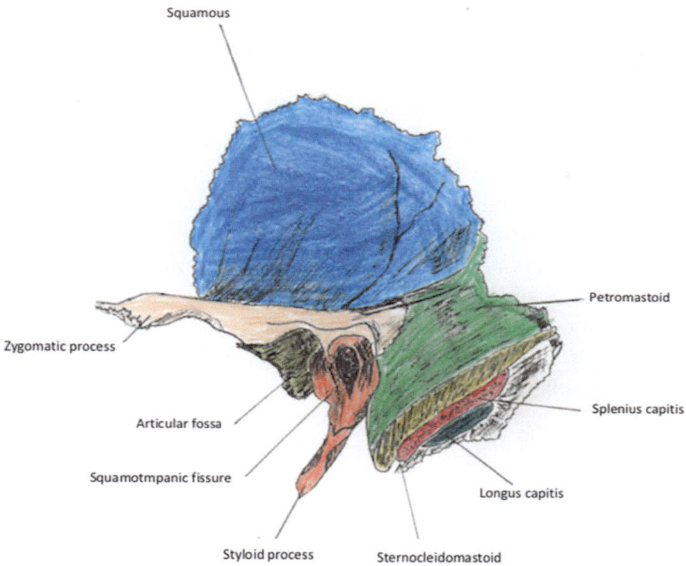

Diagram 6.6 The isolated temporal bone. Separate components (squamous, zygomatic, petromastoid and tympanic) are shown. The shaded area of the zygomatic process gives origin to the masseter muscle and the styloglossus (anterior) and stylohyoid (posterior) origins are also shown on the sides of the styloid process. The external auditory meatus and the articulation for the temporomandibular joint are seen. The *squamotympanic fissure* (also called the *petrotympanic fissure*) lying between the tympanic bone and the articular surface holds the *chorda tympani* before it joins the lingual nerve

and the spheno-occipital suture. It is a point where emissary veins may enter from the pterygoid plexus into the cavernous sinus. It can also aberrantly sometimes transmit the greater or deep petrosal nerves, the entire nerve of the pterygoid canal, the artery of the pterygoid canal (from the third part of the maxillary artery) and a branch of the ascending pharyngeal artery. The foramen is of little clinical significance although the ICA runs directly over the top.

The petrous temporal demonstrates the cylindrical internal acoustic meatus, articulating medially with the sloping part of the occipital bone (clivus). Here there is an impression for the inferior petrosal sinus. The clivus and the two petrous temporal bones form the front part of the posterior cranial fossa. The base of this pyramidal part is the mastoid and the area fans superiorly as the squamous temporal from which emanates the zygomatic process. Inferiorly is the mandibular fossa for temporomandibular joint (TMJ) articulation. Below lies the external acoustic meatus, the tympanic part of the temporal bone meeting the squamous part at the squamo-tympanic fissure which is medially separable into petro-squamous and petro-tympanic parts. The petrotympanic fissure transmits the chorda tympani.

This fissure passes up into the middle ear (tympanic cavity) and houses the anterior ligament of the malleus and transmits the chorda tympani in its medial and anterior opening, the anterior canaliculus.

Below and projecting from the petrous temporal bone and lying between the jugular fossa and the external auditory meatus is the styloid process with the stylomastoid foramen behind the styloid base where Cranial VII exits the skull. More medially lies the carotid canal lies which is a circular opening within the petrous temporal bone that transmits the ICA along with its SNS plexus (the carotid nerve) emerging over the top of the foramen lacerum before twisting as the carotid siphon against the body of the sphenoid.

Take the opportunity to examine the temporal bone and its surrounds in an intact skull. Note the four parts of the temporal bone:

- Petrous (or petromastoid)
- Squamous
- Zygomatic process and
- Tympanic part (along with the styloid process).

The mastoid is grooved deeply by the digastric notch which is the origin of the posterior belly of the digastric muscle. Above it gives attachment to the occipital belly of occipitofrontalis and auricularis posterior. This area is often perforated posteriorly by a *mastoid foramen* which transmits an emissary vein from the suboccipital triangle to the sigmoid venous sinus. On the styloid, the stylopharyngeus (IX) arises high up and medially, the stylohyoid (VII) high up but more posteriorly and the styloglossus (XII) low down and anteriorly. All of this represents the styloid apparatus near the stylomastoid foramen (transmitting Cranial VII and the stylomastoid branch of the posterior auricular artery). The styloid process also gives attachment to the stylohyoid and stylomandibular ligaments. The clinical relevance here is that the styloid process is covered by the lower part of the parotid gland with Cranial VII crossing its base and the ECA its tip (both lying within the parotid substance). Deeply the origin of the IJV is separated from the styloid by the stylopharyngeus muscle. In patients undergoing a carotid endarterectomy for transient ischaemic attacks, if the carotid bifurcation is high, access to clamp the ICA can be very limited and additional room can be created in this digastric triangle by dividing the posterior belly of the digastric (ligating the occipital artery below and the posterior auricular artery above) and by forcibly blindly snapping the styloid process. This is distinct from the rare circumstance of an elongated styloid process associated with ICA compression and facial or throat pain due to trigeminal and/or glossopharyngeal neuralgia (Eagle syndrome).[5]

The ridge of bone between the jugular foramen and the carotid canal is perforated by small foraminae that transmit the tympanic branches of IX and the caroticotympanic SNS branches from the ICA (carotid nerve). Note the termination of the spine of the sphenoid. This area of bone has grown downwards from the middle ear and is referred to as the tegmen tympani dividing into a medial part behind the spine with the petrosquamous fissure lying in front and a petrotympanic fissure lying behind.

SCALP

One additional area of consideration at this point is the scalp and its basic neurovascular layout. The scalp covers the vault of the skull and extends down between the right and the left temporal

[5]Eagle syndrome named after Watt W. Eagle (1898–1980) an American otolaryngologist who described the syndrome in 1937.

lines, the eyebrows and the superior nuchal lines. The mnemonic SCALP reminds of its individual layers which are important in performance of a craniotomy. The mnemonic includes: **S**kin, **C**utaneous tissue, the **A**poneurosis (or galea aponeurotica:t: Galea = helmet, also known as the epicranial aponeurosis), **L**oose areolar tissue and the **P**eriosteum (pericranium). The galea is the tendon uniting the frontalis and the occipitalis muscles with the skin, with both fixed to the galea by dense vertical strands. The nerves and the blood vessels lie within this superficial space and deep to the aponeurosis there is a relatively avascular layer which can slide freely upon the pericranium. Bleeding from scalp lacerations can be excessive (and even life threatening) and is readily controlled by haemostat forceps placed on the galea which lift it up and tamponade vessels emergently without the initial need to find the vessels individually. In neurosurgical procedures these vessels are controlled by compression clips.

In the scalp the temple (or the temporal fossa) is situated between the temporal line and the zygomatic arch, housing the temporalis muscle, the temporal fascia and an extension of the epicranial aponeurosis from which the extraauricular muscles originate. This region has a motor innervation by Cranial VII, a sensory innervation from the front to the vertex by the supraorbital and supratrochlear branches of the frontal nerve (V_1) and posteriorly by the dorsal sensory rami of C2 and C3 spinal nerves respectively as the *greater occipital* and *third occipital* nerves. The *greater occipital nerve* is the thickest nerve in the body with no sensory component of the dorsal C1 ramus. The *third occipital* fills in the area on the nape of the neck as far as the external occipital protuberance. Additional SNS supply to the precapillary sphincters, the sweat glands and the arrectores pili are derived from the superior cervical ganglion. The lesser occipital nerve (ventral rami of C2,3 from the cervical plexus) fills in the area of supply to the posterior ear lobe.

The scalp has a very rich arterial anastomotic network. These are the branches of the ECA except for the forehead which receives the supraorbital and the supratrochlear arteries originating from the ophthalmic artery. The ECA arteries here include the superficial temporal artery which originates in the depth of the parotid gland running alongside the auriculotemporal nerve.

There is in addition a transverse facial artery running forwards over the masseter below the zygomatic arch, a middle temporal artery at the root of the arch running above the external auditory meatus and there may be a zygomatico-orbital artery which can form an anastomosis with branches of the ophthalmic artery under the temporalis fascia. The remaining arteries include the posterior auricular and the occipital arteries.

The veins of the scalp accompany these arteries but there are different drainage points. The supraorbital and supratrochlear veins unite at the medial angle of the eye to form the angular facial vein which has direct communications with the orbital veins. The superficial temporal vein joins the middle temporal vein and forms the retromandibular vein at the root of the zygomatic arch. The retromandibular vein is joined by the transverse facial vein and the maxillary veins coming from the depth of the face to form the anterior branch. This anatomy may however be quite variable. The anterior branch of the retromandibular vein joins the facial vein and drains into the IJV whereas the posterior branch of the retromandibular vein joins the posterior auricular vein to form the external jugular vein (EJV). Posteriorly, the occipital vein joins the suboccipital venous plexus deep to semispinalis capitis muscle. There is frequently a connection between the sigmoid sinus and an emissary vein in the region of the mastoid as well as a further connection between parietal foraminae and the superior sagittal sinus (See Chap. 10).

Muscles of the scalp and the temporal fossae are the occipitofrontalis and the temporalis muscles. The occipital bellies of the occipitofrontalis are shorter and narrower than the frontal bellies. Occipitalis arises from the highest nuchal line and passes forwards into the aponeurosis fading out laterally by blending with the temporalis fascia. Frontalis arises in the aponeurosis and ends its attachment in the orbicularis oculi and the skin of the eyebrow. The frontalis muscles meet one another but the occipitalis muscles are separate. Facial nerve innervation is via the posterior auricular nerve posteriorly and the zygomatic and temporal branches anteriorly. There are no lymph nodes located on the scalp with lymphatic drainage to occipital and posterior auricular nodes and to preauricular and parotid nodes.

Temporal Fossa and the Zygomatic Arch

Examine a skull where two wavy temporal lines can be seen laterally, a superior and an inferior which emerge from a common origin at the border of the zygomatic process. The temporal fossa is bounded by these lines above and the zygomatic arch below. The landmark of the pterion is located here and the temporal fossa is filled in with the temporalis muscle and temporalis fascia. Deeply this fossa (at the level of the greater wing of the sphenoid) becomes continuous with the deeper infratemporal fossa. The temporal fossa is formed by the zygomatic process of the frontal bone, the zygomatic arch and the maxilla (Diagram 6.6).

The temporalis fascia is attached here at the superior temporal line passing down to the zygomatic arch with its deeper layer running under the arch continuous with the deep fascia overlying the masseter muscle. This territory carries the superficial temporal vessels and the auriculotemporal nerve which are superficial to the temporal and zygomatic branches of Cranial VII.

Temporalis

This fan-shaped muscle takes origin from the inferior temporal line and inserts by a stout tendon into the coronoid process of the mandible extending a little on to the front of the ramus and partly on to the mandibular notch. These attachments are relevant as this insertion needs to be removed in order to adequately display the infratemporal fossa and the base of the skull (permitting good visualization of the maxillary artery, the middle meningeal artery and the mandibular nerve). The attachment of temporalis can extend as far as the attachment of the buccinator and to the retromolar fossa. The blood supply comes from the temporal branches of the second part of the maxillary artery and the motor supply via branches of the mandibular nerve). The temporalis powerfully shuts the jaw but it is also the only muscle to retract the condyle of the TMJ (via its posterior fibres).

An appreciation of the anatomy of the temporalis fascia assists in management of a fractured malar. The structure of the malar (cheekbone) is as a triradiate bone with zygomaticofrontal and arch sutures so that when the cheekbone is broken this block of bone can move up, out, or inwards. In some cases it can impact directly onto the coronoid process. Normally as part of this injury the mouth cannot be widely opened (trismus) because of masseteric spasm. But in a case where the malar is impacted against the coronoid process the jaw cannot be opened making intubation for reduction of this fracture difficult. The Gillies approach[6] is to make a small vertical temple incision and to place a periosteal elevator just under the zygomatic arch (and hence under the dense white temporalis fascia). This blindly lifts the fractured zygoma up and into position.

The *superficial temporal* artery (along with the maxillary artery) is the termination of the ECA. It is approached for a biopsy in the condition temporal arteritis. In the past this procedure was performed in front of the tragus, however, because of its proximity to the auriculotemporal nerve Duplex ultrasound is used to make a small incision near the forehead hairline. The superficial temporal artery usually has a parietal branch in front of the temporalis fascia which anastomoses with the posterior auricular and occipital arteries. The frontal branch is tortuous and may anastomose with the supraorbital and frontal arteries (a point of ECA-ICA anastomosis).

Q and A: Chap. 6 (Answers at the End of This Chapter)

1. Concerning the osteology of the skull
   (a) The nuchal line is the surface marker of the tentorium cerebelli
   (b) The pterion is an H-shaped area at the lateral end of the coronal suture comprising the frontal, the lesser wing of the sphenoid bone, and the parietal bone
   (c) The perpendicular plate of the palatine bone contributes to the point of transmission of the pharyngeal branch of the pterygopalatine ganglion

[6]Named after the UK plastic surgeon Sir Harold Gillies (1882–1960).

   (d) The orbital process of the palatine bone forms the floor of the orbit.
2. The pterygoid hamulus
   (a) Arises from the lateral pterygoid plate
   (b) Gives indirect origin to the superior constrictor and the buccinator
   (c) Attaches to the pharyngobasilar fascia
   (d) Provides part of the origin of the tensor veli palatini
3. The petrotympanic fissure
   (a) Transmits the Geniculate ganglion
   (b) Connects to the capsule of the temporomandibular joint via the anterior ligament of the malleus
   (c) Is separable from the tegmen tympani
   (d) Runs between the borders of the petrous and tympanic parts of the temporal bone
4. The foramen lacerum
   (a) Is an ossific gap between the petrous and sphenoid bones
   (b) Transmits the lesser petrosal nerve
   (c) Can connect the pterygoid plexus with the cavernous sinus via an emissary vein
   (d) Lies anteromedial to the foramen ovale
5. The calvarium is made up of:
   (a) Frontal bone
   (b) Sphenoid bone
   (c) Ethmoid bone
   (d) Occipital bone
   (e) Wormian bones
6. The occipital bone forms an articulation with:
   (a) Petrous bone
   (b) Atlas
   (c) Sphenoid bone
   (d) Clivus
   (e) Parietal bone
   (f) Temporal bone
7. Foraminae evident in the sphenoid include:
   (a) Foramen lacerum
   (b) Carotid canal
   (c) Pterygoid canal

(d) Palatovaginal canal
(e) Foramen spinosum
(f) Foramen Vesalii

8. The orbital walls are formed by:
   (a) The lesser wing of the sphenoid
   (b) The maxillary bone
   (c) The lacrimal fossa
   (d) The parietal bone
   (e) The palatine bone

Answers

1. a, c, d
2. b
3. b, d
4. a
5. a, e
6. b, c, e, f
7. c, d
8. b, c, e

References

1. Niibo T, Takizawa K, Sakurai J, Takebayashi S, Koizumi H, Kobayashi T, Kobayashi R, Kuris K, Gotou S, Tsuchiya R, Kamiyama H. Sphenoparietal sinus transposition technique: optimization of the surgical corridor with preservation of prominent bridging veins between the brain and the cranial base during aneurysm clipping via the pterional approach. J Neurosurg. 2021;134:999–1005.
2. Di Ieva A, Bruner E, Haider T, Rodella LF, Lee JM, Cusimano MD, Tschabitscher M. Skull base embryology: a multidisciplinary review. Childs Nerv Syst. 2014;30(6):991–1000.

The Cranial Nerves and Their Central Connexions

7

Contents

Brief Overview of Brainstem Orientation and Cellular Structure............ 137
Individual Cranial Nerve Pathways.. 143
Ophthalmic Division—V_1.. 150
Maxillary Division—V_2: (Maxillary Nerve)... 151
Mandibular Division—V_3: (Mandibular Nerve)................................... 153
Intracranial Course of IX.. 160
Take Home Points.. 163
Q and A: Chap. 7 (Answers at the End of This Chapter)......................... 167
Answers.. 168

Beyond the detailed description of the extracranial course and innervation of each of the cranial nerves, it is also important to understand how the different types of receptive cells are arranged into functional groups within the brainstem.

Brief Overview of Brainstem Orientation and Cellular Structure

Briefly, some developmental aspects of the brain stem mirror those in the spinal cord with a separation into a dorsal alar lamina (sensory afferent cells) and a ventral basal lamina (motor efferent), with a third type of brain cell in each lamina (the branchial afferent and efferent) cells. The make-up of the cranial nerves that

A. Zbar, *Anatomy--Head and Neck*,
https://doi.org/10.1007/978-3-031-69538-4_7

supply the derivatives of the branchial arches that lies between these dorsal and ventral cell types formulate the autonomic or visceral cells and are distinct from the somatic cells.

There are central stations of these nerves for the pharyngeal arches that are included in Cranials V, VII, IX and X. These cells become reorientated more like an opened-out spinal cord such that the motor cells lie medial and the sensory cells lateral with the autonomic cells intervening. The very specialist functions lead to special afferents and efferents. The separation is thus into:

Somatic motor nuclei (to the orbit and the tongue muscles).

Branchial motor function (also called the Visceral motor function which includes the PSNS cardiac, the visceral muscles and glands).

The Visceral (branchial) afferents for taste.

The Somatic Efferents (Cranial V).

Special Somatic Afferent (Cranial VIII).

Table 7.1 shows this cell differentiation categorized as afferent or efferent. These can be separated into general and special with a further division into visceral and somatic. The motor side of the branchial arches are all referred to as *visceral*. Special senses include vision and hearing. Visceral afferents include taste and visceral efferents innervate the muscles of the branchial arches

Table 7.1 Cell subtypes in the brainstem nuclei

	Visceral		Somatic	
	General	Special	General	Special
Afferent **Cell type**	Baroreceptors[a] Chemoreceptors[a] **GVA**	Taste (IX, VII, X) **SVA**	Somatic sensory (V) **GSA**	Special senses (II, VIII) **SSA**
Efferent **Cell type**	PSNS **GVE**	Branchial motor (VII) **SVE**	Somatic motor (III, IV, VI, XII) **GSE**	No cell type

[a]Transmitted in the Cranial IX—Carotid sinus nerve

Legend: *GVA* General visceral afferent; *SVA* Special visceral afferent; *GSA* General somatic afferent; *SSA* Special somatic afferent; *GVE* General visceral efferent; *SVE* Special visceral efferent; *GSE* General somatic efferent

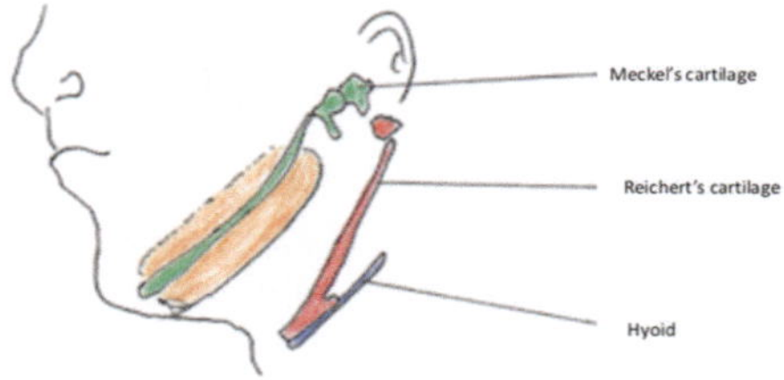

Diagram 7.1 Primitive facial cartilages. Meckel's cartilage (including the brown shaded area of the mandible). Includes the malleus and the incus. Reichert's cartilage for lesser wing and body of the hyoid. The remainder of the hyoid (greater wing) is formed from the third branchial arch (Blue)

including the first (Meckel's) arch (V motor to the muscles of mastication), the second (muscles of facial expression and the motor output of Cranial VII) and the third arch (Stylopharyngeus, the only motor output of Cranial IX).

The embryological make up is shown in Table 7.1. In summary this includes:

First arch cartilage—(Meckel's cartilage)—Diagram 7.1.

Gives origin to:

- Malleus, incus, frontonasal prominence, maxilla, zygomatic, squamous temporal, vomer, palatine, mandible
- The artery is the maxillary and
- its nerve is Cranial V.
- Gives rise to the muscles of mastication, mylohyoid, anterior belly digastric, tensor veli palatini, tensor tympani
- Sensation to: Face, inner nose and mouth and anterior 2/3 tongue

Second arch cartilage—(Reichert's cartilage).[1]

Gives origin to:

- Stapes. Styloid process, upper half and lesser wing of the hyoid bone

[1]Named after Karl Bogislaus Reichert (1811–1883), a German anatomist.

- Has two arteries—the stapedial artery (an artery regressing as a connexion between the ICA and the middle meningeal) and the hyoid artery
- The associated nerve is Cranial VII
- Innervating the muscles of facial expression, stapedius, stylo-hyoid, posterior belly digastric and platysma
- Special sensation via the chorda tympani part if the VII brings taste from the anterior 2/3 of the tongue

Third arch cartilage –
Gives origin to:

- The lower body of the hyoid and greater horn
- The third arch artery is the CCA and the take-off of the ICA
- The relevant nerve is Cranial IX
- Motor innervation to the stylopharyngeus
- The sensation is taste and general sensation to the posterior 1/3 of the tongue

Diagram 7.2a:
Diagram 7.2a: The orientation of the sensory and motor columns in the brainstem.

Diagram 7.2 Anatomy of the brainstem—nuclei and cranial nerve take-off after brain extraction
(**a**) The *right-hand side* of the image shows the motor nuclei. The *left-hand side* shows the sensory nuclei. The Edinger-Westphal nucleus lies close to the cluster of Cranial III nuclei in the mid-brain. Both the superior and inferior salivatory nuclei are shown. The nucleus ambiguus is branchiomotor lying near the dorsal motor nucleus of the vagus. On the sensory side the spinal nucleus of V is afferent for pain and temperature. It connects to the chief nucleus which is afferent for touch and proximally the mesencephalic nucleus which is afferent for proprioception. These sensory nuclei lie close to the V motor for a local reflex arc of chewing proprioception and jaw closure. The gustatory-taste nucleus (nucleus of the tractus solitarius) is connected to the vestibulocochlear nuclei and distally to the cardiorespiratory centre
(**b**) Ventral surface of the brainstem (vessels removed). The trochlear (Cranial IV) is often torn on brain removal and is not shown

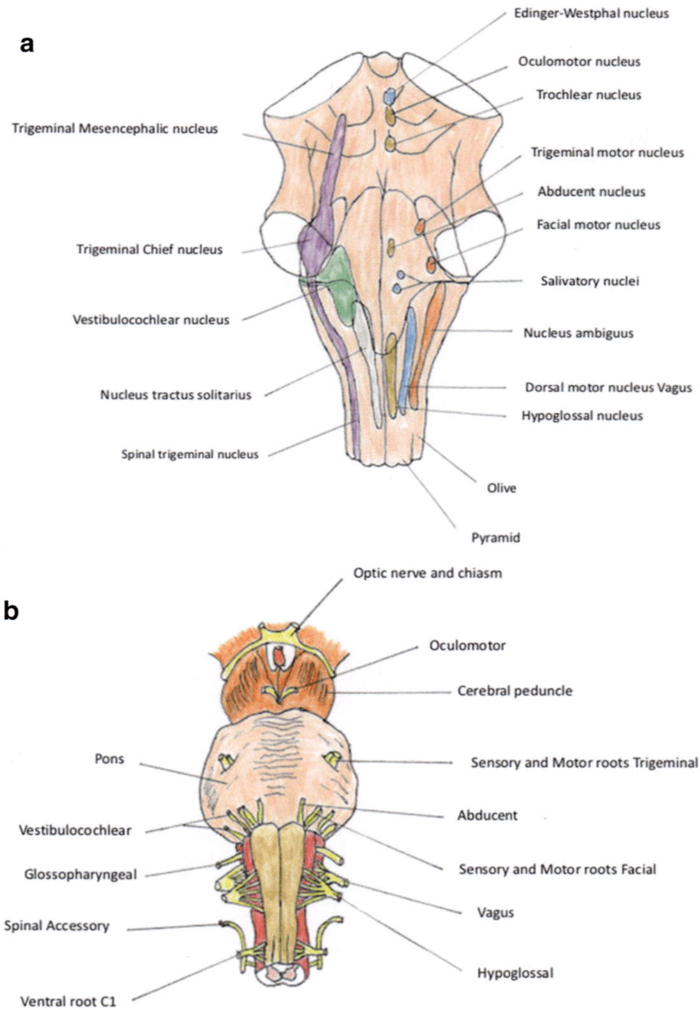
a
Edinger-Westphal nucleus
Oculomotor nucleus
Trochlear nucleus
Trigeminal Mesencephalic nucleus
Trigeminal motor nucleus
Abducent nucleus
Facial motor nucleus
Trigeminal Chief nucleus
Salivatory nuclei
Vestibulocochlear nucleus
Nucleus ambiguus
Nucleus tractus solitarius
Dorsal motor nucleus Vagus
Hypoglossal nucleus
Spinal trigeminal nucleus
Olive
Pyramid
b
Optic nerve and chiasm
Oculomotor
Cerebral peduncle
Pons
Sensory and Motor roots Trigeminal
Abducent
Vestibulocochlear
Sensory and Motor roots Facial
Glossopharyngeal
Vagus
Spinal Accessory
Hypoglossal
Ventral root C1

Diagram 7.2b: Positional take-off of the Cranial nerves from the brain stem and pons after removal of the brain.

Sensory columns: These include:

- The GSA (General systemic afferents) which convey pain, temperature, touch and proprioception. They synapse through the spinal nucleus of Cranial V and the other sensory V nuclei (mesencephalic and chief nuclei).
- The SSA (special somatic afferents) are for special sensation including vision (Cranial II) and hearing/balance for the vestibulocochlear apparatus (Cranial VIII).
- Although it is not a particularly good term all branchial arches are called viscera and their SVA cells (special visceral afferents) bring in taste fibres.
- The other sensory cell type is the GVA (General Visceral Afferents) which relay just below the taste fibres of the tractus solitarius to the cardiorespiratory centres and which bring in the reflexes that are part of the carotid and aortic sinuses and bodies (baroreceptors and chemoreceptors). In the head and neck these are afferent fibres in the carotid sinus nerve (part of Cranial IX). This area in the brain stem is part of a crowded relay so that the taste fibres run rostrally to the gustatory (solitary) nucleus and the *cardiorespiratory fibres in the distal part of the same nucleus.*

Motor Columns: These include:

- The GSE (General Systemic Efferents) which go to the voluntary muscles derived from somites (including the tongue and the extraocular muscles via Cranials III, IV and VI and in Cranial XII)
- The GVE (General Visceral Efferents) which are the autonomic outflow (PSNS) to the smooth and cardiac muscles. In the midbrain and the pons these include the Edinger-Westphal nucleus, the superior and inferior salivatory nuclei and the dorsal X autonomic nucleus.
- The SVE (Systemic Visceral Efferents) are the motor supply to the muscles which are derived from the pharyngeal arch meso-

derm (the branchial arches) as the muscles of mastication and the muscles of facial expression. The SVE relay in the motor nuclei of V and VII and in the nucleus ambiguus (located deep in the medullary reticular formation and containing the cell bodies that innervate the muscles of the soft palate, pharynx and larynx and which are concerned with speech and swallowing coordination).

A simple way of remembering this is to construct Table 7.1 dividing the cell bodies into General and Special functions. Within each of these there are afferent and efferent cell types with a separable division into Visceral and Somatic.

Individual Cranial Nerve Pathways

Images are provided of the pathways of Cranials V, VII and IX.

I—OLFACTORY NERVE: Like the optic nerve this is an outdrawn part of the CNS. There are approximately 20 olfactory nerves which pass from the specialized neuroepithelium in the upper nose through the cribriform plate of the ethmoid and which end in the olfactory bulb. The first order neurons are scattered bipolar cells which synapse in the bulb with mitral cells which then pass in the olfactory tract as medial and lateral olfactory striae to the anterior perforated substance and to the uncus.

II—OPTIC NERVE: (Diagram 7.3) The nasal fibres of the optic nerve (Cranial II) decussate in the optic chiasm (which are second order ganglion retinal cells). As a result, the right optic tract contains fibres from the right half of each retina: i.e. the nasal field of the right eye and the temporal field of the left eye. Following the optic chiasm the optic tracts pass around the midbrain (the cerebral peduncles) to end in three destinations: the lateral geniculate nucleus in the thalamus, the pretectal nuclei and the superior colliculus. The former relays from the lateral geniculate nucleus to the posterior (occipital or visual) cortex. The pretectal nuclei control the ipsilateral and contralateral pupillary

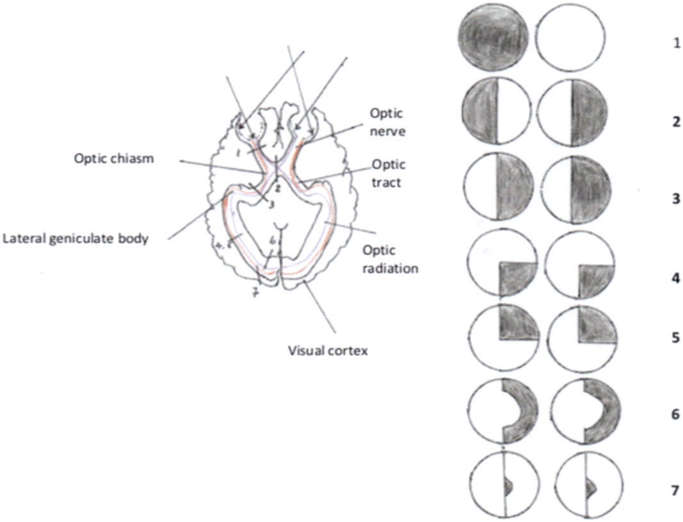

Diagram 7.3 The visual pathway. The arrows show the direction of light (right and left visual fields) to each retina. The numbers correspond to specific lesions affecting vision

Number	Lesion	Consequence
1	Left optic nerve	Blind left eye
2	Optic chiasm	Bitemporal hemianopia
3	Left optic tract	Right homonymous hemianopia
4	Upper left optic radiation	Right lower quadrantic homonymous hemianopia
5	Lower left optic radiation	Right upper quadrantic homonymous hemianopia
6	Anterior left visual cortex	Similar to 3 but with macular sparing
7	Tip of occipital lobe	Homonymous macular defect

1 may occur with optic neuritis; 2 with a pituitary lesion; 3 with a cerebrovascular accident; 4 with a parietal lobe lesion; 5 with a temporal lobe abscess; 6 with occlusion of the posterior cerebral artery; 7 with occlusion of the middle cerebral artery supplying the tip of the occipital lobe that represents the macula

reflex (See Diagram 5.4, Chap. 5). The superior colliculus controls the body reflexes to light.

The optic nerve as an extension is covered in the arachnoid and the subarachnoid allowing ophthalmoscopy to reflect intracranial pressure (papilloedema). The vascular supply of the optic tract is by the anterior choroidal and the posterior communicating arteries (See Chap. 9). The optic chiasm and the intracranial part of the optic nerve is supplied by the anterior cerebral artery. In the orbit, the arterial supply is from the ophthalmic and more distally by the central artery of the retina.

A knowledge of this basic anatomy allows an appreciation of the different visual defects: (Diagram 7.3).

- A complete lesion of the optic nerve results in complete blindness
- Compression of the optic chiasm results in a bitemporal hemianopia (a feature of an enlarging pituitary tumour)
- A lesion of the left optic tract will result in a right homonymous hemianopia
- A lesion of the lower fibres of the left optic radiation leads to a right upper quadrantic hemianopia (e.g. a result of a temporal lobe abscess)
- A lesion of the upper fibres of the left optic radiation leads to a right lower quadrantic hemianopia (e.g. a result of a parietal lobe lesion)
- A lesion of the anterior visual cortex leads to a right homonymous hemianopia (e.g. a posterior cerebral artery occlusion). This usually spares the macula (which is supplied by the middle cerebral artery)
- Traumatic damage to the tip of the left occipital lobe results in a right homonymous macular defect

To recapitulate: Pupillary size is an interplay between PSNS and SNS function. In the direct reflex, the optic tract leads back to the pretectal nucleus stimulating the EW nucleus on both sides. The cross-over of the chiasm also ensures that both pretectal nuclei are stimulated. Pupillary fibres lie on the dorsal surface of the optic nerve with their blood supply in the sheath so that they are highly susceptible to pressure. Note that the convergence (accommodation or so-called "near") reflex is part of a different pathway not involving the pretectal nuclei but rather the EW nucleus and the III nuclei for medial rectus convergence.

III—OCULOMOTOR NERVE: The nerve is a combination of somatic (to the striated ocular muscles) and visceral (to the smooth muscle in the eye) fibres with the Edinger-Westphal (accessory oculomotor) nucleus which lies cranial to the somatic nuclei. The Cranial III passes forwards from the midbrain just above the pons between the posterior cerebral and the superior cerebellar artery lying below and lateral to the posterior communicating artery. Cranial III lies just below the free margin of the tentorium cerebelli and passes the interpeduncular cistern below the floor of the third ventricle, piercing the arachnoid and the dura mater in the roof of the cavernous sinus at the point of the carotid siphon.

Cranial III is attached to the lateral part of the wall of the cavernous sinus just above Cranial VI where III collects SNS fibres from the carotid plexus destined for the smooth muscle in the levator palpebrae superioris. At the anterior pole of the cavernous sinus Cranial III splits into a superior and an inferior root inside the muscle ring (See Diagram 6.5a; Chap. 6) and traverses the superior orbital fissure between the nasociliary and the abducent nerve medially. The remainder of the structures passing through the superior orbital fissure are extraconal (lacrimal, frontal and trochlear). The superior division of III carries the SNS along with the somatic innervation to the superior rectus muscle. The inferior division of III breaks up into three branches to the medial and inferior rectus muscles and to the inferior oblique. All of the preganglionic PSNS fibres from the Edinger-Westphal nucleus lie in the proximal part of the inferior III division leaving to enter the ciliary ganglion via the short ciliary nerves (See Diagram 5.3a; Chap. 5).

Anatomical aspects of III nerve palsy:

- Complete ptosis of the lid
- When the lid is lifted, the eye looks *down and out* (as a result of the unopposed actions of the lateral rectus (VI) and the superior oblique (IV)
- Diplopia is less severe when looking outwards.

- The pupil is dilated (mydriasis) and does not react to light or constrict on accommodation. The consensual reflex in the opposite eye is preserved.

IV—TROCHLEAR NERVE: The somatic efferent (destined for the *superior oblique* muscle) emerges behind the inferior colliculus just below the free edge of the tentorium cerebelli and between the posterior cerebral and superior cerebellar arteries. The nerve pierces the roof of the cavernous sinus just behind Cranial III where Cranial VI lies uppermost entering the superior orbital fissure lateral to the tendinous ring (extraconal) as shown in Diagram 6.5a; Chap. 6). A lesion of this nerve means that the eye cannot look downwards when turned inwards leading to diplopia in practice particularly when reading or going downstairs. In this circumstance patients will tilt their head back towards the opposite shoulder to compensate for this in an attempt to realign the visual axis.

V—TRIGEMINAL NERVE (See both Diagrams 7.2a and 7.2b).

The Trigeminal nerve and its intracranial/extracranial course is shown in Diagram 7.4.

The motor nucleus of Cranial V is located in the upper pons and is destined for the branchial muscles of the first arch (muscles of mastication). The sensory part of Cranial V is somatic and is divided into three discrete areas running the length of the brainstem into the upper segments of the spinal cord. These include:

- The *Mesencephalic nucleus i*n the midbrain near the periaqueductal grey matter. The nucleus is proprioceptive from the muscles of mastication. Interacting with motor V it creates a local reflex arc that prevents the muscles from biting down too hard during chewing.
- The *Chief nucleus* is the main sensory nucleus in the upper pons responsible for touch.
- The *Spinal nucleus* is an onion-skin like area that is inverted and which works backwards from the mouth with the most inferior representation the ophthalmic region.

Diagram 7.4 Course and coverage of the Trigeminal Nerve (Cranial V)
(**a**) *Top Left Image:* The three segments of the Cranial V for the face show how and where V_3 is pulled up. Below the mandible sensation is covered by the cervical plexus. As the cranial cavity expands during development, the facial skin is drawn upwards with the beard skin drawn up like a smile over the temple. This explains how the auriculotemporal nerve is distributed and the way that the neck skin is drawn up to replace this area. The only area of facial skin not supplied by Cranial V is the angle of the mandible which is the territory of the great auricular nerve (C2, 3). The muscles of the face are also supplied by proprioceptive fibres from these cutaneous nerves which frequently have functional connections with filaments of Cranial VII
Legend: Ophthalmic nerve (V_1), Maxillary nerve (V_2), Mandibular nerve (V_3)
Top Right Image: The brainstem attachments of the Trigeminal ganglion. The motor root (to the special visceral efferents (to the muscles of mastication) are mixed with general somatic afferents to the mesencephalic nucleus (proprioceptive), the chief nucleus (touch) and the spinal nucleus (pain and temperature)
Bottom Image: Cranial V leaves the pons and divides into an ophthalmic division (V_1) via the superior orbital fissure, the maxillary division (V_2) via the foramen rotundum and the mandibular division (V_3) as a large anterior sensory root and a small motor root via the foramen ovale
(**b**) Trigeminal branches
V_1: Frontal—Supraorbital (SO) and supratrochlear (ST)
Lacrimal
Nasociliary—Infratrochlear (IT), Anterior ethmoidal (AE), Posterior ethmoidal (PE)
V_2: Terminates as infraorbital nerve. Posterior, Middle and Anterior Superior alveolar nerves, zygomatic nerve (dividing into zygomaticofacial and zygomaticotemporal)
V_3: Nervus spinosus (to dura mater of the middle cranial fossa)
Buccal
Lingual (assisted by Chorda tympani for taste to the anterior 2/3 tongue)
Inferior alveolar (plus Nerve to mylohyoid; also innervating anterior belly digastric) and terminates as mental nerve
Foraminae coloured red; PSNS ganglia coloured green
Note V_2–V_1 connexion from the zygomaticofacial branch to the lacrimal nerve transmitting PSNS postganglionic fibres from the pterygopalatine gland for lacrimation

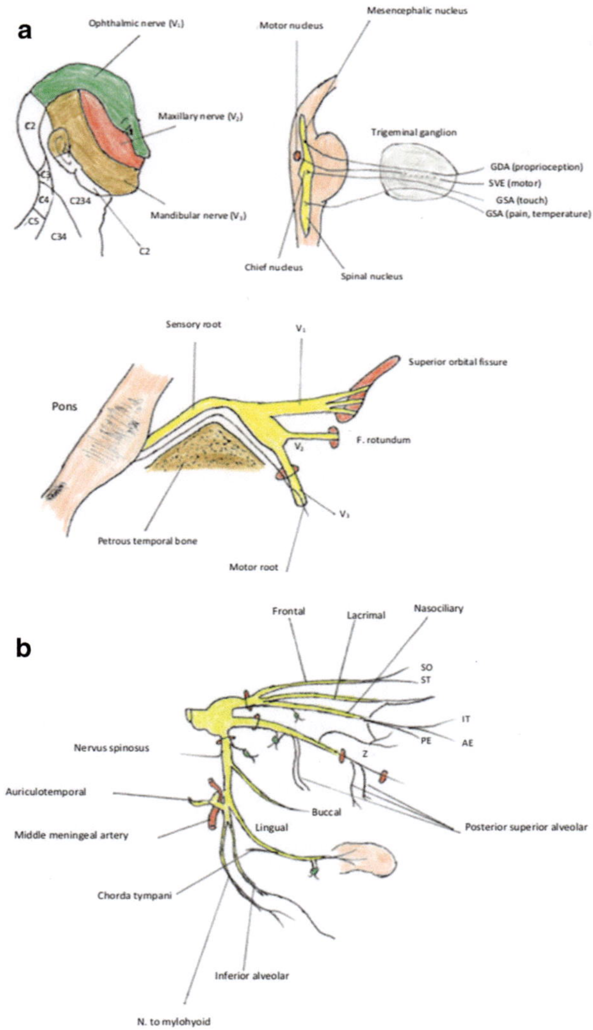
a
Ophthalmic nerve (V_1)
Maxillary nerve (V_2)
Mandibular nerve (V_3)
C2
C3
C4
C5
C234
C34
C2
Motor nucleus
Mesencephalic nucleus
Trigeminal ganglion
GDA (proprioception)
SVE (motor)
GSA (touch)
GSA (pain, temperature)
Chief nucleus
Spinal nucleus
Sensory root
V_1
Superior orbital fissure
Pons
F. rotundum
V_2
V_3
Petrous temporal bone
Motor root
b
Frontal
Lacrimal
Nasociliary
SO
ST
IT
AE
PE
Z
Nervus spinosus
Auriculotemporal
Middle meningeal artery
Buccal
Lingual
Posterior superior alveolar
Chorda tympani
Inferior alveolar
N. to mylohyoid

The motor root of Cranial V emerges cranially and medial to the larger sensory root with the fusion of the dura in such a way that the posterior roots of the V ganglion are bathed in cerebrospinal fluid. The first two branches (V_1 and V_2) pass forward in the lateral wall of the cavernous sinus. The mandibular (V_3) division passes with the motor root to the foramen ovale.

Ophthalmic Division—V_1

This nerve is sensory (pain, thermal) for the upper face and the eye. In the formation of these sensory areas, the orbit and forehead are innervated by V_1, the middle one-third of the face and sinuses by V_2 and the mandibular region by V_3. The side of the face and the temple region are pulled up and bunched up to include V_3 during development as shown in Diagram 7.4a.

The ophthalmic nerve picks up SNS fibres from the cavernous plexus (destined for the dilator pupillae) and gives off meningeal branches (tentorial nerves) and then its individual branches:

- Lacrimal
- Frontal and
- Nasociliary

The ***lacrimal nerve*** is joined by the zygomaticofacial nerve (PSNS) which hitchhikes along the lacrimal nerve to supply the lacrimal gland. The lacrimal nerve has a lateral palpebral branch for sensation of the palpebral and ocular surfaces of the lateral conjunctiva.

The ***frontal nerve*** is quite large running on top of the levator palpebrae superioris and which runs through the supraorbital fissure (or foramen when present) to become the *supraorbital nerve* and the *supratrochlear nerve*. The supraorbital nerve covers sensation from the frontal sinus, the upper eyelid and the conjunctiva as well as the skin and soft-tissues extending over the frontal scalp as far backwards as the vertex. The supratrochlear nerve supplies an area of skin running towards the forehead from the midline up to the hairline.

The ***nasociliary nerve*** is sensory to the eyeball and the paranasal sinuses as well as to the mucous membrane of the nasal cavity and the external skin of the nose. This nerve carries SNS fibres to the dilator pupillae. It changes name to become the *anterior ethmoidal nerve* sensory to the anterior and middle ethmoidal air cells and then descends alongside the crista galli into the root of the nose innervating the antero-superior quadrant of the lateral wall and that segment of the nasal septum. After this the nerve is renamed the *external nasal nerve* where it sensorily innervates the tip of the nose. One of the branches of the nasociliary is the *infratrochlear nerve* which innervates the skin and conjunctiva of the medial upper eyelid and the area below that on the bridge of the nose. A further branch is the *posterior ethmoidal nerve* (before the take-off of the infratrochlear nerve) which sensorily innervates the posterior ethmoidal air cells and adjacent sphenoid sinus and which is transmitted via the posterior ethmoidal foramen. This nerve does not reach the nasal cavity and in some cases is absent.

There is in addition a communicating branch to the ciliary ganglion (the *sensory root of the ciliary ganglion*; See Diagram 5.3a, Chap. 5). The postganglionic PSNS pupillo-constriction fibres travel via the short ciliary nerves. The long ciliary nerves are sensory to the eye (cornea but not conjunctiva) entering the sclera independently and carrying SNS fibres.

Maxillary Division—V_2: (Maxillary Nerve)

This is the nerve of the middle third of the face running in the upper and outer part of the cavernous sinus and then out of the middle cranial fossa via the foramen rotundum which forms part of the roof of the pterygopalatine fossa (See Chap. 8). The maxillary nerve runs past the inferior orbital fissure and ends as the infraorbital nerve.

The maxillary nerve innervates the nasal mucosa, palate upper teeth, lacrimal gland and the skin of the face between the eye and the mouth (middle third territory). The pterygopalatine ganglion functions as a central relay station for transmission of arteries, sensory elements, SNS and PSNS distribution to the nose, palate, pharynx, orbit and middle third of the face. Only PSNS fibres synapse in this ganglion.

Nasal branches are: the nasopalatine and the posterior superior nasal.

Palatine branches are: the greater palatine (running forward on to the hard palate) and the lesser palatine (running backwards on to the soft palate).

A pharyngeal branch running backwards to the pharynx (near the opening of the auditory tube and the tubal tonsil) via the palatovaginal canal.

Orbital branches. The PSNS system for lacrimation is distributed via the maxillary nerve jumping to the lacrimal branch of the ophthalmic division.

The *nasopalatine nerve* (previously called the *long sphenopalatine nerve*) enters the nose via the sphenopalatine foramen, crossing the roof of the nose and supplying the postero-inferior half of the nasal septum. It is transmitted through the incisive canal to innervate the hard palate and the gingiva behind the two incisor teeth. The *posterior superior lateral nerve* (formerly called the *short sphenopalatine nerve*) and the medial nasal nerves supply the postero-superior quadrant of the lateral nasal wall and the nasal septum (the remaining antero-superior part of the nose and septum Is innervated by the anterior ethmoidal nerve with the posterior ethmoidal nerve innervating the posterior-superior part). See Chap. 12. Further innervation of this highly sensitive area is via the posterior lateral nasal nerve and the greater palatine nerve (to the postero-inferior nose and the maxillary sinus).

The *zygomatic nerve* arises in the pterygopalatine fossa entering the inferior orbital fissure and running along the lower lateral wall of the orbit carrying the postganglionic PSNS sudomotor fibres to the lacrimal gland and joining the lacrimal nerve. The *zygomaticofacial nerve* supplies the local skin and the *zygomaticotemporal nerve* pierces the temporalis fascia to supply the skin above the zygomatic arch (hairless temple skin). There are also posterior superior alveolar nerves in the pterygopalatine fossa. These divide and enter the posterior wall of the maxilla above the maxillary tuberosity to innervate the maxillary sinus and most of the sensory innervation to the three molar teeth (except the buccal part of the first molar) as well as the gum of the vestibule alongside the three molars.

The *infraorbital nerve* supplies the maxillary sinus, giving off the *middle superior alveolar nerve* to the two premolars and the anterior buccal root of the first molar. The *anterior superior alveolar nerve* innervates the canine and the two incisors and goes as far as the inferior part of the nose including the nasolacrimal duct and nasal floor ending on the nasal septum. The infraorbital nerve emerges from the infraorbital foramen between the levator labii superioris and the levator anguli oris muscles where it may communicate with radicals of Cranial VII. The infraorbital terminates as *palpebral branches* to the lower eyelid and conjunctiva and *labial branches* to the upper lip skin and mucous membrane from the midline to the second premolar tooth.

The infraorbital nerve may be blocked intraorally by infiltrating local anaesthetic against the upper lip after working forwards of the bony maxillary buttress. It is a painless intraoral block which is underutilized but which is ideal for small lacerations or dog bites around the upper lip and the base of the side of the nares.

Mandibular Division—V_3: (Mandibular Nerve)

This nerve passes into the infratemporal fossa (See Chap. 8) between the upper head of the lateral pterygoid muscle and the tensor palati muscle. The nerve divides as a leash into an anterior group of branches which are all motor except one branch and a posterior group of branches which are all sensory except for one branch. Before this break the main nerve gives off a meningeal branch (the *nervus spinosus*) which travels via the foramen ovale or the foramen spinosum and which innervates the cartilaginous portion of the Eustachian tube. The nerve runs posteriorly to also innervate the mastoid antrum and the mastoid air cells. The second nerve given off before division is the nerve to the medial pterygoid which has a separate branch given off near the otic ganglion (and traversing the ganglion) to supply the two tensors (tympani and palati).

The 6 Anterior branches are:

- Two nerves to the *lateral pterygoid* muscle (one per head)
- Two *deep temporal nerves* to the temporalis
- *Nerve to masseter*
- *Buccal nerve* which runs between the two heads of the lateral pterygoid to supply sensation for the mucosa over the buccinator and below the zygomatic arch as well as for the vestibular

gum of the three mandibular molar teeth. This nerve also carries PSNS sudomotor fibres for minor buccal and molar glands

The buccal nerve should not be confused with the buccal branch of Cranial VII.

Note also that the nerve to the masseter follows Hilton's Law (namely that a motor nerve to a muscle tends to give a branch of supply to the joint on which the muscle acts as well as another branch to the skin (or mucosa in this case) over the joint. In this instance the buccal nerve sends a sensory twig to the temporomandibular joint capsule.[2]

The 3 Posterior branches are:

- *Auriculotemporal nerve*—This nerve has two roots which envelop the middle meningeal artery. This nerve transmits postganglionic fibres from the otic ganglion destined for the parotid gland. The nerve is sensory to the TMJ and the parotid, dividing into an auricular branch innervating sensation of the external auditory meatus and the EAM and the external ear (auricle) above this point and a temporal branch. The latter runs over the root of the zygomatic process and supplies the hairy skin of the scalp (the first area to grey).
- *Inferior alveolar* (*dental*) *nerve*. This nerve lies on the medial pterygoid between the mandible and the sphenomandibular ligament. It enters the mandibular foramen in front of the inferior alveolar artery and vein. The main inferior alveolar nerve supplies the posterior five teeth (three molars and two premolars) and terminates as the incisive branch (canine and both incisors) with some central overlap. It terminates as the *mental nerve* (which is transmitted through the mental foramen) to innervate sensation to both surfaces of the lower lip and to the gum from the midline to the second premolar. There are some additional minor otic ganglion fibres distributed to minor labial glands. Just before the inferior alveolar nerve enters the mandibular foramen a motor branch (*Nerve to mylohyoid*) is given

[2]John Hilton (1805–1878) a British surgeon articulated this 'law' in a series of lectures delivered between 1860 and 1862.

off to innervate the mylohyoid and the anterior belly of digastric by piercing the sphenomandibular ligament.

- The *lingual nerve* is joined by the chorda tympani just below the skull base and curves on the medial pterygoid a centimetre in front of the inferior alveolar nerve. The lingual nerve passes under the free lower border of the superior constrictor muscle just below the last molar tooth against the mandible giving off a gingival branch which supplies the lingual gum to the midline. The lingual nerve swerves around the submandibular duct on the surface of the hyoglossus muscle and supplies **sensation and taste to the anterior 2/3 of the tongue**.

VI—ABDUCENT NERVE:

The nerve arises at the lower pons as a somatic motor nucleus near the motor nucleus of Cranial VII (overlying as the facial colliculus). Cranial VI emerges above the pyramid of the medulla and enters the pontine cistern above the anterior inferior cerebellar artery to pierce the dura over the clivus to enter the inferior petrosal sinus at the apex of the petrous temporal bone and then by bending forward under the petroclinoid ligament to pass through the cavernous sinus. The Cranial VI passes from the most medial part of the superior orbital fissure to enter the cone of muscles and move laterally to innervate the *lateral rectus muscle.*

An **abducent nerve lesion or palsy** results in an eye that cannot look outwards and which is turned in (intorted) by the unopposed action of the medial, superior and inferior recti (all innervated by Cranial III). An abducent palsy may be a non-localizing sign of raised intracranial pressure (with a brain tumour for example) by virtue of its relatively long intracranial course.

***VII—FACIAL NERVE*:** (Diagram 7.5).

The main nerve contains a motor root (for the muscles of the second branchial arch), visceral efferents (PSNS) for the submandibular and sublingual glands, lacrimal glands and glands in the nose, palate and pharynx, special visceral afferents for taste to the anterior 2/3 of the tongue (and soft palate) and a small insignificant area of somatic afferent sensation near the skin of the external auditory meatus and nearby tympanic membrane.

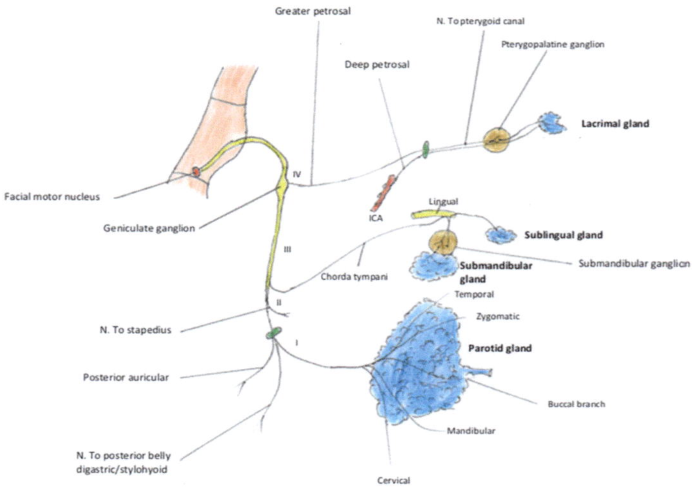

Diagram 7.5 Course and coverage of the Facial Nerve (Cranial VII). I-IV represent sites of potential facial nerve lesions. (See main text and Table 7.2 in this chapter). The main VII exiting the skull travels via the stylomastoid foramen. The autonomic nerve supply to the middle one-third of the face and for lacrimation travels via the pterygoid canal (Both foraminae are shown in *green*). ICA -internal carotid artery. The connected ganglia are shown in *brown*—pterygopalatine, submandibular

A thorough knowledge of the anatomy allows an understanding of specific VII nerve lesions.

The *Facial nucleus* is located in the lower pons where the fibres make a genu on the surface of the VI nerve nucleus, emerging above the olive. The secretomotor nucleus of the *nervus intermedius i*s the superior salivatory nucleus which lies nearby. The sensory nucleus (gustatory nucleus of the *tractus solitarius*) lies in the medulla and receives the central processes of taste cell bodies lying in the *geniculate ganglion.* The small area of sensation in the tympanic membrane has its receptive cell bodies in the spinal V nucleus.

The nervus intermedius part of VII emerges at the lower border of the pons with the inferior cerebellar peduncle near Cranial VIII. The nervus intermedius enters the internal acoustic meatus at the pontocerebellar angle and the point of the pontine cistern. In the inner ear, Cranial VII takes a right-angled curve forming the geniculate ganglion and runs near the lateral semicircular canal to emerge from the skull via the *stylomastoid foramen* where it is a pure motor nerve.

Intracranial branches of VII located in the petrous temporal bone include:

- Greater petrosal nerve
- Tympanic branches to the middle ear
- The motor nerve to the stapedius muscle and the
- Chorda tympani.

The *greater petrosal nerve* is secretomotor to the lacrimal gland, the glands of the palate and nose and pharynx and a few taste fibres to the palate (cell bodies lie in the geniculate ganglion). The greater petrosal nerve joins the deep petrosal nerve derived from the superior cervical ganglion to form the nerve of the pterygoid canal (See Chap. 5).

Small *tympanic branches* are sensory joining the tympanic plexus in the middle ear with some drifting to the auriculotemporal territory near the skin of the external auditory meatus.

The *nerve to stapedius* is given off in the facial canal and reaches the muscle via a minute canaliculus.

The *chorda tympani* leaves in the facial canal and passes through the posterior wall of the middle ear near the neck of the malleus. It emerges at the petrotympanic fissure and grooves the medial aspect of the spine of the sphenoid to join the lingual nerve just above the lateral pterygoid muscle.

Once outside the stylomastoid foramen, extracranial branches of VII include:

The posterior auricular nerve which innervates the occipital belly of the occipitofrontalis muscle.

The nerve to the posterior belly of digastric.

The nerve to stylohyoid and

The terminal nerves to the muscles of facial expression and platysma (temporal, zygomatic, buccal branch, mandibular and cervical) (See Chap. 3, also Diagram 3.5 - middle image).

Table 7.2 Manifestations of an ascending cause of VII nerve palsy. A dry mouth may not be noticed by the patient as there is still salivation from the parotid and the contralateral salivary glands. The symptoms can be traced as one moves from the stylomastoid foramen to the exit point of Cranial VII from the lower pons. Examples of causes for each level are included as diagnoses

Diagnosis	Bell's palsy	Hyperacusis	Dry mouth	Loss of taste	Loss of hearing	Loss of lacrimation
Ramsay-hunt Syndrome	+					
Middle ear Disease	+	+				
Acoustic Neuroma	+		±	+	+	
Cerebello-Pontine angle Tumour	+		±	+	+	+

By following Cranial VII as it enters the skull we can anatomically locate specific lesions (Table 7.2):

***VIII—VESTIBULOCOCHLEAR NERVE*:** This is a wholly sensory, special somatic afferent (SSA) for sound reception and balance. It includes the *Cochlear nerve* afferent from the hair cells of the spiral organ (*Organ of Corti*) which enters the lower cerebellar peduncle at the lower end of the pons (Diagram 7.2b). These fibres run via the tegmentum to the inferior colliculus (as reflex responses to sound) and then via the lateral lemniscus (which includes tectal reflexes that are responsive to head and neck and body/limb positioning). This then relays in the medial geniculate body via the auditory radiation to the auditory area within the lateral cortical sulcus (Chap. 16). By contrast, the vestibular nerve is triggered by the neuroepithelium of the hair cells in the maccule of the utricle and saccule and in the ampullae of the semicircular canals (which relay static and kinetic balance, respectively). These then relay through the vestibular nuclei in the medial geniculate body.

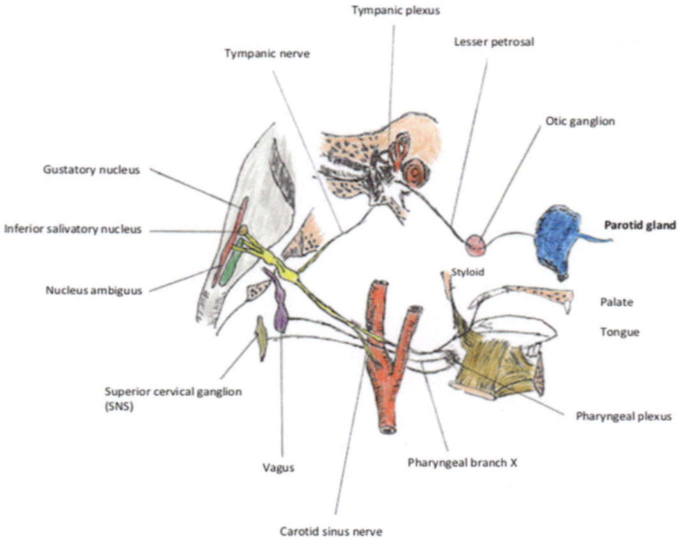

Diagram 7.6 Course of the Glossopharyngeal nerve (Cranial IX). Central relay is separately to the nucleus ambiguus, the nucleus of the tractus solitarius (gustatory) and the inferior salivatory nucleus. The only muscle innervated by motor fibres of IX is the stylopharyngeus

IX—THE GLOSSOPHARYNGEAL NERVE: (Diagram 7.6): The nuclei lie in the medulla (and the lower pons) and define the nerve of the third branchial arch. Cranial IX is therefore visceral (branchial) and mixed sensory (somatic and taste) as well as sudomotor.

Branches of IX include:

- The **branchial** fibres which are limited, corresponding to the nucleus ambiguus as a motor branch directed to only one muscle, the *stylopharyngeus*.
- The **secretomotor** supply is derived from the inferior salivatory nucleus in the lowest part of the pons lying just rostral to the dorsal nucleus of Cranial X. These preganglionic fibres are destined for the parotid gland entering the otic ganglion via the *lesser petrosal nerve*.

- Taste is supplied to the **posterior 1/3 of the tongue**
- Sensation is supplied to the inner ear as part of the **tympanic plexus** via the tympanic canaliculus and to the palate, pharynx, Eustachian tube and posterior 1/3 of the tongue as part of the pharyngeal plexus with the motor branches of X as General Somatic Afferents (GSA)
- General visceral afferents (GVA) traveling in the **carotid sinus nerve** from the carotid sinus and carotid bodies (Glomus Type I cells) synapsing in the reticular formation below the gustatory nucleus.[3]

Central relay for taste is in the nucleus of the tractus solitarius (gustatory nucleus), whereas those for sensation of the palate, pharynx and posterior tongue synapse in the spinal nucleus of V.

Intracranial Course of IX

The nerve rootlets of IX emerge between the olive and inferior cerebellar peduncle, joining as a single nerve at the pontine cistern to enter the anterior compartment of the jugular foramen (separated from X and XI by a septum of fibrous dura). Cranial IX deeply notches the inferior border of the petrous bone just below the internal acoustic meatus and at this point as it perforates the dura and the arachnoid, it swells to form the inferior (petrous) ganglion. Proximal to this is a superior (jugular) ganglion (or ganglia) which is a sensory peripheral ganglion (innervation to the middle ear and tympanic membrane). Axons form the tympanic nerve combined with the preganglionic PSNS fibres. The superior IX ganglion is smaller than the inferior IX ganglion. Cranial IX gains access to the jugular foramen passing between the sigmoid sinus and the inferior petrosal sinus in the front end of the foramen. The inferior ganglion is also a sensory ganglion sitting in the jugular foramen but providing a wider range of pseudounipolar

[3] The carotid sinus nerve is also called Hering's nerve after Heinrich Hering, (1866–1948) a German born Czech pathologist who also described the central cardiac pacemaker.

cells responsible for taste, sensory innervation of the pharynx, palate and the cells involved in baroreceptor and chemoreceptor function.

Cranial IX extracranially runs between the ICA and the ECA and around the substance of the stylopharyngeus to pass into the pharynx between the superior and middle constrictor muscles deep to hyoglossus and deep to the styloid process and its connected muscles (See Diagram 3.6; Chap. 3). It forms the pharyngeal plexus on the substance of the middle constrictor muscle. The *stylopharyngeus* is the longest of the three styloid muscles, arising from the inner upper surface of the styloid process near its root. It blends within the pharynx with the palatopharyngeus with which it is partly inserted into the epiglottis. It lifts the larynx and pulls the base of the epiglottis upwards and backwards during swallowing and speaking.

The tympanic branch passes into the middle ear via the tympanic canaliculus forming the tympanic plexus from which emerges the lesser petrosal nerve running typically through the foramen ovale to the otic ganglion. It runs with two slender carotico-tympanic branches which are derived from the SNS plexus on the surface of the ICA.

X—VAGUS**:** (*Specific aspects of the Cranial X and its branches are considered elsewhere in this volume as well as in other volumes of this series*).

The Vagal nuclei lie in the upper medulla and comprise branchial or visceral branches (afferent and efferent) and somatic afferents to the:

- palate) which are provided by the cranial accessory fibres which join the Cranial X (*vide supra*).
- The dorsal motor nucleus of the X (lying below the X trigone) supplies cardiac and bronchial and gut smooth muscle.
- The nucleus of the tractus solitarius receives afferent fibres from the heart and thorax as well as the abdominal viscera along with a few taste fibres from the epiglottis. (General sensation fibres -GSA—arising from parts of the pharynx and larynx and relaying in the spinal nucleus of V).

- There is a small auricular branch of Cranial X which may relay here (covering sensation of the mastoid process, the lower half of the tympanic membrane and the external auditory meatus) which is transmitted via the tympanomastoid fissure.

The Cranial X leaves the medulla (just below Cranial IX) by a series of delicate rootlets emanating from the sulcus between the olive and the inferior cerebellar peduncle. Cranial X unites in the middle compartment of the jugular foramen forming a small superior ganglion (containing the cell bodies of the meningeal and auricular branches) and a longer, larger inferior ganglion just below the skull base (housing the cell bodies of all the other sensory fibres in Cranial X). The cranial root of XI sends all of its nucleus ambiguus fibres (motor to skeletal muscle of the pharynx, larynx, palate and upper oesophagus) to X at the level of the inferior ganglion. The physical structure of this connexion somewhat mimics the way in which any spinal motor root joins the spinal nerve distal to the dorsal root sensory ganglion.

Vagal branches include:

- Head and Neck—*meningeal*, *auricular* and *carotid body*
- The *pharyngeal branch* running between the ICA and the ECA
- The *superior laryngeal* branch running deep to the CCA and dividing into an *external laryngeal* branch (which pierces the thyrohyoid membrane to supply the mucosa of the pharynx and larynx) and which is motor to the cricothyroid muscle and an *internal laryngeal* nerve. The internal laryngeal nerve also pierces the thyrohyoid membrane and sensorily innervates the pirform recess
- The *right recurrent laryngeal nerve* (RLN) hooks around the subclavian artery and runs in the trachea-oesophageal groove by passing under the inferior constrictor muscle. The RLN supplies all of the intrinsic muscles of the larynx ***except for the cricothyroid muscle.*** The RLN also innervates sensation to the laryngeal mucosa below the level of the vocal folds. On the left side, in the thorax, the left RLN hooks around the ligamentum arteriosum and runs under the aortic arch at the level of the

sternal angle. If this is traced back this level finishes at the T4–T5 vertebral junction and is a useful marker on axial CT scans for the identification of structures which potentially can be involved in a lung cancer. Both the main X and the RLN give off additional cardiac branches, as well as tracheal and oesophageal branches which contribute to the oesophageal plexi in front of and behind the oesophagus before these coalesce to form the anterior and posterior vagal trunks.

- Cervical and cardiac branches (upper and lower on the right and lower on the left) which join the deep part of the cardiac plexus. That on the right joins the superficial cardiac plexus.

Take Home Points

- The internal laryngeal nerve in piercing the thyrohyoid membrane runs with the superior laryngeal branch of the superior thyroid artery.
- Structures running between the ICA and ECA all have a '*pharyngeal*' title and include: the Glossopharyngeal (IX) nerve, the pharyngeal branch of the Vagus and the stylopharyngeus muscle.
- The cricothyroid is the only intrinsic muscle of the larynx not innervated by the RLN (but rather by the external laryngeal branch of the superior laryngeal nerve).

In general, concerning the X branches to the gut and its derivatives, these are motor to smooth muscle and secretomotor to glands but do not carry pain afferents. Pain fibres from the abdominal viscera run with the SNS fibres, however, in the thorax Cranial X is sensory to the thoracic viscera (oesophagus, trachea and lungs). Vagal fibres also carry afferents from the pelvic organs (Diagram 7.7).

***XI—THE ACCESSORY NERVE*: ** (Diagram 7.8).

Cranial XI has cranial and spinal roots. The *cranial root of XI* is best considered part of the Cranial X and innervates the striated muscles of the pharynx and palate (and oesophagus and larynx).

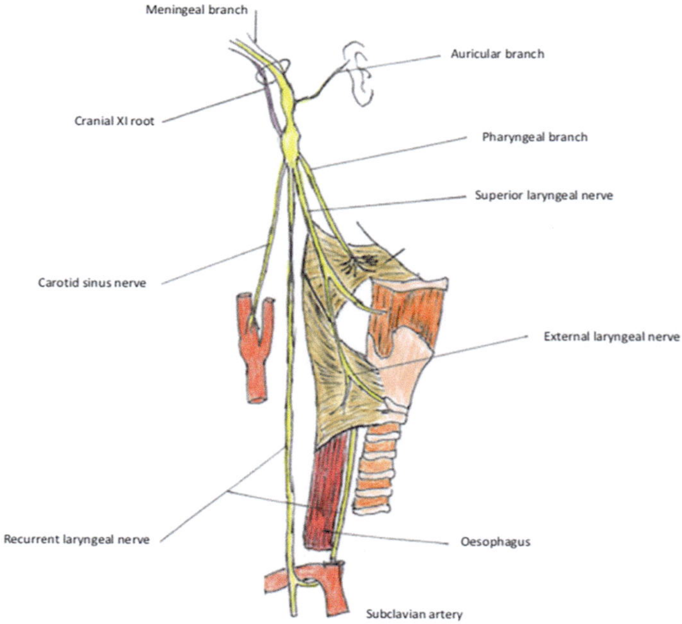

Diagram 7.7 Course and connexions of the Vagus nerve (Cranial X). Head and neck branches include: a meningeal branch to the dura of the posterior cranial fossa, an auricular branch, the pharyngeal branch (contributed to the skeletal musculature via the Cranial XI), the superior laryngeal nerve (external and internal laryngeal), a similar nerve to that of IX (carotid sinus/body nerve) and the recurrent laryngeal nerve (RLN)

These fibres emanate from the nucleus ambiguus, leaving the medulla as a series of rootlets below those rootlets of Cranial X between the olive and the inferior cerebellar peduncle (Diagram 7.2a, b) uniting into a single cranial root that is joined by the spinal root of XI coming up into the pontine cistern through the foramen magnum.

The *spinal root of XI* emanates from the spinal accessory nucleus formed in the anterior horn of the upper 5 or 6 cervical segments (mainly C2,3,4). These do not leave the anterior horn but rather emerge behind the denticulate ligament as a series of root-

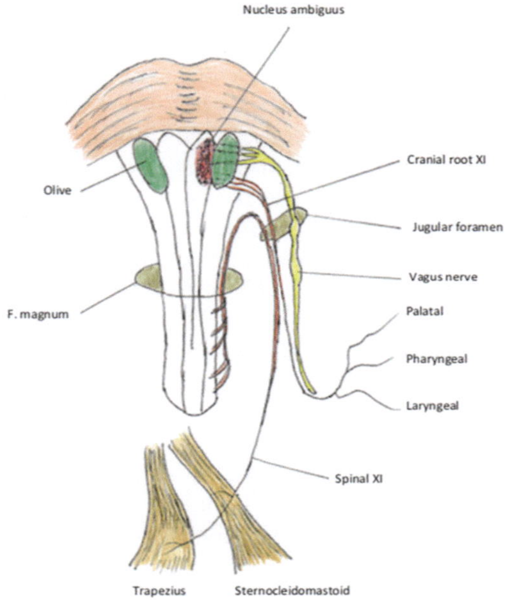

Diagram 7.8 Course and connexions of the Accessory nerve (Cranial XI) The cranial root of XI passes with Cranial X through the jugular foramen and is destined for somatic innervation to the pharynx, palate and larynx. The spinal root arises from C1–C5 and enters via the foramen magnum before exiting the skull for distribution to the sternocleidomastoid and the trapezius muscles

lets that then form a single nerve which joins the cranial nerve root. In reality, these two roots have nothing to do with one another, but pass together through the jugular foramen before parting company for different functions. Cranial XI lies caudal to Cranial X and passes through the middle compartment of the jugular foramen.

In the neck, spinal XI is wholly motor, running over the lateral mass of the atlas on top of the IJV and then passing into the sternocleidomastoid and then descending over the levator scapulae into the trapezius.

XII—HYPOGLOSSAL NERVE: The XII nucleus is located in the medulla lying in the floor of the fourth ventricle with motor fibres passing ventrally out between the olive and the pyramid, joining into two roots that enter the hypoglossal (anterior condylar) canal in the occipital bone. This then passes forwards above the atlanto-occipital joint as a single nerve which pierces the arachnoid and dura. Cranial XII spirals laterally behind the inferior ganglion of Cranial X and extracranially runs directly over the front of the CCA bifurcation below the posterior belly of the digastric. Here it is related to the *ansa cervicalis* and is covered by the common facial vein and the investing layer of deep cervical fascia. This is a point where there is branching of the ECA (posteriorly as the occipital and anteriorly as the lingual). The Cranial XII follows the pathway of migration of the suboccipital myotomes forming the muscles of the tongue. It runs deep to mylohyoid on the surface of the hyoglossus and supplies all of the intrinsic muscles of the tongue and all the extrinsic muscles of the tongue (viz; all muscles with '*glossus*' in their name—styloglossus, hyoglossus and genioglossus) **except palatoglossus**. Both geniohyoid and thyrohyoid are innervated by C1 traveling along with Cranial XII.

It is easier to remember if we think of it where the palatoglossus is considered more as a depressor palati (that attaches to the tongue rather than primarily moves it) and then this muscle should be innervated by the pharyngeal branch of the Vagus (and is not part of the XII development or innervation). Hypoglossal branches before it reaches the tongue are all derived from C1 nerve fibres joining at the XII canal.

The fibres from the XII nucleus have no supply outside of the tongue.

There is also a meningeal branch off the mainstem for the innervation of the dura mater in the posterior cranial fossa near the foramen magnum. The upper root of the ansa cervicalis (superior root C1 + inferior root C2, 3) is embedded in the anterior felt-like substance of the carotid sheath. The slender nerve to thyrohyoid (C1) comes off as the main XII nerve lies on the lingual artery and the last branch to geniohyoid (C1) is given off in the mouth above the mylohyoid. Lesions of Cranial XII (as may occur from a cerebrovascular accident) result in tongue muscle wasting on the side of the lesion and when the tongue is poked out it deviates towards affected side.

Q and A: Chap. 7 (Answers at the End of This Chapter)

1. The accessory nerve
   (a) Has a cranial segment which supports the Vagus and provides pharyngeal and palatal innervation
   (b) Has spinal segments which arise below the medulla
   (c) Runs between the scalenus anterior and the scalenus medius
   (d) Exits the skull via the foramen magnum
2. The glossopharyngeal (IX) nerve
   (a) Has no motor root
   (b) Carries sympathetic fibres to the otic ganglion
   (c) Forms a pharyngeal plexus on the inferior constrictor
   (d) Has a carotid sinus branch
3. The trochlear (IV) nerve
   (a) Emerges above the tentorium cerebelli
   (b) Is lateral to the oculomotor (III) nerve in the superior orbital fissure
   (c) Enters the orbit extraconally
   (d) Controls an extraocular muscle which depresses the eye more purely in extorsion
4. Concerning the Cranial nerves
   (a) The central nucleus of the VIII (vestibulocochlear) crosses the pons and medulla
   (b) The motor nucleus of V is pontine
   (c) The XII nucleus lies below the dorsal vagal nucleus
   (d) The nasal fibres of II decussate in the optic chiasm
5. A nasopharyngeal carcinoma of the Sinus of Morgagni may present with:
   (a) Palatal asymmetry
   (b) Hyperacusis
   (c) Loss of lacrimation
   (d) Trismus in advanced cases
   (e) Paralysis of the tongue musculature

6. An accessory nerve injury in the neck is suggested if:
   (a) The patient cannot extend their neck against resistance
   (b) Is unable to shrug their shoulder on the affected side
   (c) Cannot raise their arm on the affected side
   (d) Complains of numbness over the back of the neck
7. A cerebellopontine angle tumour may present with:
   (a) Neural deafness
   (b) Loss of taste to the posterior one-third of the tongue
   (c) A very dry mouth
   (d) An ipsilateral dry eye
8. An oculomotor nerve palsy presents with
   (a) Partial ptosis
   (b) Diplopia on looking inwards
   (c) Mydriasis
   (d) Sluggish or absent direct and consensual pupillary response

Answers

1. a, b
2. d
3. b
4. a, b, d
5. a, d
6. b
7. a, d
8. c, d

The Infratemporal and Pterygopalatine Fossae

8

Contents

Infratemporal Fossa........ 169
Mandibular Nerve........ 173
Maxillary Artery (Diagram 8.3)........ 174
Regional Muscles: Masseter, Lateral and Medial Pterygoid........ 178
Masseter........ 178
Lateral Pterygoid........ 179
Medial Pterygoid........ 179
Pterygopalatine Fossa (Diagram 8.4)........ 180
Input Recap........ 183
Output Recap (Diagram 5.3c; Chap. 5) [4]........ 183
Q and A: Chap. 8 (Answers at the End of This Chapter)........ 184
Answers........ 186
References........ 186

Infratemporal Fossa

Earlier chapters of this book have covered both the autonomic nervous system of the head and neck and the osteology of the skull as it pertains to the temporal fossa. This naturally leads into the infratemporal and pterygopalatine fossae. The infratemporal fossa is a complicated region at the skull base deep to the masseter muscle acting as a relay station for vascular entry and exit to the deep face and for sensory and autonomic distribution to the V_2 region with infraorbital, nasal, palatal and pharyngeal innervation and secretion. The fossa is wedge-shaped deep to the zygomatic

A. Zbar, *Anatomy--Head and Neck*,
https://doi.org/10.1007/978-3-031-69538-4_8

arch that directly communicates with the temporal fossa antero-superiorly and deeply with the pterygopalatine fossa (PPF). The lateral connection of the infratemporal and pterygopalatine fossae is via the pterygomaxillary fissure. The boundaries are bony and muscular. It is wise here to examine an intact skull from the side if available (after removing the mandible).

- Laterally is the condylar process and the ramus of the mandible
- Medially is the lateral pterygoid plate along and above the tensor and levator palati muscles with the superior constrictor below
- The anterior limit is the posterior border of the maxilla (the infratemporal crest) behind the origin of the maxillary sinus displaying the foraminae for the posterior superior alveolar nerves and vessels. The inferior orbital fissure represents the natural gap between the greater wing of the sphenoid and the maxilla
- The posterior limit is the carotid sheath, the tympanic plate, the mastoid and the styloid processes.
- The roof is that part of the greater wing of the sphenoid housing the foraminae (rotundum, ovale and spinosum)
- The temporal and infratemporal fossae meet under the zygomatic arch

This area dissected in the cadaver or in prosected specimens is bets seen with the majority of the zygomatic arch resected and by removal of the head of the mandible along with removal of the coronoid process and its attaching temporalis tendon. The mandible may be split length ways where the inferior alveolar nerve is displayed with its mylohyoid branch just before the mandibular foramen.

The area examined lies just below the skull base and demonstrates the mandibular nerve (V_3) running out of the foramen ovale. The maxillary artery is dissected off the substance of the lateral pterygoid and here gives off the middle meningeal artery.

Diagram 8.1 shows the bony disposition of this region. Take an intact skull and try and identify the starting point which is the

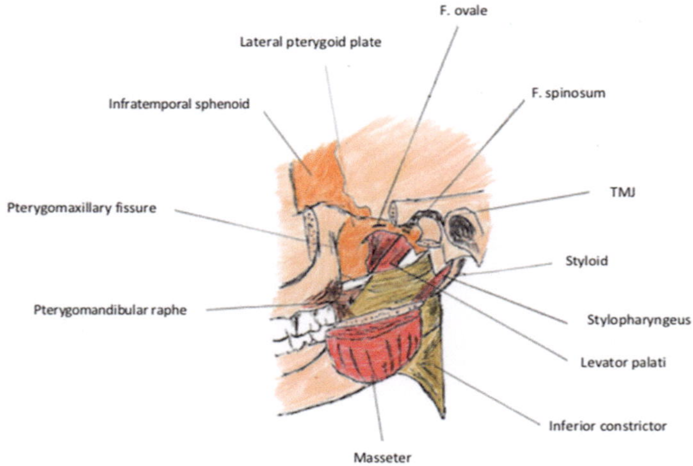

Diagram 8.1 Lateral view of the skull base showing the bony landmarks. The orientation is the deep lateral pterygoid plate. The pterygoid muscles and the maxillary vessels have been removed. The hamulus of the medial pterygoid plate attaches the pterygomandibular raphe (*arrow*) which gives partial origin to the superior constrictor muscle (running backwards to join its fellows in the pharyngeal raphe) and the buccinator muscle which runs forwards (shown in *red* also taking origin from the alveolar margins of the maxilla and mandible)

lateral entry to the deep face, the pterygomaxillary fissure. From here internally you can see the sharp lateral pterygoid plate which is the support for the pterygoid musculature and which leads into the pterygopalatine fossa.

The contents of this fossa are (Diagram 8.2):

- The two heads of the lateral pterygoid
- Internally the medial pterygoid
- The mandibular nerve with a large anterior (sensory) ne*rve and a smaller motor nerve.* Branches here include the *Auriculotemporal* nerve, the *Buccal* nerve, the *Lingual* nerve

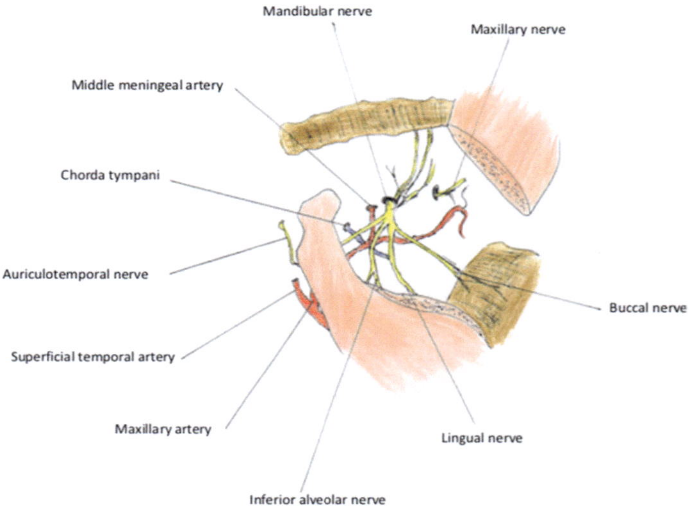

Diagram 8.2 In this view the pterygoids have been removed to show the neurovascular arrangement at the skull base. To see this infratemporal fossa, the zygomatic arch must be widely removed along with the coronoid process of the mandible and the insertion of temporalis. The neck of the mandible can be cut or the head and neck can be removed to expose the temporomandibular joint. The foraminae and nerves of V_3 should be identified. Here we can see the buccal nerve running forward, the lingual nerve running deep to the mandible and the inferior alveolar nerve running into the substance of the mandible. The nerve to mylohyoid is visible in take-off just before the inferior alveolar nerve enters the mandibular foramen. The mandibular (first) part of the maxillary artery has its leading branch the middle meningeal travelling towards the foramen spinosum

and the *Inferior alveolar* nerve. Included here is the *nerve to mylohyoid*. The Lingual nerve runs inside the mandible with the inferior alveolarnerve more superficially running in the substance of the mandible.

- The chorda tympani joins the lingual nerve near the posterosuperior limit of the fossa
- Pterygoid venous plexus
- The first (mandibular) part of the maxillary artery and its branches
- Otic ganglion

Mandibular Nerve

The main trunk is divided into a sensory and a motor branch. The main nerve provides a meningeal branch (*nervus spinosus*) which re-enters the middle cranial fossa (via the foramen ovale or occasionally via the foramen spinosum) to innervate the dura mater over the posterior half of the middle cranial fossa as well as the mastoid antrum and air cells and small twigs to the cartilaginous portion of the auditory tube. The main trunk also gives off the *nerve to medial pterygoid.* This also supplies a 'motor root' to the otic ganglion (which traverses the ganglion but which does not synapse there) and which is responsible for the innervation to the tensor muscles (tympani and palati).

The anterior division of the mandibular nerve is largely motor with one sensory branch. Motor supply is to the temporalis (usually as two separate and sometimes three branches), a masseteric branch (which also supplies the temporomandibular joint), a branch to both heads of the lateral pterygoid and the sensory buccal nerve (running forward on the buccinator supplying the muscle with proprioceptive branches and supplying part of the external cheek and its inner mucous membrane). It innervates territory between the second premolar and the mental foramen.

By contrast, the posterior division is largely sensory with one motor element. The three sizeable branches visible are the *auriculotemporal,* the *inferior alveolar* and the *lingual*. The *auriculotemporal* nerve appears as two rootlets which embrace the origin of the middle meningeal artery with the nerve passing backwards between the mandibular neck and the sphenomandibular ligament. There is a sensory branch to the temporomandibular joint with the nerve running upwards in front of the zygomatic process as an auricular branch innervating the tragus of the ear and the upper pinna and external auditory meatus and the outer surface of the tympanic membrane. The temporal branch innervates the skin and soft-tissues over the greying area of the temple and carries postganglionic PSNS fibres to the parotid gland derived from the otic ganglion synapse.

The *inferior alveolar* nerve lies on the medial pterygoid entering the mandibular foramen in front of the maxillary vessels with the nerve to mylohyoid piercing the sphenomandibular ligament beforehand. The inferior alveolar nerve supplies the three molar and two premolar teeth and has a mental and an incisive branch, the latter supplying the pulp and periodontal membrane of the canine and incisors with some midline cross-over. The *lingual* nerve runs between the medial pterygoid and the mandible and runs directly against the mylohyoid line against the third molar and runs into the mouth on the mylohyoid muscle joined by the chorda tympani.

The pterygoid plexus of veins is often evident forming over the substance of the lateral pterygoid. It is usually dissected and removed in prosected specimens and is poorly shown in cadavers because it is partly intramuscular. The plexus drains inferior ophthalmic veins from the inferior orbital fissure and deep facial veins permitting communication with the angular facial vein at the medial canthus of the eye and then drainage into the cavernous sinus. Further communication to the cavernous sinus is directly via an emissary vein through either the foramen ovale or the foramen Vesalii. The plexus terminates as a pair of stout maxillary veins which join the superficial temporal vein to form the retromandibular vein. An alternative method of drainage is via deep facial veins. The plexus has valves drawing blood from incompressible territory (the facial skeleton and the orbit) with the lateral pterygoid acting as a peripheral pump of stagnant blood during yawning.

Maxillary Artery (Diagram 8.3)

It is not important to know all of the individual branches of the maxillary artery but rather how the artery is clinically and anatomically divided and about its important branches that are of

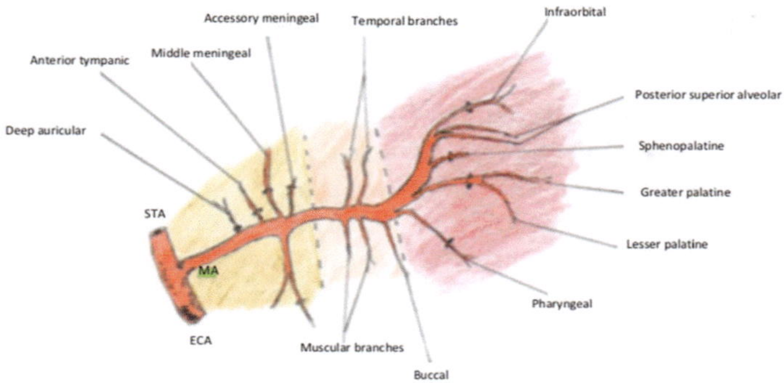

Diagram 8.3 Isolated branches and segments of the maxillary artery. Different colours have been used to show the different parts (mandibular, pterygoid and pterygopalatine). See Table 8.1 for corresponding foraminae. An additional artery to the pterygoid canal (Vidian artery) arising from the third part of the maxillary artery is not shown. The maxillary artery enters via the pterygomaxillary fissure (with the veins draining). The terminations travel to the infraorbital region as the infraorbital artery, to the nasal cavity (sphenopalatine artery) to the pharynx (pharyngeal artery) and to the oral cavity (descending palatine artery with greater palatine branches for the hard palate and lesser palatine branches for the soft palate).
Legend:
ECA External carotid artery
STA Superficial temporal artery
MA Maxillary artery

clinical significance. The maxillary artery is divisible into three component parts, the first (mandibular), the second (pterygoid) and the 3rd (pterygopalatine) portions. This separation is based on its relation to the pterygoid musculature (which has often been removed along with the pterygoid venous plexus) to show this branching anatomy.

The first part runs typically between the neck of the mandible and the sphenomandibular ligament on the lower border of the lateral pterygoid muscle. There are five branches to this mandibular part with the main artery usually running on top of the lateral pterygoid (however, in a little less than half of cadavers it can sometimes run deep to the lateral pterygoid and on or in the substance of the deeper lying medial pterygoid) [1].

Branches can be easily remembered with two straddling the tympanic membrane, the more superficial of which is called the deep auricular and the deeper of which running on the inner side of the membrane is the anterior tympanic. Next is the middle meningeal which enters the skull at the middle cranial fossa by traversing the *f. spinosum*. There may also be an accessory meningeal (which can traverse the *f. ovale* or the *f. Vesalii*) and which typically provides the blood supply to the trigeminal ganglion in the middle cranial fossa. Lastly there is the inferior alveolar artery which runs with the inferior alveolar nerve into the mandibular foramen. This terminates on the chin and lower lip as the mental artery. A small mylohyoid artery running with the nerve to mylohyoid anastomoses with a submental branch of the facial on the surface of the mylohyoid muscle or in the substance of the anterior belly of the digastric.

The vital branch of this mandibular section is the middle meningeal artery since it is implicated in fractured skull with life-threatening extradural haematomas. The middle meningeal ascends between the roots of the auriculotemporal nerve, posterolateral to the main V_3 lying on the lateral surface of the tensor palati which separates it from the auditory tube. As a reminder of its intracranial course, it runs on the floor of the middle cranial fossa dividing into a frontal and a parietal branch on the greater wing of the sphenoid. The parietal branch passes towards the lambda with the larger frontal branch running towards the lesser wing of the sphenoid over the surgical landmark of the pterion (confluence of the greater sphenoid wing, the frontal and parietal bones). The artery does not cross the subdural space and has no role in the arterial supply to the brain or the pia/arachnoid mater. On occasion, the accessory meningeal artery and even the anterior tympanic can arise from the middle meningeal artery.

The second (pterygoid) part of the maxillary artery provides muscular branches as it lies on or in the lateral ptyerygoid. These are therefore temporal, pterygoid (both lateral and medial) and buccal (to buccinator). There are often two large temporal branches making five separate branches in this pterygoid section although this can be quite variable.

The third (pterygopalatine) section of the maxillary artery is unseen here as it turns between the two heads of the lateral pterygoid. This part of the artery follows the branching of the pterygopalatine ganglion (See Chap. 5). Additional aspects of this artery will be considered in Chap. 12 on the nose and paranasal sinuses and in Chap. 13 on the mouth and palate. As connexions occur to the nose, hard and soft palate, pharynx and infraorbital region (where the maxillary artery terminates), these branches are therefore: sphenopalatine, greater palatine, lesser palatine, pharyngeal, posterior superior alveolar and infraorbital, respectively. Typically the infraorbital artery will also provide additional middle superior and anterior superior alveolar arteries to cover this part of the maxilla, teeth and gingival margin before the infraorbital reaches the soft-tissues of the middle one-third of the face. The anterior superior alveolar typically supplies the incisor/canine area and the middle superior alveolar supplying a similar region but often rudimentary and in some cases absent (Table 8.1).

Branching order variations of the maxillary artery may occur and have been classified by Ikakura such that: in Type 1 the order is the middle meningeal, the inferior alveolar, the posterior deep temporal, buccal, anterior deep temporal, posterior superior alveolar, infraorbital, descending palatine and sphenopalatine. In Type II the order of the middle meningeal and the inferior alveolar is reversed and in Type III the buccal artery is absent. Variations of the origin of the posterior superior alveolar and infraorbital are subclassified [2]. Further classifications (Fujita) have been made between the position of the maxillary artery and the mandibular nerve dependent upon whether the artery runs superficial or deep to the lateral pterygoid. Maeda et al. [3] have shown a relationship between the origin of the middle meningeal artery and the course of the maxillary artery with considerable variation in the origin of the inferior alveolar artery. It has been suggested that these vessels originate from the foetal stapedial artery however, the extent of variation in the inferior alveolar artery in particular likely means that it has additional vascular origins (most likely from the ECA).

Table 8.1 Branches and foraminae of the maxillary artery

Branch	Foramen
1st Part (Mandibular)	
Deep auricular	Squamotympanic fissure
Anterior tympanic	Petrotympanic fissure
Middle meningeal	F. spinosum
Accessory meningeal	F. ovale
Inferior alveolar	Mandibular foramen
2nd Part (Pterygoid)	
Temproal br	
Pterygoid br	
Buccal br	
3rd Part (Pterygopalatine)	
Pharyngeal	Palatovaginal canal
Palatine	Descending palatine canal
Hard palate—Greater palatine	
Soft palate—Lesser palatine	
Sphenopalatine	Sphenopalatine foramen
Artery of the pterygoid canal	Pterygoid canal
Posterior superior alveolar	Minor foraminae
Infraorbital	Infraorbital foramen/notch
Also middle superior alveolar	
Anterior superior alveolar	

Regional Muscles: Masseter, Lateral and Medial Pterygoid

Masseter

This is a quadrilateral robust muscle with two heads, the larger superficial arising from a tough aponeurosis around the zygomatic bone and the inferior and anterior 2/3 of the arch with the fibres passing inferiorly and posteriorly to insert into the angle of the mandible and the lateral ramus. The insertion of the medial pterygoid over a similar locale on the inner aspect of the mandible provides some evidence of the balance of these muscles. The slender, far less substantial deep head of the masseter arises from the posterior aspect of the lower border of the inner surface of the zygomatic arch and is inserted into the upper half of the ramus as far as the coronoid process. The posterior masseter is covered by the parotid gland.

The muscle acts to elevate the mandible—to shut the mouth, paralleling the medial pterygoid although the masseter is much stronger. Some of the more superficial fibres may protrude the jaw.

Lateral Pterygoid

This muscle also has two heads but demonstrates some variability. The upper head is the smaller one, originating superficially from the infratemporal crest part of the greater wing of the sphenoid bone and inserting into a depression just beneath the medial end of the mandibular head called the pterygoid fovea. Part of the insertion attaches to the fibrous capsule of the TMJ and its articular disk. The lower head of the lateral pterygoid arises from the full length of the lateral pterygoid plate up to the skull base and inserts on to the neck of the condyloid process of the mandible.

The primary function of the muscle is to pull the head of the condyle out of the mandibular fossa and along the articular eminence so that the mandible may be protruded. A single unilateral muscle action acts with the medial pterygoid to produce an excursion to the other side; a slewing action during chewing (think of it like a camel chewing as both the lateral and the medial pterygoid are well developed in ruminants). The lateral pterygoid is effectively the only muscle of mastication that depresses the mandible and that opens the jaw. This initiation can be assisted by the digastric, mylohyoid and geniohyoid muscles to some extent.

Medial Pterygoid

This muscle also consists of two interlocking heads with most of its substance arising as a deep head from the medial (inner) surface of the lateral pterygoid plate (and the pterygoid fossa between pterygoid plates) and with a smaller, superficial slip that arises from the maxillary tuberosity (as well as a small pyramidal process from the back of the palatine bone). The medial pterygoid muscle passes backwards and downwards and is inserted as a tendinous lamina into the medial surface of the ramus and the angle of the mandible right up to the mandibular foramen.

The function is for a combination of the masseter and the medial pterygoid (referred to in some textbooks as the pterygomasseteric sling) to act so as to close the jaw. The inner surface of the muscle lies closely related to the tensor palati, the styloglossus and the salpingopharyngeus muscles so that they separate the medial pterygoid from the superior constrictor (Diagram 8.1). As a reminder, the medial pterygoid is innervated by the nerve to the medial pterygoid which is also a central relay station for the innervation of the tensor tympani and the tensor palati and which usually runs through the otic ganglion as a definitive motor root. The sphenomandibular ligament passing down from the spine of the sphenoid to the lower margin of the mandibular foramen is the remaining perichondrium of Meckel's cartilage with its dorsal end forming the malleus and incus (Diagram 7.1; Chap. 7).

Pterygopalatine Fossa (Diagram 8.4)

This small but discrete space lies between the back of the maxilla and the front of the pterygoid process of the sphenoid bone, directly communicating with the infratemporal fossa. It is best considered as a room or a corridor with entry points and exit windows whose task is to act as a relay station concerned with the nerve and the blood supply to the middle third of the face. This area is not visible in the intact skull but it communicates with the lateral depth of the face at the pterygomaxillary fissure.

Boundaries: The borders are made up of the palatine and sphenoid bones and the maxilla. The back of the maxilla and the lower part of the lateral pterygoid process are interposed by a small part of the pyramidal process of the palatine bone. Anteriorly is the posterior wall of the maxillary sinus. On the lateral nose the maxilla is separated from the medial pterygoid plate and inferiorly lies the palatine bone and the descending palatine canal. Posteriorly, is the pterygoid process and root of the sphenoid (that part which contains the pterygoid canal and the foramen rotundum). Medially, lies the perpendicular plate of the palatine bone which forms the sphenopalatine foramen and anteriorly is the back wall of the maxilla. The roof is comprised of the body of the sphenoid and the orbital process of the palatine bone.

To recap:

- The entry and exit for deep facial vessels is the pterygomaxillary fissure
- Superiorly, the entry of the maxillary nerve via the foramen rotundum continues on via the inferior orbital fissure to reach the infraorbital groove (or foramen)
- The pterygoid canal (also in the posterior wall and roof) passes near the foramen lacerum but is (from behind) below and medial to the foramen rotundum transmitting the Vidian nerve
- The nasal exit is via the sphenopalatine foramen for the sphenopalatine vessels and nerve (nasopalatine nerve)
- The palatal exit is via the descending palatine foramen moving forward into the hard palate as the greater palatine neurovascular bundle and posteriorly into the soft palate as the lesser palatine neurovasculature
- The palatovaginal canal in the roof of the nose takes the pharyngeal artery and nerve

The contents include:

- Maxillary nerve
- Maxillary artery
- Pterygopalatine ganglion

The maxillary nerve after giving off a meningeal branch to the dura mater over the front aspect of the middle cranial fossa passes via the foramen rotundum to the pterygopalatine fossa and ends as the infraorbital nerve. The zygomatic nerve enters the orbit via the inferior orbital fissure. In the fossa the maxillary nerve gives off numerous branches which include

- Infraorbital
- Zygomatic
- Nasopalatine
- Posterior superior alveolar
- Pharyngeal
- Greater and lesser palatine nerves

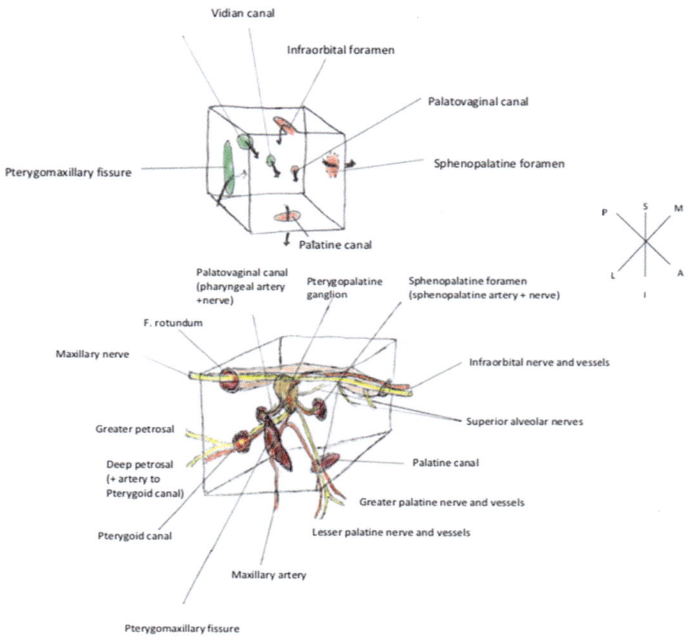

Diagram 8.4 Schematic view of the walls of the pterygopalatine fossa. This region may be considered as a corridor with a roof and a floor and side walls as well as entry and exit doors. The foramen rotundum enters through the roof from the middle cranial fossa, carrying the maxillary nerve. The entry point at the back is via the pterygoid canal and from the outer side via the pterygomaxillary fissure. The fossa is exited at the back via the palatovaginal canal and at the front through small posterior superior alveolar foraminae. The terminal continuation is into the middle 1/3 of the face as the infraorbital territory

The maxillary nerve will directly communicate with the pterygopalatine ganglion via two small trunks, the pterygopalatine nerves which suspend the ganglion. The ganglion relays pontine fibres from the superior salivatory nucleus to the lacrimal gland and mucous and serous glands in the palate, nose and paranasal sinuses. (One way of thinking of it is as the "*ganglion of Hay Fever*")

Input Recap

1. PSNS root via the nerve of the pterygoid canal (greater petrosal nerve from the nervus intermedius)
2. SNS root from the superior cervical ganglion via the deep petrosal nerve
3. Sensory root from a branch of V_2 with cell bodies in the V ganglion

Output Recap (Diagram 5.3c; Chap. 5) [4]

1. To the lacrimal gland (zygomatic and lacrimal nerves) and to the mucous glands in the nose, nasopharynx and palate
2. Some taste fibres from the palate (running in the greater petrosal nerve with their cell bodies in the geniculate ganglion of VII)
3. Nasopalatine nerve (formerly known as the long sphenopalatine nerve)
4. Lateral posterior superior nasal nerve (formerly known as the short sphenopalatine nerve) to innervate the postero-superior lateral nose quadrant (See Chap. 12).
5. Greater palatine (nasal branches supply the postero-inferior quadrant of the lateral nose) and the medial wall of the maxillary sinus (See Chap. 12)
6. Lesser palatine nerves innervating the soft palate and the palatine tonsil
7. Pharyngeal nerve innervating part of the Eustachian tube and adjacent nasopharynx

8. One or two very fine orbital branches which travel via the inferior orbital fissure to innervate some of the orbital periosteum, the mucous membrane of the sphenoidal and ethmoidal sinuses and the orbitalis muscle (a rudimentary non-striated muscle covering the inferior orbital fissure).[1]

Q and A: Chap. 8 (Answers at the End of This Chapter)

1. The pterygopalatine fossa
   (a) Connects to the pterygomaxillary fissure
   (b) Is not connected to the palatine bone
   (c) Joins to the pharynx via the palatovaginal canal
   (d) Is the origin of the middle and anterior superior alveolar nerves
2. A cerebellopontine tumour can be associated with
   (a) An absence of lacrimation on the affected side
   (b) Reduced salivation
   (c) A supranuclear facial nerve palsy
   (d) No disruption of taste
3. The boundaries of the pterygopalatine fossa
   (a) Anteriorly run against the maxillary sinus
   (b) Is separable from the palatine canal
   (c) Lies medially against the perpendicular plate of the palatine bone
   (d) Lies superiorly against the superior orbital fissure
4. The pterygopalatine fossa contains:
   (a) the middle superior alveolar nerves
   (b) the lesser palatine nerve
   (c) the pterygopalatine nerves
   (d) the nasopalatine nerve

[1] This small muscle also known as Müller's muscle was described by Heinrich Müller (1820–1864), a German retinal anatomist who discovered the rod photopigment rhodopsin. The muscle has no known function in humans but in animals is thought to control orbital volume and autonomic vascular regulation of the orbital contents.

5. The maxillary artery
   (a) Terminates as the greater palatine artery
   (b) Sends a sphenopalatine artery to the lower orbit
   (c) Does not supply the lacrimal gland
   (d) Has a posteriorly running pharyngeal branch
   (e) Does none of the above
6. Concerning the canals of the middle cranial fossa
   (a) The pterygoid canal runs through the lateral pterygoid plate
   (b) The pharyngeal canal connects via the palatovaginal canal to supply the mucosa of the nasopharynx near the Eustachian tube
   (c) Has the superior orbital foramen communicating the pterygopalatine fossa with the orbit as a space between the maxilla and the sphenoid
   (d) The greater palatine canal represents an articulation between the bottom end of the pterygopalatine fossa with the palatine bone and the maxilla
   (e) The sphenopalatine foramen connects the sphenoid with the perpendicular plate of the palatine bone
7. The muscles of mastication not associated with jaw closure are:
   (a) Masseter
   (b) Temporalis
   (c) Stylopharyngeus
   (d) Lateral pterygoid
   (e) Medial pterygoid
   (f) Buccinator
8. A local chewing reflex involves
   (a) Spinal afferents in the V nucleus
   (b) Motor afferents in the mid-brain
   (c) Cells in the mesencephalic nucleus
   (d) Cells in the nucleus tractus solitarius

Answers

1. a, b, c
2. a, b
3. a, c
4. c, d
5. d
6. b, d, e
7. d
8. a, c

References

1. Uysal II, Buyukumumcu M, Dogan NU, Seker M, Ziylan T. Clinical significance of maxillary artery and its branches: a cadaver study and review of the literature. Int J Morphol. 2011;29(4):1274–81.
2. Otake I, Kageyama I, Mataga I. Clinical anatomy of the maxillary artery. Okajimas Folia Anat Jpn. 2011;87(4):155–64. https://pubmed.ncbi.nlm.nih.gov/21516980/
3. Maeda S, Aizawa Y, Kumaki K, Kageyama I. Variations in the course of the maxillary artery. Anat Sci Int. 2012;87:187–94.
4. Ruskell GL. Orbital passage of pterygopalatine ganglion efferents to paranasal sinuses and nasal mucosa in man. Cells Tissues Organs. 2003;175(4):223–8.

The Arterial Circulation 9

Contents

External Carotid Artery (ECA) and Its Branches.................................... 192
Ascending Pharyngeal Artery.. 193
Superior Thyroid Artery.. 194
Lingual Artery.. 195
The Facial Artery... 196
The Occipital Artery.. 197
The Posterior Auricular Artery.. 198
The Vertebral Artery.. 199
The Basilar Artery.. 202
The Circle of Willis: The Circulus Arteriosus (Diagram 9.4)...................... 203
Q and A: Chap. 9 (Answers at the End of This Chapter).............................. 207
Answers.. 208

Before assessing the branches of the external carotid artery (ECA) and the course of the internal carotid artery (ICA) and the vertebral artery, it is well to review the carotid sheath (as covered in Chap. 2). The sheath is a vertically disposed neurovascular bundle of the neck lying on each side of the median airway and foodway extending from the root of the neck to the base of the skull. It lies on the sympathetic chain and the prevertetbral muscles where it contains the internal jugular vein (IJV) with the common carotid artery (CCA) situated medial with Cranial X placed behind and between the main artery and vein. The carotid bifurcation is typically located at the upper border of the thyroid notch where it

A. Zbar, *Anatomy--Head and Neck*,
https://doi.org/10.1007/978-3-031-69538-4_9

divides into an ICA which inclines upwards and forwards lying on the surface of the pharynx to get to the carotid canal higher up and running together with the internal carotid nerve (a bundle of sympathetic fibres derived from the superior cervical ganglion). The bifurcation level is normally at the C3/4 vertebral junction (also at the level of the greater horn of the hyoid bone) which acts as a landmark. This bifurcation level is of critical surgical importance in the procedure of carotid endarterectomy or in the vascular approach to excision of a carotid body tumour (chemodectoma) that develops from the chemoreceptor cells at the bifurcation. If the bifurcation is higher, extra room may be achieved by dividing the posterior belly of the digastric muscle, ligating the occipital and posterior auricular arteries coming from the back of the ECA below and above the muscle respectively and by blindly fracturing the styloid process as it lies deep to the vessels. The need to perform these additional procedures in order to gain access to a high carotid bifurcation may also be required for a level III carotid vascular injury.

The IJV is discussed in further detail in Chap. 10 but briefly, it descends vertically from the jugular foramen where it is formed just below the skull base with the confluence of the inferior petrosal sinus. The jugular bulb (before this) exits with Cranials IX, X, and XI and with Cranial XII exiting the hypoglossal canal a little more medially. High up in the neck, Cranial XII lies behind the ICA but as it descends closely applied with Cranial X, the hypoglossal nerve receives a branch from the C1 ventral ramus with the superior root of the ansa cervicalis remaining inside the sheath. Cranial XII then runs laterally over the carotid bifurcation acting as a landmark where the nerve is held down and in place against the carotid sheath by a posterior branch of the occipital artery, the sternomastoid branch of the occipital (Diagram 9.1).

Students should note that the ECA is the artery with branches since **the ICA has no branches in the neck**. This anatomical point is obviously vital for identification in penetrating neck trauma and during a carotid endarterectomy. At the bifurcation the ECA is usually more superficial than the ICA and lies anteromedial but parallel to the ICA (which ascends on the pharyngeal wall

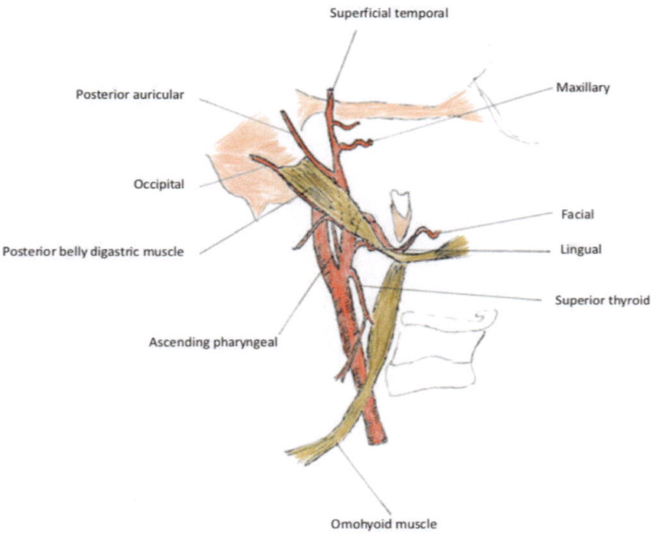

Diagram 9.1 Branches of the external carotid artery (ECA). The image shows a sternomastoid branch of the occipital and superior thyroid arteries. Above the maxillary artery a transverse facial may be given off as shown

giving branches to the foodway and the airway). Both arteries run through the carotid triangle and into the digastric triangle by passing under the posterior belly of the digastric and the stylohyoid muscle. Above this point, the ECA turns more laterally and leaves the ICA by entering the deep surface of the parotid gland where at the back of the neck of the mandible it divides into the superficial temporal artery and the maxillary artery (Diagram 9.1). The relationship between the lower cranial nerves and the carotid bifurcation and ECA branches is shown in Diagram 9.2. The maxillary artery is considered in Chap. 8.

Since the ECA has been displaced laterally, the styloid process and part of its apparatus, (stylopharyngeus, Cranial IX and the pharyngeal branch of the X) all pass between the ICA and the ECA. A simpler way of thinking about this is that the structures going to the pharynx (and with *'pharyngeus'* in their

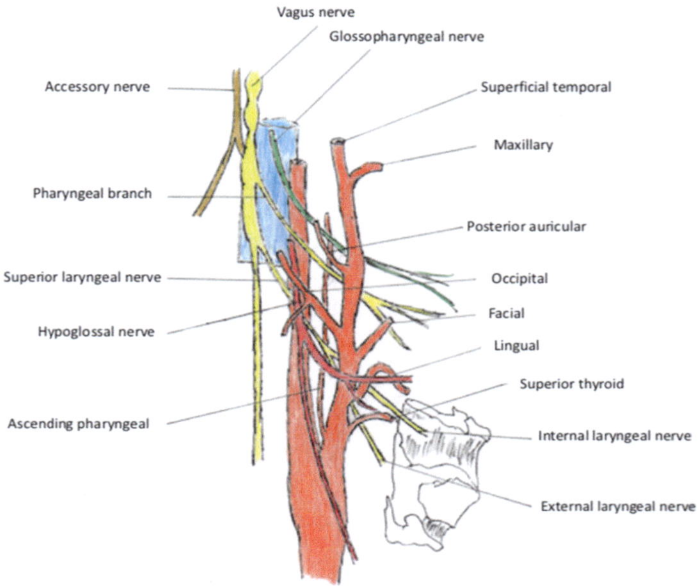

Diagram 9.2 Detail of the Common carotid artery bifurcation and its relationship to the lower Cranial nerves. Cranial XII is held down by the sternomastoid branch of the occipital artery. Running between the ICA and the ECA are the pharyngeal branch of X, Cranial IX and the stylopharyngeus muscle. The X shows both the superior and inferior ganglia. At the skull base the IJV lies behind the ICA

name) need to pass backwards between the ICA and ECA. This is also the passageway for a congenital branchial fistula. The commonest variant of such a fistula is as a remnant of the second branchial arch with a central connection that connects the tonsillar fossa by running between the ECA and the ICA over Cranial nerves XII and IX.

The task of the ECA is the supply in the neck of the structures of the foodway and the airway. The task of the subclavian artery is the supply of the remainder of the neck, namely the muscles and bones. The task of the ICA is the arterial supply of the brain (with a shared task with the verterbal) as well as the orbital contents, the forehead, the anterior scalp and parts of the external and internal nose. The rest of the head has an ECA supply.

A brief recap of the carotid sheath shows it running from the base of the skull where at its upper point it is attached to the petrous bone and to the lower part of the tympanic portion of the temporal bone (See Chap. 6). Contained is the IJV, the ICA and the last four cranial nerves with the pharynx applied medially and above the styloid process with its three sloping muscles and with the infratemporal fossa lying anteriorly. Reviewing the skull, the carotid canal lies immediately in front of the jugular foramen with the hypoglossal canal medially (See Chap. 6). At the base of the skull therefore, the IJV lies behind the ICA but ultimately the IJV slopes laterally so that lower down it lies lateral to the CCA. The Cranial X maintains its posterior position in the groove between the Carotid and the IJV with Cranial IX and XI emerging between the artery and the vein to diverge from one another and with Cranial XII passing from a medial position through the sheath by curling behind the inferior X ganglion to emerge between the CCA and the IJV. Passing deep to both carotids is the *superior laryngeal nerve* and both of its branches (the *external laryngeal nerve* and the *internal laryngeal nerve*).

To remind of the CCA pathway and position in the neck. The right CCA arises from the brachiocephalic trunk behind the sternoclavicular joint, the left arising from the arch of the aorta and asymmetrically ascending to enter the neck posterior to the left sternoclavicular joint. In the neck, the CCA ascends on the subclavian and the vertebral arteries to meet the prevertebral fascia on the transverse process of C6 (Chassaignac's tubercle). The CCA lies anterior to the inferior thyroid artery (ITA) with the recurrent laryngeal nerve (RLN) posteriorly located and with the thoracic duct turning anterolaterally between the left inferior thyroid artery (ITA) and the vertebral artery.

Below the thyroid cartilage, the thyroid gland separates the carotids from the pharynx, larynx, trachea and oesophagus. Dissection of the crook of the carotid bifurcation shows the dilated section of the ICA, the carotid sinus as well as the carotid body. Briefly, the carotid sinus is a gentle dilatation of the upper part of the CCA and the adjacent origin of the ICA acting as a pressoreceptor with heavy innervation and where local distension of the wall stimulates the afferent (the carotid sinus branch of IX) which then is relayed in the medulla at the cardiorespiratory centre (as GVA cells) with an efferent closure of the reflex via Cranial X to slow the heart and to reduce blood pressure. Some vascular surgeons during a carotid endarterectomy inject this region with prilocaine as the bifurcation is manipulated so as to inhibit carotid sinus reactivity and reduce the risk of intraoperative hypotension. By contrast, the carotid body is more embedded in the bifurcation although it has a similar nerve supply which also includes the Cranial X and the SNS. The carotid body responds to decreased oxygen tension or increased CO_2 resulting in reflex respiratory changes. The carotid body consists of two types of cells, the glomus cells (type 1 as peripheral chemoreceptors and type 2 sustentacular or supportive cells). The Glomus type I cells are neural crest derived and release a range of neurotransmitters (Ach, ATP and dopamine) that influence the respiratory centre. Tumours of these cells are quite specific and include those of the aortic body, carotid body, glomus jugulare tumours and non-chromaffin paraganglionomas. These rare tumour groups consist of histologically round or ovoid hypochromatic cells that are often grouped into an alveolus like pattern with scant stroma and thin-walled large vascular channels. The afferents of similar aortic bodies are via the Cranial X.

External Carotid Artery (ECA) and Its Branches

In the carotid triangle the ECA ascends directly on the surface of the pharynx over the top of the branches of the superior laryngeal nerve. The facial and lingual veins lie superficial as does Cranial XII. These points are critical to identify in a carotid endarterectomy operation. On the ECA surface there is an external carotid plexus arising as SNS fibres from the superior cervical ganglion akin to the vertebral and subclavian plexi. As mentioned, the ECA is at first medial to the ICA, then the ECA slopes upwards in front of the ICA lying initially against the pharynyx until that position is adopted by the ICA which then lies against the pharynx right up to the skull base. So effectively, as the ECA divides into its terminal branches within the deep part of the parotid, it is that part of the gland that separates the ECA and the ICA along with what we have already labelled as the 'pharyngeal structures' (stylopharyngeus, Cranial IX, and the pharyngeal branch of the X). At the commencement of the ECA the IJV is typically lateral but higher up the IJV runs deep to the artery because the jugular foramen is more posterior than the carotid canal.

Before entering the parotid gland there are typically six branches of the ECA; three from the front, two from behind and one medially. The three front ones are the *superior thyroid*, the *lingual* and the *facial*. The two from behind run below and above the posterior belly of the digastric as the *occipital* and the *posterior auricular* respectively. The medial one running alongside the pharynx is the *ascending pharyngeal*.

Ascending Pharyngeal Artery

Some textbooks regard this artery as the first branch of the ECA. The ascending pharyngeal artery runs deep to the ICA supplying the pharyngeal wall and the soft palate (and the tonsil), the Eustachian tube and the medial wall of the tympanic cavity and provides meningeal branches through nearby foramina (most notably the *f. lacerum*, the jugular foramen and the hypoglossal canal). On occasion there are additional meningeal branches to the dura near Cranials IX, X and XII. So this rather seemingly insignificant vessel actually has an important distribution. It is not commonly considered in many textbooks but it has three branches that contribute to the blood supply of the pharynx, prevertebral muscles, middle ear and dura mater which are the *pharyngeal*, *inferior tympanic* and *meningeal* branches.

The ascending pharyngeal forms anastomoses with the ascending palatine branch of the facial artery near the palatine tonsil and with an ascending cervical branch of the vertebral artery. The latter creates a naturally pre-existing vascular anastomotic network between the ECA and the subclavian artery. The pharyngeal branches of the ascending pharyngeal reach the soft palate between the superior constrictor and the levator palati and the inferior tympanic travels to the middle ear through the tympanic canaliculus. One of the meningeal branches reaching as far as the cerebellar fossa via the jugular foramen is labelled as the posterior meningeal artery. This artery is strictly the terminal branch of the ascending pharyngeal. On occasion the ascending pharyngeal can arise from the occipital artery, the CCA, the facial artery and even rarely from the base of the ICA rather than from the ECA.

Superior Thyroid Artery

This artery along with its special relationship to the external laryngeal nerve has been considered in Chap. 3. The superior thyroid artery runs vertically downwards from its ECA take-off to the thyroid gland where it splits on the upper pole of the gland and forms an anastomosis with the ITA. In many textbooks the superior thyroid artery (STA) is considered the first branch of the ECA. Branches of the STA include a large infrahyoid (*superior laryngeal*) artery which pierces the thyrohyoid membrane with the internal laryngeal nerve. Another important branch of the STA is its *sternomastoid branch* to the lower part of the muscle. (This small artery can occasionally arise directly from the ECA). There may also be muscular branches of the STA to the infrahyoid muscle group and sometimes a separate infrahyoid artery which joins its fellow below the thyrohyoid membrane. This latter variant is a remnant of the second aortic arch and when present will run along the lower border of the hyoid bone. Deep to the sternothyroid muscle the STA will also give off a *cricothyroid branch* which runs across the front of the cricothyroid and anastomoses with its fellow on the cricothyroid membrane. On occasion this cricothyroid artery runs more superficially in front of the sternothyroid with the branches of the ansa cervicalis. The artery can be a source of troublesome haemorrhage during an emergency cricothyroidotomy designed to maintain the airway.

Lingual Artery

The artery often forms a short upward loop off of the front of the ECA passing forwards towards the tongue along the upper border of the hyoid bone and then runs under the back free end of the hyoglossus muscle accompanied by the deep lingual vein. Cranial XII may cross in front of it along with a companion vein which can open into the facial vein so that the facial vein overlies the loop of the lingual artery running deeply and Cranial XII at this point. It is the marker for the carotid bifurcation. There are several discrete branches:

1. The suprahyoid is the homologue of the STA infrahyoid. It joins with its opposite side and is a soft tissue vessel.
2. The dorsal lingual artery (arteries) are 2–3 branches which arise beneath the hyoglossus muscle ascending to the dorsum of the tongue and supplying the glossopalatine arch, the soft palate and as far as the epiglottis with contralateral anastomosis. This is also part of the palatine tonsillar supply (See Chap. 13).
3. The deep lingual artery(so-called ranine artery) is the terminal part of the lingual artery after a sublingual artery is given off. It runs very tortuously on the under surface of the middle of the tongue in the substance of the intrinsic longitudinal muscle. It is tortuous to allow give and flexibility to occur when there are protruding movements of the tongue. It lies on the lateral genioglossus with the lingual nerve but it is deep to hyoglossus so that it separates from the lingual nerve in both height and plane. It may anastomose at the tongue tip with the opposite deep lingual artery with each running on either side of the frenulum.
4. At the front of the hyoglossus a sublingual artery is given off running between genioglossus and mylohyoid to the sublingual gland. One part may pierce the mylohyoid and anastomose with the submental branch of the facial artery.

A common faciolingual trunk is present in about 20% of cadavers and a thyrolingual common trunk in about 7% of cases.

The Facial Artery

This usually arises above the lingual artery from the front of the ECA and runs upward on the superior constrictor muscle deep to the digastric and stylohyoid grooving the back and under surface of the submandibular gland in the way described in Chap. 2. As it is lying on the superior constrictor it gives off a *tonsillar branch* to the tonsil and the soft palate. It runs around the edge of the mandible where it gives off a sizeable submental artery in front of the masseter which accompanies the nerve to mylohyoid supplying the muscles and the skin of the submental triangle but sending perforators deep through the floor of the mouth to anastomose with the sublingual artery. Its branches include for completeness:

1. The ascending palatine which hooks over the upper border of the superior constrictor and which descends on to the palate with the levator palati muscle passing between the styloglossus and the sylopharyngeus. Close to the levator it divides into two branches one of which pierces the superior constrictor to get to the auditory tube and the palatine tonsil. This is supplemented by branches of both the lesser and the greater palatine arteries. It will then anastomose with the ascending pharyngeal artery as well as the tonsillar branch of the facial artery. The other branch runs with the levator palati and passes over the upper edge of the superior constrictor to get to the soft palate and anastomoses with the descending palatine branch of the maxillary artery. So this is a natural collateral network between branches of the ECA.
2. The tonsillar artery is superficial to the styloglossus (actually ascending between the styloglossus and the medial pterygoid muscle) although it perforates the superior constrictor to reach the palatine tonsil.
3. Small glandular branches to the submandibular gland.

4. The submental artery (supplying the submandibular and sublingual glands and adjacent muscles and skin). It is the largest of the cervical branches of the facial artery. It divides into a superficial and a deep branch with the superficial anastomosing with the inferior labial artery and the deep branch anastomosing with the inferior labial and the mental branch of the inferior alveolar artery (i.e. another facial maxillary connection).

The arteries on the face (as well as the superficial temporal artery at the termination of the ECA) include the inferior and superior labial, lateral nasal and angular branches.

The Occipital Artery

This arises from the back of the ECA level with the facial artery running on the lower surface of the posterior belly of the digastric and grooving the mastoid lateral to the rectus capitis lateralis muscle to pass through the posterior neck triangle (anterior to the ICA, the IJV, the X and XI) and supply the back of the scalp. Before doing so it gives off one or two branches to the sternocleidomastoid. The upper branch can be a guide to Cranial XI and holds down at its origin Cranial XII. It pierces the trapezius about 2–3 cm off the midline with the greater occipital nerve. The artery has extensive muscular branches and connexions. There is a mastoid branch supplying the bone and meningeal branches to the dura mater. There is also a descending branch which passes deep to semispinalis capitis and which anastomoses with a deep cervical artery from the costocervical trunk (second portion of the subclavian artery - (SCA)). For completeness, formal branches include: a sternomastoid, auricular, (supplying the posterior neck and ear and posterior scalp and pericranium) mastoid, occipital, meningeal, (dura around the jugular foramen, parietal foramen, foramen magnum, condylar canal), a descending branch and muscular branches (to the regional muscles including the digastric, rectus capitis lateralis, stylohyoid, superior and inferior obliques, the rectus capitis posterior major and minor, the semispinalis capitis and the splenius capitis). Rarely the occipital artery can arise from the ECA directly, or the thyrocervical trunk, the ITA or the vertebral artery. In 15% of cases, there is a common occipitoauricular trunk for the origin of the occipital and the posterior auricular arteries. Moreover, in 20% of cases, the posterior meningeal artery which we remember was a branch of the ascending pharyngeal may arise from the occipital and this makes sense to supply the dura around the posterior skull foraminae.

The Posterior Auricular Artery

It runs above the posterior belly of digastric crossing the surface of the mastoid and is often a source of bleeding in the back of a Blair parotidectomy incision. It has pinna branches, a stylomastoid branch which enters the stylomastoid foramen and which supplies Cranial VII and a stapedial artery which supplies the stapedius and which is the remnant artery of the second branchial arch. More formally its branches include: a stylomastoid artery, a posterior tympanic, auricular branches, occipital branch, a parotid branch and some perforating muscular branches. It supplies part of the external auditory meatus (EAM), tympanic cavity and tympanic membrane as well as the semicircular canals and the mastoid antrum cells. To rcap the branches include:

1. The stylomastoid artery
2. The posterior tympanic artery (supplying the back of the tympanic membrane) contrasted with the anterior tympanic from the maxillary so that there is a vascular circle over the inner tympanic membrane.
3. The auricular branch for the medial surface of the auricle, the extrinsic auricular muscles (auricularis anterior, superior and posterior).
4. The occipital branch for the posterosuperior auricle and the occipitofrontalis.
5. A parotid branch
6. There are often perforators to the SCM, digastric and stylohyoid.

We next move on to the ICA:

INTERNAL CAROTID ARTERY IN THE NECK: Starts off lateral to the ECA at its origin but soon slopes up posteriorly to occupy a more medial and a deeper level alongside the pharynx with no branches to the carotid canal anterior to the IJV and the jugular foramen. Behind outside the sheath is the sympathetic chain and the longus capitis. The superior laryngeal branch of X runs behind to its medial side and the ascending pharyngeal artery is also medial. The IJV is lateral with Cranial X positioned in between. The ICA is crossed by the lingual and the facial veins as well as by the occipital artery and Cranial XII with the superior root of the ansa cervicalis running down along it embedded in the sheath. Higher up it is crossed by the posterior belly of digastric, the stylohyoid and the posterior auricular artery as well as by those structures that separate it from the ECA, (the stylopharyngeus, Cranial IX and the pharyngeal branch of X).

Orientation of the vessels and nerves near the carotid bifurcation are shown in Diagram 9.2.

The Vertebral Artery

The posterior circulation of the brain (supply to the occipital lobes, cerebellum and brainstem) consists of the *vertebral* and *basilar a*rteries. The first branch of the subclavian artery, the vertebral artery, ascends towards the foramen transversarium of C6 by passing between the longus colli and the scalenus anterior, posterior to the CCA, the ITA and the vertebral vein but anterior to the ventral rami of the seventh and eighth cervical nerves. In the standard orientation of vein, artery and nerve, the stellate ganglion can be found lying partially behind and medial to the artery sending filaments as a plexus around the artery (vertebral plexus). On the left side the thoracic duct crosses in front of the vertebral artery. Superiorly, the vertebral artery joins its fellow to form the basilar artery supplying the upper part of the spinal medulla, the medulla oblongata, the pons, the cerebellum, the midbrain and the posterior cerebrum.

The vertebral artery has four parts:

1. The first (pre-foraminal) part is the branch of the first part of the subclavian artery
2. The second (foraminal) part passes through the foramina transversaria with the vertebral veins and the SNS plexus anterior to the ventral rami of the cervical nerves and between the transverse processes. The artery turns laterally in the f. transversarium of the axis and then bends upwards to enter the foramen transversarium of the atlas which is the most laterally orientated. At this point a spinal branch is given off into each intervertebral foramen.
3. The artery appears on the superior surface of the atlas between the rectus capitis lateralis and the superior articular process of the atlas curving horizontally with the ventral ramus of C1 and grooving the posterior arch of the atlas in the depths of the suboccipital triangle (Diagram 9.3). The artery lies above C1 and leaves this triangle by passing medially in front of the posterior atlanto-occipital membrane. In the depth of this triangle the vertebral artery lies between the superior and inferior oblique muscles on the posterior arch of the atlas. To approach the vessel, the incision needs to split the trapezius, splenius and semispinalis (in order) so as to expose it below the inferior oblique, lateral to the superior oblique and superior to the rectus capitis posterior major. Here the artery appears bowed backwards in order to permit flexibility during movement of the atlantoaxial joint. This third part has been labelled 'Atlantic', or 'extradural'.
4. The artery then turns superiorly and pierces the dura mater and the arachnoid (fourth part or intradural/intracranial part) where it enters the cranial cavity via the f. magnum in front of the uppermost ligamentum denticulatum. Here the vertebral artery runs on the surface of the medulla oblongata between the rootlets of the first cervical nerve and Cranial XII. At the lower border of the pons it unites with the opposite vertebral artery to form the basilar artery which runs in the basilar cistern until it divides into the two posterior cerebral arteries. These give off a posterior communicating which anastomoses with the middle cerebral artery so that there is a vertebral/ICA communication.

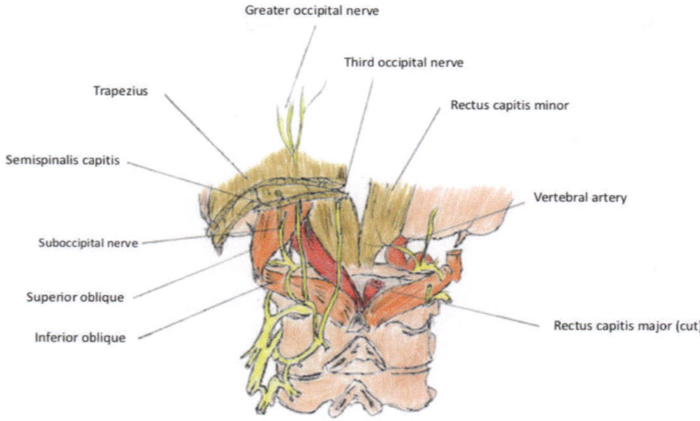

Diagram 9.3 Course of the vertebral artery through the suboccipital triangle. Before becoming intracranial, the vertebral artery snakes around the transverse process of the atlas to pierce the atlanto-occipital membrane before passing through the foramen magnum to join its fellow as the basilar artery (artery of the pons). The vertebral artery lies very deeply in this triangle which requires division of the trapezius, spinalis and semispinalis in order to demonstrate the borders (medially the rectus capitis major, inferiorly the obliquus inferior and laterally the obliquus superior). In this image there is a variable anastomosis between the dorsal rami of C1–3 which is called Cruvelhier's plexus (after Jean Cruvelhier—1791–1874—a French anatomist and pathologist)

To summarize:

- There are no branches of this vessel from the first part.
- Segments are pre-foraminal, foraminal, extradural (from the transverse foramen of the axis to the vertebral canal) and intradural (to the inferior border of the pons).
- Branches include the anterior and posterior spinal, (with the latter sometimes arising from the posterior inferior cerebellar), the posterior inferior cerebellar (PICA), meningeal, medullary and basilar. The PICA is the largest and most tortuous branch insinuating the rootlets of Cranial XII, X and IX nerves. It supplies the medulla oblongata, the choroid plexus of the fourth ventricle and the cerebellum and it varies inversely in size with

the anterior inferior cerebellar artery (although it is usually much larger than the AICA).

- There are spinal and muscular branches from the second and third parts (forming anastomoses with the occipital artery and with branches of the deep cervical artery)

A plexus of veins coalesces around the third part of the artery, these forming from the union of the internal vertebral venous plexus and the veins of the suboccipital triangle. There is a rich anastomosis with the deep cervical veins to create a couple of stout tributaries which pass from the sixth of seventh f. transversarium in front of the subclavian artery and which enter the brachiocephalic vein.

The Basilar Artery

This artery runs in front of the pons lying against the dorsum sellae of the sphenoid where it gives off the anterior inferior cerebellar artery and many pontine branches. The labyrinthine artery may either be a branch of the anterior inferior cerebellar or arise directly from the basilar artery. The basilar artery ends at the upper pons as the posterior cerebral arteries after giving off a superior cerebellar branch. The anterior inferior cerebellar artery supplies Cranial VI, VII and VIII as well as the antero-inferior part of the cerebellum. The labyrinthine artery supplies Cranial VIII (and VII). The superior cerebellar artery winds around the pons and the middle cerebellar peduncle to supply the upper part of the midbrain. There is extensive cerebellar supply with the posterior cerebral artery supporting the midbrain via the posterior perforated substance and then supplying the occipital lobe through a posterior choroidal which supplies the choroid plexus near the lateral and the third ventricles. There are additional vessels to the temporal, occipital, calcarine and collateral sulci. Above this area both the posterior cerebral and superior cerebellar supply the upper and lower parts of the midbrain along with the Cranial III and IV nuclei.

The Circle of Willis: The Circulus Arteriosus (Diagram 9.4)

This area is discussed in detail in Volume 6 of this series on the Central Nervous System. There is an arterial circle which is formed from the posterior cerebral artery (PCA), the posterior communicating (running through the interpeduncular cistern to

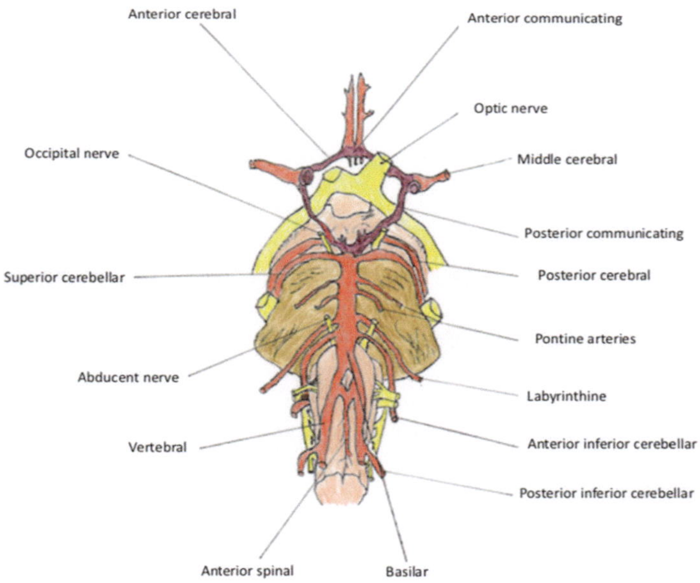

Diagram 9.4 The Circle of Willis. The circle (*purple*) is derived as a continuation of the intracranial ICA (as the anterior and middle cerebral arteries). The relationship is shown between the cranial nerves and the communicating vessels. A third nerve palsy is a typical (and the commonest) presentation of a posterior communicating artery (berry) aneurysm. When a 'medical' third nerve palsy occurs because of damage to the vasa vasorum of the nerve, pupillary involvement is often not present whereas it is an early and usual feature of third nerve compression.
Legend:
IJV Internal jugular vein
ICA Internal carotid artery
CA External carotid artery

join the ICA at the anterior perforated substance), the anterior cerebral and the anterior communicating artery (which unites the anterior cerebral arteries in the chiasmatic cistern below the rostrum of the corpus callosum). Blood that enters this system (either via the ICA or the basilar artery) is distributed to any part of the cerebral hemispheres. The branches from this circle pass through the anterior and posterior perforated substance although without any significant anastomoses within the brain substance itself. By contrast, the cortical branches ramify over the surface of the cortex but anastomose fairly freely on the pia mater entering the cortex at right angles via multiple branches which then do not anastomose within the brain substance. As a result it is damage to the perforating vessels rather than these surface pial vessels which have significant consequences, the effect of which are altered by the impact of a very extensive SNS network running on these small vessels.

In summary, both the cerebral hemispheres as well as the diencephalon are supplied by the ICA and the vertebral artery with the grey matter heavily supported by a superficial cortical arterial network and with more tenuous perforators supplying the subcortical nuclei. The ICA and vertebral systems anastomose around the optic chiasma and the infundibulum of the pituitary stalk as this Circle of Willis (also known as the polygon of Willis) permitting an equalization of blood flow between the two hemispheres.[1] Clinically, about 90% of spontaneous non-traumatic subarachnoid haemorrhages arise from rupture of an aneurysm of the circle vessels with congenital aneurysms located more frequently on the carotid side and more commonly at branching points (such as the junction of the anterior cerebral and the anterior communicating or at the ICA and the posterior communicating or middle cerebral junction points). These are anatomically the sites of greatest weakness within the arterial tunica media.

[1]Thomas Willis (1621–1675) described the circle of cerebral anastomosis in his 1664 book *Cerebri anatome*. He was an anatomist working at Oxford University who employed Sir Christopher Wren (1632–1723) as his principal illustrator. Afterwards, Wren went on to design about 50 London churches including St. Paul's Cathedral following the great fire of London in 1666 and then to be one of the longest serving Presidents of the Royal Society.

The *posterior communicating* passes posteriorly across the crus cerebri sending minute branches to the crus, the optic tract, the pituitary gland and to the hypothalamus. One of the branches the anterior choroid artery turns above the temporal lobe just above the posterior communicating artery take-off to enter the choroid plexus of the inferior horn in the lateral ventricle.

The *anterior cerebral* artery joins its fellow with the short anterior communicating just in front and above the optic chiasm. The anterior cerebral then bends upwards running against the medial hemisphere providing before this a few slender hypothalamic branches as well as some supply to the optic chiasm and the optic nerve. Some recurrent vessels circle back to the anterior perforated substance sending medial striate branches into the brain substance.

The *middle cerebral* artery is by comparison a large vessel which is the direct continuation of the ICA (hence within the field of embolic trash). This artery runs laterally out of the field of view within the stem of the lateral sulcus, breaking up on the insula separating the temporal from the frontal and parietal lobes. It is here that most of the sensory and the motor cortex is supplied as well as the auditory cortex.

In summary:

- The cerebral blood supply is via the anterior, middle and posterior cerebral arteries
- There is additional (non-cortical) support from the anterior choroidal
- Although there is extensive anastomosis across the cerebral hemispheres, the perforating vessels are end arteries.
- Larger surface vessels have a SNS innervation but intracortical arteries do not
- The middle cerebral artery territory supplies the motor and sensory areas for the opposite half of the body as well as the auditory and speech cortices. (This excludes the leg and the perineum which are supplied along with the micturition and defaecation centres by the anterior cerebral artery).

- Because of the anastomosis with the anterior communicating, one ACA territory can be sustained by the contralateral ICA. In these cases an occlusive stroke results in ipsilateral blindness and contralateral hemiplegia (ischaemia to the sensory capsule + the ophthalmic artery)
- Occlusion of the posterior cerebral artery affects the contralateral visual cortex although the middle cerebral artery may supply the macular part of the visual area (Diagram 7.3; Chap. 7).
- Long central (striate) branches supply the internal capsule and the thalamus and basal nuclei. These vessels are named including lenticulostriate, thalamostriate and thalamolenticular branches
- Variations are common most often hypoplasia or aplasia of one posterior communicating artery, aplasia of the first segment of the anterior cerebral artery or fenestration of the anterior communicating artery. A complete circle only occurs in 25% with posterior anomalies more common than anterior variants.

Typical patterns of stroke can include:

Occlusion	Presentation
Anterior cerebral artery	Total contralateral hemiplegia and hemianaesthesia (leg arm and face)
Distal to recurrent Heubner branch[a]	Behavioural changes, contralateral hemiparesis (face, arm leg), dysarthria, visual neglect
Middle cerebral	Total contralateral hemiplegia and hemianaesthesia/Aphasia (left-sided lesions)
Posterior cerebral	Contralateral hemianopia and hemianaesthesia
Anterior choroidal	Contralateral hemiplegia, hemianaesthesia, hemianopia.

[a]Heubner's recurrent artery (a branch of the anterior cerebral) is a distal medial striate artery that supplies the anterior limb of the internal capsule and the caudate nucleus. Named after Johan Otto Leonard Heubner (1843–1926), the 'father' of German paediatrics

Q and A: Chap. 9 (Answers at the End of This Chapter)

1. The ascending pharyngeal artery
   (a) Supplies the Eustachian tube
   (b) Is a vascular supply of the VIII cranial nerve
   (c) Has no anastomosis with the vertebral artery
   (d) The vessel enters the pharynx at the upper end of the middle constrictor muscle
2. The facial artery
   (a) Runs deep to the superior constrictor muscle
   (b) Supplies part of the auditory tube
   (c) Does not anastomose with the ascending pharyngeal artery
   (d) Does not supply the sublingual glands
3. The occipital artery:
   (a) Arises from the posterior surface of the external carotid artery and typically runs along the upper surface of the posterior belly of the digastric muscle
   (b) Has a sternomastoid branch which holds down the XII (Hypoglossal) nerve as it runs over the carotid bifurcation
   (c) Gives off a mastoid branch which supplies part of the dura of the posterior cranial fossa
   (d) Does not anastomose with terminal branches of the subclavian artery
4. The superior thyroid artery
   (a) Is given off the external carotid artery at the level of the greater cornua of the hyoid bone
   (b) Supplies the infrahyoid muscles
   (c) Does not anastomose with the inferior laryngeal artery
   (d) Has a cricothyroid branch
5. The maxillary artery
   (a) Does not contribute to dural blood supply
   (b) Is the main arterial supply to the maxilla
   (c) Enters the deep face at the pterygomaxillary fissure
   (d) Winds around the front of the temporomandibular joint
   (e) Passes between the neck of the mandible and the sphenomandibular ligament
   (f) Forms an anastomosis around the tympanic membrane

Answers

1. a
2. b
3. b, c
4. b, d
5. b, c, e, f

The Venous Drainage and Sinuses

10

Contents

Internal Jugular Vein........ 209
Venous Drainage of the Brain: A Brief Overview [1]........ 212
Anatomy of the Venous Sinuses (Diagram 10.2a– c)........ 215
Cavernous Sinus (Diagram 10.4)........ 219
Relations........ 220
Entry Points........ 221
Exit Points........ 221
Vertebral Venous Plexi........ 224
Q & A: Chap. 10 (Answers at the End of This Chapter)........ 228
Answers........ 229
References........ 230

In this section the formation and anatomy of the IJV is considered along with the dural venous sinuses and the anatomical mechanics of CSF drainage.

Internal Jugular Vein

The IJV forms **extracranially** just below the skull base combining the jugular bulb of the sigmoid sinus with the draining inferior petrosal sinus. (In the jugular fossa the upper end of the vein dilates to form a superior bulb usually with a two or three cusped valve).

A. Zbar, *Anatomy--Head and Neck*,
https://doi.org/10.1007/978-3-031-69538-4_10

Initially located behind the ICA, the IJV comes to lie on the lateral mass of the atlas where it is crossed by the spinal branch of Cranial XI. The posterior relations of the IJV include the cervical plexus lying on the levator scapulae, the scalenus medius and the phrenic nerve lying on the front of the scalenus anterior (passing from lateral to medial). On the left-hand side, the thoracic duct crosses behind the left IJV at the C7 vertebral level. The IJV then descends vertically in the neck applied usually to the lateral (superficial) side of the ICA and then subsequently the CCA with both enclosed with the Cranial X within the carotid sheath (See Chap. 2). The IJV joins the subclavian vein behind the sternoclavicular joint to form the brachiocephalic vein. On the right-hand side the right CCA recedes a little distance from the IJV but these two structures lie together much more closely on the left-hand side.

Typically, the right IJV is larger than the left as it tends to drain blood from the superior sagittal sinus. (If one examines the internal skull grooves for the transverse and the sigmoid sinuses on a dried skull this is usually evident as these markings make larger impressions). It is noted that developmentally the mass that includes the jugular foramen, the hypoglossal canal, the occipital condyle, the styloid process and the stylomastoid foramen is separable from that mass of more anteriorly located bone containing the carotid canal and the petrous temporal bone. At the jugular foramen, the IJV lies posterolateral to the ICA with the last four cranial nerves (IX, X, XI and XII) intervening. Below this, the structures that are in contact with the IJV are those that contact the ICA above and the CCA below but with both arteries separating the IJV from those medial structures. Nerves crossing the ICA are then medial to the vein (Cranial IX, the pharyngeal branch of the X, Cranial XII and the superior root of the ansa cervicalis). The inferior root and superior root join at a variable level in front of the vein. The spinal branch of Cranial XI tends to run anterior to the upper part of the IJV with the inferior root of the ansa cervicalis either lateral or medial to the lower IJV.

The vein is lateral to the arteries which means that the IJV is anterior to the roots of the cervical plexus and hence to the prevertebral muscles and phrenic nerve. The terminal IJV lies between the sternal and the clavicular heads of the sternocleidomastoid and is a percutaneous entry landmark for central line catheterization. The vein is approached (with or without ultrasound guidance) 5 cm above the clavicle at the posterior border of the SCM directed towards the jugular notch or more commonly 2 cm above the clavicle between the sternomastoid heads in a slightly backwards and lateral direction of entry.

The surface marking of the IJV joins the lobule of the ear to the sternal end of the clavicle. The visible JVP pulse reflects the RA pressure with its 'a' (atrial contraction), 'c' (ventricular contraction) and 'v' (venous filling) waves.

Remember that veins do not have branches, they have tributaries. The tributaries of the IJV are (Diagram 10.1):

- The inferior petrosal sinus (remember this is the first IJV tributary).
- The pharyngeal plexus (usually draining into the upper IJV by a couple of stout veins).
- The facial, lingual and superior thyroid veins (entering the IJV in the carotid triangle usually at the level of the tip of the greater horn of the hyoid bone).
- The middle thyroid vein (a useful landmark when present which needs to be ligated in order to expose and lift up the thyroid lobe).
- Occasionally a jugular lymph trunk can enter at the root of the neck (of importance in chylous leaks).

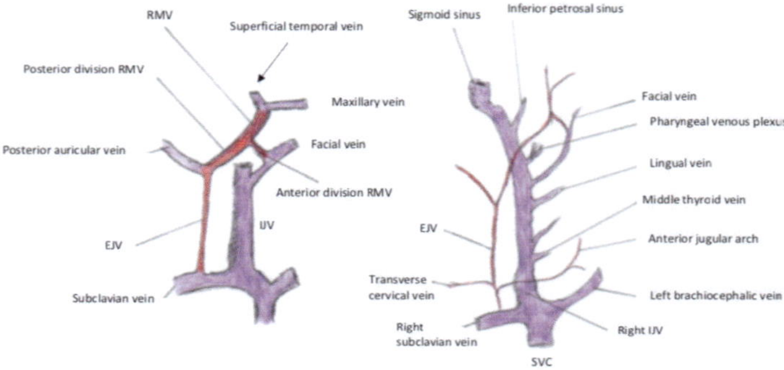

Diagram 10.1 The *left-hand* image shows the formation of the external jugular vein by separation of the retromandibular vein in the substance of the parotid gland (the faciovenous plane with branches of Cranial VII superficial). The anterior division of the retromandibular vein drains into the facial vein and ultimately the internal jugual vein (IJV). The posterior division of the retromandibular vein joins the posterior auricular vein to become the external jugular vein (EJV). The EJV pierces the investing layer of deep cervical fascia to *drain into the subclavian vein.*
Legend:
IJV Internal jugular vein
EJV External jugular vein
RMV Retromandibular vein
The right-hand image shows the formation and tributaries of the IJV. The highest tributary is the inferior petrosal sinus. The arrangement is highly variable and in this image the EJV tributaries have been overlain.
Legend:
SVC Superior vena cava

Venous Drainage of the Brain: A Brief Overview [1]

This topic is covered in more detail in Volume 6 of this series. In a broad overview here, the majority of the veins of the cerebral hemispheres lie on the surface in the subarachnoid space and these surface veins drain into the venous sinuses by crossing the subarachnoid and subdural spaces and by piercing the arachnoid and the dura mater. The superior cerebral veins for example converge on the superior sagittal sinus (anterior and posterior) with most of the inferior cerebral veins converging on the middle cerebral vein and those from the occipital lobe passing inferiorly into the transverse sinus.

The veins carry about 70% of the cerebral blood volume with drainage either via the cerebral veins or the dural venous sinuses. Cerebral veins are valveless traversing the pia into the surface veins and thence into the sinuses. The system of veins includes the superficial venous system, the deep system and the veins of the posterior fossa. The superficial veins (also known as the cortical veins) include superior, middle (or Sylvian) and inferior veins with connectors such as Trolard's great vein (running in the postcentral sulcus and joining the superior sagittal sinus and the middle cerebral vein) and the veins of Labbé which is the largest lateral superficial vein linking the temporal lobe to the transverse sinus.[1] These latter connecting veins take on significance if there is cavernous sinus thrombosis. The deep venous system drains the corpus callosum, the basal ganglia and part of the brainstem to the paramedian basal vein of Rosenthal which originates on the medial temporal lobe and which drains into the great vein of Galen that empties into the inferior sagittal sinus.[2] The vein of Rosenthal is closely applied to the posterior cerebral artery and Cranial IV. The veins of the posterior fossa drain upwards into the Galenic vein, anteriorly into the petrosal sinuses and posteriorly into the sigmoid sinus. Anastomotic venous connexions drain anteriorly to superficial cerebral veins, posteriorly to the basal vein and via direct communications to the sinuses (superior petrosal, straight and transverse).

After separating the hemispheres and dividing the corpus callosum the medial surface is drained by the great vein of Galen emerging at the splenium of the corpus callosum to enter the inferior sagittal sinus and form the straight sinus (Diagram 10.2a–c). Joining

---

[1] Named after Jean Baptiste Paulin Trolard (1842–1910) a French neuroanatomist. The vein of Labbé was named after Charles Labbé (1851–1889) who described the vein as a third year medical student.

[2] Named after Friedrich Christian Rosenthal (1780–1829) a German anatomist and physician. Named after Claudius Galen of Pergamon (129–216 AD) considered the father of anatomy was personal physician to the Emperor Marcus Aurelius (121–180 AD).

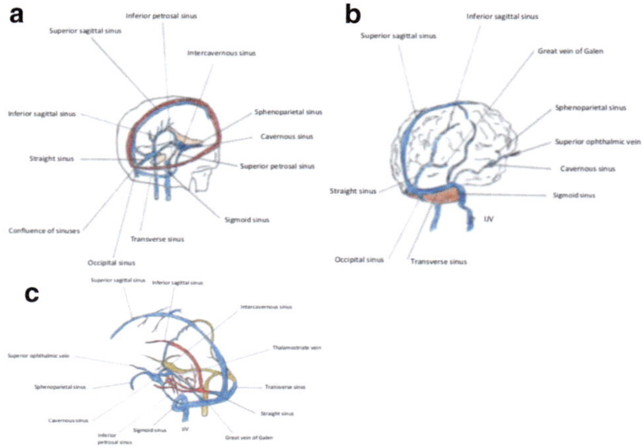

Diagram 10.2 The arrangement of the dural venous sinuses
(**a**) shows the appearance with the brain removed
(**b**) leaves the brain *in situ*
(**c**) shows a more detailed isolated view of the sinuses. In this image the great vein of Galen is shown draining into the straight sinus and itself receiving the basal vein of Rosenthal (*not marked*)

the great cerebral vein are a leash of midbrain and inferior cerebellar tributaries as well as the basal veins which curl around the midbrain. The basal vein is formed by the confluence of the anterior cerebral (which travels with the corresponding artery), a deep middle cerebral vein lying in the depths of the insula and a striate vein emanating from the anterior perforated substance. Those veins of the brainstem and the cerebellum drain backwards to enter the basal and the great vein as well as nearby sinuses. The veins of the medulla oblongata connect to those within the spinal medulla.

To recap on the basic design:

- The cerebral pattern of venous return (like the heart) does not follow the arteries (arteries travel deeply, veins superficially)
- A more 'arterial pattern' can be adopted by veins that are anterior or basal

- Superior drainage is usually into the superior sagittal sinus, middle cerebral veins empty into the cavernous sinus, posterior and inferior veins join the superior sagittal and transverse sinuses
- Medial and inferior regions drain via the inferior cerebral veins into the nearest sinus (except anteriorly where the anterior cerebral vein does run with its corresponding artery towards the basal vein).
- The insula and the depth of the lateral sulcus lie far from sinuses necessitating unique bridging veins
- The basal vein passes around the cerebral peduncle receiving blood from the thalamus and the posterior perforated substance joining the great vein below the splenium to drain the basal ganglia and to drain into the internal cerebral vein
- The internal cerebral vein receives blood from the chorioidal vein (draining the choroid plexus of the lateral ventricle), the thalamostriate vein(s) draining the thalamus and the caudate nucleus and the veins of the septum pellucidum (draining the corpus callosum and the head of the caudate nucleus)

Anatomy of the Venous Sinuses (Diagram 10.2a– c)

The unique features of the venous sinuses pertains to their dural attachments with the outermost of the meningeal layers fusing with the endocranium except where a fold is formed between meningeal layers between major parts of the brain and in the creation of brain supports (the falx cerebri and tentorium cerebelli). The dura mater also encloses the spinal medulla from the *f. magnum* to the sacrum separated by the internal vertebral venous plexus (effectively a dural venous sinus homologue). The meningeal vessels are therefore extradural whereas the cerebral vessels lie in the subarachnoid space.

Each of the venous sinuses (except for the inferior sagittal sinus and the straight sinus) lies between an inner and an outer layer of dura mater where one of the layers is endosteal. The inferior sagittal and straight sinuses are entirely meningeal. The sinuses include:

- Superior sagittal
- Inferior sagittal
- Lateral
- Cavernous (and intercavernous)
- Straight
- Sigmoid
- Occipital
- Petrosal (superior and inferior)

These sinuses may be divided into postero-superior (superior and inferior sagittal, lateral, sigmoid and occipital) and antero-inferior groups (superior and inferior petrosal, cavernous). The confluence of the sinuses (also known as the *torcular herophili*) is formed by the superior sagittal joining the straight, transverse and occipital sinuses.[3]

Superior Sagittal Sinus: travels from the *f. caecum* to the internal occipital protuberance creating a deep groove in the midline calvarium. This sinus has 3–4 lakes of blood which house the arachnoid (Pacchioni) granulations also leaving marked impressions.[4] The lacunae extend into this space the largest of which overlies the motor cortex so that many arachnoid granulations enter the lateral lacunae which accept meningeal and diploic veins directly (Diagram 10.3). The superior sinus does not drain the frontal pole of the hemisphere, draining the superior cerebral veins against the flow. Most often, the superior sagittal sinus turns to the right side to become the transverse (lateral) sinus. The falx cerebri (a sickle-shaped fold of dura mater) separates the cerebral hemispheres anteriorly where it is attached to the crista galli becoming continuous with the upper tentorium cerebelli posteri-

---

[3]Named after the Greek anatomist Herophilus (335–280 B.C.E.) *torcula Lt: to twist.*

[4]Antonio Pacchioni (1665–1726) was a student of Malpighi and Morgagni describing these bodies in 1705 in his *Dissertatio Epistolaris de Glandulis Conglobatis Durae Meningis Humanae.*

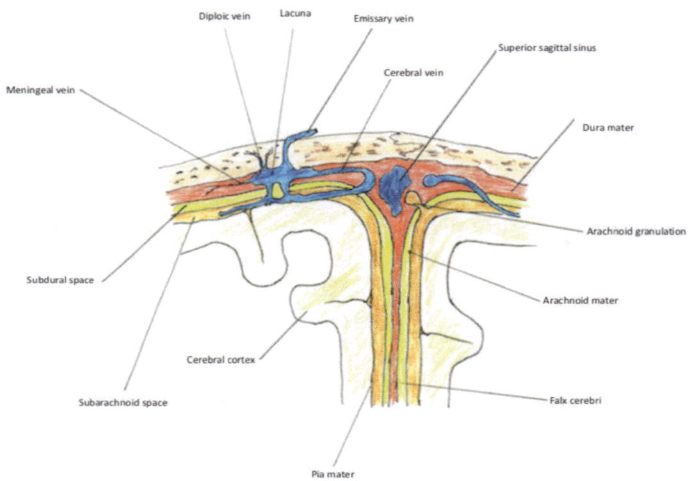

Diagram 10.3 The arachnoid (Pacchioni) granulations are tufts of arachnoid mater which sit inside the dural sinuses permitting the entry of CSF into the venous system

orly. The sinus also importantly accepts veins from the scalp so that deep-seated scalp infections can lead to superior sagittal sinus thrombosis. The lower border of the falx overhangs the corpus callosum housing the inferior sagittal sinus in its free margin and the straight sinus in that part attaching the tentorium cerebelli. The inferior sagittal sinus drains the lower parts of the medial surface of each hemisphere, the corpus callosum and the cerebellum.

Transverse (lateral) Sinus[5]*:* commences at the internal occipital protuberance and runs laterally between the two layers of the tentorium cerebelli grooving the occipital bone and the mastoid angle to curve downward and become the sigmoid sinus. One sinus is larger than the other. This is the sinus receiving the superior sagittal sinus (usually the right-side) so that in effect the

[5]In some textbooks the transverse and sigmoid sinuses are collectively referred to as the lateral sinus.

transverse sinus looks like a direct continuation of the superior sagittal sinus.

The right transverse sinus, (usually) the right sigmoid sinus and the right jugular vein contain blood from the superficial parts of the brain with the left transverse sinus, left sigmoid sinus and left internal jugular vein containing blood mostly from the deep parts of the brain draining the internal cerebral, basal and great veins. Each of these lateral sinuses effectively has two portions (transverse and sigmoid) so that drainage is from the posterior cerebrum, cerebellum and brainstem but also drainage from the middle ear which can be of clinical importance in middle ear infection and mastoiditis.

Straight Sinus: receives the inferior sagittal sinus anteriorly, the right and left basal cerebral veins and the great cerebral vein.

Sigmoid Sinus: curves downwards and sinuously forwards to the posterior edge of the jugular foramen connecting with a mastoid emissary vein that also joins the suboccipital venous plexus. The sigmoid sinus drains the superior petrosal sinus at its upper end and the occipital sinus inferiorly also draining the mastoid air cells.

Occipital Sinus: runs down from the start of the transverse sinus to the *f. magnum* and drains into the lower part of the sigmoid sinus communicating with the sigmoid sinuses and the *posterior internal vertebral plexus.* Here it receives cerebellar and medullary tributaries and drains the choroid plexus of the fourth ventricle. The occipital sinus is the smallest of the dural sinuses.

Basilar Sinuses: are a network of veins lying between the layers of dura covering the clivus and connecting the two inferior petrosal sinuses to receive drainage from the lower pons and the front of the medulla. Thrombosis of this venous system is fatal. It should be noted that no veins accompany the vertebral and basilar arteries with the basilar sinuses communicating with the internal vertebral venous plexus through the *f. magnum.*

Cavernous Sinus (Diagram 10.4)

This sinus has great clinical importance because of its proximity to structures which can be involved in infections and/or thrombosis (and with caroticocavernous fistula). The architectural arrange-

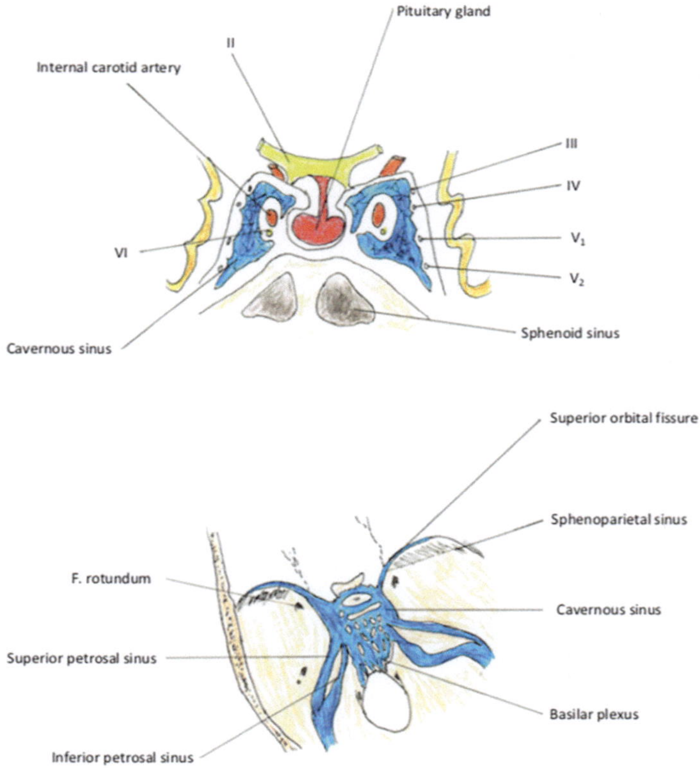

Diagram 10.4 Cavernous sinus. The relations are shown in the top image. The internal carotid artery (ICA) and the abducent nerve (Cranial VI) lie within the sinus with the oculomotor (Cranial III), the trochlear (Cranial IV), the ophthalmic (Cranial V_1) and the maxillary (Cranial V_2) lying against the dural sinus border.
The bottom image shows the drainage of the superior and inferior petrosal sinuses and the rich venous network over the clivus in front of the pons that communicates via the *f. magnum* with the internal vertebral venous plexus

ment permits the spread of such infection centrally (intracranially) via emissary veins (*see below*) connecting the dural venous sinuses with the pharynx, orbits, deep face and scalp. The cavernous sinus is a series of venous channels that are incompletely fused lying alongside the body of the sphenoid and extending from the medial aspect of the superior orbital fissure towards the apex of the petrous temporal bone.

The pituitary gland is located medially and the sphenoid sinus infero-medially. Meckel's cave is lateral with the Vth ganglion and V_2 and V_1 as well as Cranials III and IV lying superiorly n the lateral wall of the sinus. Within the sinus although separated from it by endothelium is the ICA and Cranial VI. Each cavernous sinus receives blood from three sources

(a) the orbit
(b) the vault bones and
(c) the cerebral hemisphere

There are entry and exit veins (similar to the pterygopalatine fossa with entry and exit doors). Each cavernous sinus drains via three exiting venous channels

(a) The superior petrosal sinuses
(b) Inferior petrosal sinus and
(c) a small connecting (or emissary vein) to the pterygoid plexus.

The two cavernous sinuses communicate via an inter-cavernous sinus.

The total capacity of this vital area is only about 1.5 mL.

Relations

Because of its key position the cavernous sinus acts as a topgraphical clinical landmark. The sinus lies between the periosteum of the body of the sphenoids and a fold of inner dura mater. Medially at the roof of the sinus the side of the pituitary fossa and the diaphragma sellae meet with the roof attaching to the anterior and middle clinoid processes and perforated anteriorly by the emerging ICA. Laterally is a dural ridge where the tentorium cerebelli extends as far as the anterior clinoid process. The roof (*as* defined) is invaginated laterally by Cranials III and IV as well as more posterolaterally by V_1 and V_2. The lateral wall of the sinus extends onto the floor of the middle cranial fossa. Anteriorly past the anterior clinoid processes the dura extends to the free edge of the lesser wing of the sphenoid. Lateral extension of the dura fuses with that of the greater wing of the sphenoid at the lateral margin of the *f. rotundum*. The floor is a narrow strip of endosteum along the base of the greater wing of the sphenoid and the medial wall is simply the endosteum of the body of the sphenoid. The dura separates the sinus from the pituitary fossa. There very narrow posterior wall extends to the *f. ovale* and the equally narrow anterior wall is plugged at the medial superior orbital fissure by the superior ophthalmic veins.

To recap:

Entry Points

1. Superior ophthalmic vein passes in the superior orbital fissure
2. Inferior orbital vein enters at the front but a lot of this blood will drain across the inferior orbital fissure to the pterygoid plexus. There is an emissary vein draining via the *f. ovale* (or *f. Vesalii*).
3. Superficial middle cerebral vein
4. Sphenoparietal sinus draining blood from the bones over the temporal vault (middle meningeal artery territory) running in the free edge of the lesser wing of the sphenoid

Exit Points

1. Superior petrosal sinus feeding back to the commencement of the sigmoid sinus
2. Inferior petrosal sinus (which is larger than the superior petrosal sinus) exiting the cavernous sinus beneath the petroclinoid ligament under which Cranial VI lies. The inferior petrosal sinus grooves the side of the clivus to enter the anterior com-

partment of the jugular foramen as the highest tributary of the IJV.

3. Communication with the pterygoid plexus via the *f. ovale* and the sphenoidal emissary foramen (when present)
4. Communication with the pharyngeal plexus via the carotid canal

The clinical significance of this anatomy bears witness in cavernous sinus thrombosis. In this circumstance, venous occlusion can extend to the hemisphere via the superficial middle cerebral vein. The so-called "danger area of the face" lies above the level of the deep facial vein comprising the upper lip and nose and the medial part of the cheek. This area is between the angular vein which runs into the superior ophthalmic veins and thence directly into the cavernous sinus and the deep facial vein which connects via the pterygoid plexus and ultimately into the cavernous sinus. Thrombosis can result from deep facial sepsis (starting in the nose, sinuses, face or teeth) often combined with a hypercoagulable state resulting in an ophthalmoplegia (Cranial III). Retrograde thrombosis can extend into the petrosal sinuses and towards the medullary veins where it proves fatal. Symptoms include ptosis (III palsy), Cranial IV, V and VI palsies. There is periorbital sensory loss, chemosis of the eye, an impaired corneal reflex frequently with papilloedema and retinal haemorrhages visible on ophthalmoscopy.

Superior Petrosal Sinus (Diagram 10.4): is a narrow sinus draining the back end of the cavernous sinus lying in the margin of the tentorium fixed to the petrous temporal bone and itself draining into the junction of the transverse and sigmoid sinus.

Inferior Petrosal Sinus (Diagram 10.4): lies in the groove between the basi-occiput and the petrous temporal draining the back end of the cavernous sinus into the jugular foramen in the formation of the and IJV.

Diploic veins: are wide venous spaces in marrow cavities that lie between the outer and the inner tables of the skull flat bones (Diagram 10.3). These have communications both with the venous sinuses and with emissary veins.

Meningeal Veins: drain the dura mater and run alongside meningeal arteries. They end up in the sinuses and lacunae.

As points of summary:

- Veins of the brain do not possess valves.
- Veins emerge from the subarachnoid space piercing the arachnoid mater and the dura mater to drain into the nearest available dural venous sinus.
- Superficial veins include the superior sagittal sinus and the cortical veins. These are linked by anastomotic veins (Trolard, Labbé).
- Deep veins include the transverse, straight and sigmoid sinuses and deep cortical veins. Deep systems include the internal cerebral and basal veins joining the great vein of Galen and then the straight sinus. These deep veins bring blood from the basal ganglia, corpus callosum, limbic system and thalamus. These can be divided by neurosurgeons as ventricular and cisternal landmarks.

Emissary veins: connect the venous sinuses to extracranial veins. Being also valveless, their importance lies in the inward spread of outside infections. Although variable they include parietal, condylar and sphenoidal emissary veins. In theory they can also equilibrate intracranial pressure to act as a safety valve for cerebral congestion. Well known examples of emissary veins include [2]:

- Connexion of the superior sagittal sinus with scalp veins via a parietal emissary vein.
- A connecting vein between the frontal sinus via the *f. caecum* to the superior sagittal sinus.
- The cavernous sinus has the greatest number of connexions to the exterior including communications between the superior ophthalmic and facial veins, an emissary connexion to the pharyngeal venous plexus and via the *f. ovale* (or the *f. Vesalii*) to the pterygoid venous plexus overlying the middle constrictor muscle. This sphenoidal emissary vein may also traverse the *f. lacerum*.
- A connexion between the sigmoid sinus or the transverse sinus and the occipital or posterior auricular veins via a mastoid emissary vein.

- Connexion between the vertebral venous plexus and the condylar canal (via a condylar emissary vein) which also communicates via a supracondylar emissary vein with the suboccipital venous plexus.
- A connexion between the confluence of sinuses and the occipital vein via an occipital emissary vein.
- A connexion between the IJV and the carotid canal (internal carotid venous plexus).
- Miscellaneous other internal connecting veins including a petrosquamous (joining the transverse and sigmoid sinuses with the retromandibular vein), an anterior condylar vein running with Cranial XII as a hypoglossal plexus, a temporal emissary vein and variable superficial petrosal veins connecting the middle cranial fossa and veins around the stylomastoid foramen. These latter veins are more numerous in lower mammals.

Vertebral Venous Plexi

As with the brain, the epidural space separates the periosteum of the vertebral canal from the spinal dura mater. This spinal epidural space contains loose areolar tissue, small arterial twigs and a complex venous network (the latter homologous to and continuous with the cranial venous sinuses). The small but critical spinal arteries arise from the ascending cervical (a branch of the costocervical trunk) and the vertebral artery with the vessels passing via the intervertebral foraminae to supply the spinal medulla and the nerve roots and their meninges along with the soft- and hard tissues of the intervertebral space.

The internal vertebral venous plexus extends throughout the entire length of the vertebral canal and is divisible into four subordinate longitudinal channels (two anterior and two posterior). The posterior plexi lie on the deep surface of the laminae and the ligamenta flava with the anterior plexi lying against the back surface of the vertebral bodies adjacent to the posterior longitudinal ligament. These systems have extensive communications from basivertebral veins and from the veins of the body wall (via the intervertebral foraminae). The latter include direct communications with the vertebral, posterior intercostal, lumbar and lateral sacral veins. This valveless system therefore communicates with the inferior vena cava (via lateral sacral and lumbars) and with the superior vena cava (via posterior intercostals and vertebrals). This is the likely mechanism for neoplastic embolization to the bones which is for example, a common presentation of prostate cancer.

In summary [3]:

- Large basivertebral veins drain into the internal vertebral venous plexus.
- The neural arch and muscles drain to the external vertebral venous plexus.
- The internal and external vertebral venous plexi drain into the regional segmental veins (vertebral, posterior intercostal, lumbar and lateral sacral) allowing communication with venous drainage from the pelvic viscera, (via pelvic veins) the abdomen (via the left renal vein and the hemiazygos system), in the thorax and breast (via posterior and anterior intercostals) and in the neck (via the inferior thyroid veins). The latter cases explain the spread of thyroid, breast and lung cancers to bone. But also there is a mechanism for osseous metastases in breast cancer and in uterine cancer.
- Septation of venous spaces in the internal vertebral venous plexus is similar to that of the dural venous sinuses possibly serving to prevent venous overdistension or excessive collapse as well as to regulate the direction and velocity of venous blood flow. They are also likely involved in thermoregulation.

CSF Dynamics: The anatomy of CSF flow is important in explaining the impact and cause of raised intracranial pressure. Diagram 10.3 shows the appearance of the arachnoid granulations as well as the position of diploic and meningeal veins. Diagram 10.5 demonstrates the direction of CSF flow. The CSF drains from the subarach-

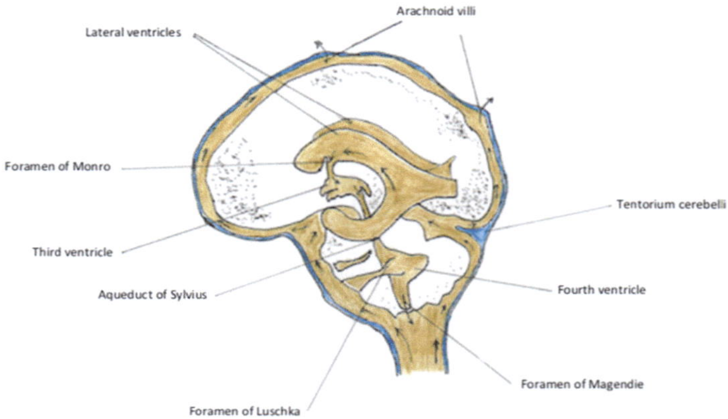

Diagram 10.5 The direction of CSF flow. CSF is produced in the choroid plexi passing from the lateral ventricles to the third ventricle via the interventricular foramen of Monro. From the third ventricle CSF passes through the cerebral aqueduct of Sylvius surrounded by periaqueductal gray matter. From the fourth ventricle, CSF flows through the central canal of the spinal cord via the obex. The fourth ventricle posses a median aperture of Magendie or via the two lateral apertures of Luschka. These apertures drain into the subarachnoid space at the cisterna magna and the cerebellopontine cistern angle respectively, with drainage from the foraminae of Luschka noted just behind the Cranial IX nerve root. CSF resorption occurs via the arachnoid granulations back into the dural venous sinuses.
Named after Alexander Monro Secundus 1733–1817, Professor of Anatomy Edinburgh Medical School who described the foramen in 1783)
Named after Franciscus Sylvius (nee Franz de le Böe), 1614–1672, a prominent Dutch physician who also described the Sylvian fissure
Named after Francois Magendie, 1783–1855 a French anatomist and vivisectionist who described the foramen in 1842
Named after Hubert von Luschka, 1820–1875, a German anatomist who described these apertures in 1855

noid space through the arachnoid granulations into the superior sagittal sinus (although there is also clearly some lymphatic drainage of the CSF). Some important points to remember are that:

- The CSF also serves as a protective fluid to the brain and spinal cord, cushioning them from mechanical injury and reducing

the brain's effective weight (the actual mass is ~1500 g while the buoyancy provided by CSF reduces its net weight to ~25–50 g).
- CSF also serves as a critical mechanism for the transport of nutrients and hormones as well as in protein clearance.
- It is estimated that around 80–90% of CSF is secreted by the choroid plexus, a highly-vascularised structure of epithelial cells located in the ventricles of the brain. The epithelial cells surrounding the capillaries create a blood-CSF barrier (BCSFB), which selectively controls the movement of solutes and water and which regulates CSF composition. This BBB consists of choroid ependymal cells (with tight cell junctions), the pia mater, the capillary endothelium and basal membrane

The normal total volume of human CSF is ~150 however, importantly, CSF production is virtually constant (0.2–0.7 mL/minute). This means that 600–700 mL of CSF is produced daily (making it replaced around four times daily). This follows the Monroe-Kellie Doctrine which states that the cerebral volume is made up of:

- The cerebral water content (cerebral blood volume/flow)
- The cerebral weight and
- The CSF volume

These combined components within the closed adult skull must be constant in total. The system is well regulated so that as cerebral volume increases (e.g. with a brain tumour) the intracranial pressure remains constant for long periods. However the P/V relationship ultimately deregulates so that small volume increases result in exponential increases in intracranial pressure (ICP). At this stage there is ultimate tentorial herniation of the temporal lobe and compression of vital cardiorespiratory centres (called coning). This understanding of basic ICP pathophysiology is due to the notion that:

$$\text{Cerebral Perfusion Pressure}\left(\text{CPP}\right)=\text{Mean Arterial BP}\left(\text{MABP}\right)-\text{ICP}$$

According to this simple formula, during coning the ICP may approach the MABP leading to cerebral non-perfusion (CPP = 0).

The basis of hydrocephalus is anatomical, divisible into disorders of increased CSF production (hypersecretory hydrocephalus), obstruction to flow (non-communicating or obstructive hydrocephalus) or impaired absorption (communicating hydrocephalus).

Q & A: Chap. 10 (Answers at the End of This Chapter)

1. The venous drainage input of the straight sinus includes:
   (a) The superior sagittal sinus anteriorly
   (b) The right and left basal cerebral veins of Rosenthal
   (c) The great cerebral vein
   (d) The thalamostriate veins
   (e) On occasion the superior cerebellar veins
2. The cavernous sinus:
   (a) Is invaginated medially by the Vth cranial nerve
   (b) Has no relationship to the trochlear nerve
   (c) Has dura mater which fuses laterally with the greater wing of the sphenoid at the lateral margin of the foramen rotundum
   (d) Is separable from the pituitary fossa by its dura
   (e) Is not invaginated by Cranial III
3. Emissary veins
   (a) Are valveless
   (b) Connect the superior sagittal sinus with the scalp
   (c) Connect the straight sinus with the vertebral venous plexus
   (d) Connect to the posterior auricular vein
4. The sigmoid venous sinus:
   (a) Does not receive diploic veins
   (b) Connects to the mastoid emissary vein
   (c) Does not connect to the suboccipital venous plexus
   (d) Does not connect to the occipital sinus

5. The mastoid emissary vein:
   (a) Connects the transverse sinus with the suboccipital venous plexus
   (b) Is rarely multiple
   (c) Connects with the external jugular vein
   (d) Tends to have right-sided dominance
6. The Great vein of Galen
   (a) Forms just below the pineal gland
   (b) Unites the internal cerebral and basal veins (of Rosenthal)
   (c) Runs around the posterior border of the splenium of the corpus callosum
   (d) Does not receive callosal veins
7. Arachnoid granulations
   (a) Contain villi
   (b) Are static in size with aging
   (c) Drain into the inferior sagittal sinus
   (d) Are located at the entrance of a superior draining cortical vein into a sinus
   (e) Have a different density on CT scanning to CSF
8. Cavernous sinus thrombosis
   (a) May present with proptosis
   (b) Most commonly presents with an abducent palsy
   (c) Can present with mandibular anaesthesia
   (d) Often presents with miosis
   (e) Rarely presents with facial pain

Answers

1. c, e
2. c, d
3. a, b, d
4. b
5. d
6. b, c
7. a, d

References

1. Jianu DC, Jianu SN, Dan FT, Munteanu G, Copil A, Birdac CD, Motoc AGM, Docu Axelerad A, Petrica L, Arnautu SF, Sadik R, Iacob N, Gogu AE. An integrated approach on the diagnosis of cerebral veins and dural sinuses thrombosis (a narrative review). Life. 2022;12:717. https://doi.org/10.3390/life12050717.
2. Mortazavi MM, Tubbs RS, Reich S, Verma K, Shoja MM, Zurada A, Benninger B, Loukas M, Cohen Gadol AA. Anatomy and pathology of the cranial emissary veins: a review with surgical implications. Neurosurgery. 2012;70:1312–9.
3. Stringer MD, Restieaux M, Fisher AL, Crosado B. The vertebral venous plexuses: the internal veins are muscular and external veins have no valves. Clin Anat. 2012;25:609–18.

The Orbit

11

Contents

Structural Anatomy of the Eyelids 234
Lacrimal Apparatus (Diagram 11.1) 237
Eye Stability 238
Structure of the Eye (Diagram 11.3a, b) 239
Retina (Diagram 11.3b) 243
Extraocular Muscles: Anatomy, Function and Dysfunction 245
Terminology 247
Actions 249
Nerves of the Orbit: A Summary 251
Vessels of the Orbit: A Summary 254
Q & A: Chap. 11 (Answers at the End of This Chapter) 255
Answers 256
Reference 256

This chapter includes consideration of the orbital osteology, the eyelid, palpebral margin and the nasolacrimal apparatus, the eye itself in brief and the function of the extraocular muscles.

The ORBIT (See Diagram 6.5b; Chap.6).

In discussion of this region there are a few caveats:

- The orbital fascia is the periosteum of the orbit which is posteriorly continuous with the dura mater and the sheath of the optic nerve.
- Accessory structures include the extraocular muscles, the eyelids, the conjunctiva and the lacrimal gland which although not completely within the orbit is considered here.

A. Zbar, *Anatomy--Head and Neck*,
https://doi.org/10.1007/978-3-031-69538-4_11

- There are a number of orbital suspensory (or support) mechanisms for the eye of which the orbital fat is probably the most important where it surrounds the optic nerve and cushion stabilizes the eye against the backward pull of the muscles. The orbital fat is not subject to weight change and dissection of the orbit is a tedious procedure because of the need for meticulous fat dissection. This is underappreciated when examining prosected specimens of the orbit.

As a recap of the bony orbit, examine a skull. The orbit is cone- (or pyramid-) shaped lying on its side. The most external part (or opening) the aditus with the narrower part at the back, the base. The smooth roof is the orbital part of the frontal bone with the lesser wing of the sphenoid completing the orbit posteriorly. On the medial side lies the frontal sinus placed between the orbital and squamous parts of the frontal bone.

There are seven bones that make up the orbit. Medially is the lacrimal bone which articulates with the nasal bone (not part of the orbit). The lacrimal bone lies against the orbital lamina of the ethmoid bone which here is rather small and which abuts against the superior part of the superior orbital fissure. When you examine this area, medially and superiorly part of the optic canal is visible. The larger bone which houses the superior orbital fissure, the optic canal and peeking through the inferior orbital fissure, is the greater wing of the sphenoid. A large part of the posterior and superior orbital margin (beyond the superior orbital fissure) is made up of the orbital process of the frontal bone. Below is the horizontal extension of the maxilla filling in the space for the inferior orbital fissure. In addition, filling in the area on the side of the maxilla and forming the lateral orbital margin is the zygomatic bone (which articulates over quite a wide area with the sphenoid). The inferior orbital fissure is incorporated here laterally. At the very medial tip of the inferior orbital fissure (between the sphenoid, the ethmoid and the maxilla) the palatine bone completes the region.

In summary: the orbit if formed by the:

- Sphenoid
- Ethmoid
- Lacrimal
- Frontal
- Maxilla
- Zygomatic and
- Palatine bones.

The posterior lacrimal crest forms a vertical ridge on the lacrimal bone with the lacrimal fossa housing the lacrimal sac that sits between this crest and a smaller anterior lacrimal crest. Inferiorly this leads into a groove for the nasolacrimal canal. At the junction of this medial wall and the roof of the orbit lie the anterior and the posterior ethmoidal foraminae with separation of the medial walls of the orbit from the ethmoidal air cells and the lateral wall of the nose. On the lateral side of the orbit, just inside the upper anterior margin is the marginal tubercle of Whitnall which lies against the greater wing of the sphenoid.[1]

The superior orbital fissure lies between the lateral wall and the roof (effectively between the greater and the lesser wings of the sphenoid which is more evident examining the open skull vault). The inferior orbital fissure diverges from the medial end of the superior orbital fissure between the lateral wall and the floor (i.e. between the greater wing of the sphenoid and the maxilla). To remind, the superior orbital fissure connects the middle cranial fossa with the orbit. The inferior orbital fissure leads into the pterygopalatine and infratemporal fossae. The lateral wall separates the orbit from the temporal fossa. Of note, the lateral wall slopes at about 45° to the sagittal plane so that the two lateral walls sit approximately at right angles to one another. The floor is the orbital surface of the maxilla grooved by the infraorbital foramen and completed laterally in front by the zygomatic bone and behind by the small

[1]Named after Samuel Ernest Whitnall (1876–1950) a British anatomist and humorist who described the tubercle in 1911 at approximately 11 mm below the frontozygomatic suture and several mm deep inside the lateral orbital margin.

orbital process of the palatine bone. The palatine bone effectively lies on its side with projecting horizontal and vertical plates. The orbital process projects off the vertical plate laterally and the sphenoidal process a medial projection.

Dissection of the orbit is achieved by chipping through the thin-ridged orbital part of the frontal bone in the anterior cranial fossa. This then permits extension into the mucoperiosteum of the ethmoid air cells medially (and into the frontal sinus). If the lesser wing of the sphenoid is removed posteriorly (leaving the medial part intact) the optic canal is isolated and the superior orbital fissure can be well demonstrated. The thin-walled cavities of the ethmoid air cells can be seen here occupying the entire ethmoid labyrinth between the orbit and the upper part of the cavity of the nose (See Chap. 12). These sinuses form three groups of which the anterior and middle empty into the middle meatus with the posterior emptying into the superior meatus.

Structural Anatomy of the Eyelids

The eyelids are covered with skin at the front and conjunctiva at the back. They are part of a skeletal framework (the orbital septum) with the thicker lid margins supported by tarsal plates. The orbicularis oculi is located at the front of the orbital septum attached to the anterior lacrimal crest with the space between the upper and lower lids (the palpebral fissure) forming a button hole between the superior and inferior tarsal plates with the medial part forming a specialized medial palpebral ligament which anchors the tarsal plates to the anterior lacrimal crest. The homologous lateral tarsal ligament is much thinner and fuses with a lateral palpebral raphé within the orbicularis oculi that attaches to Whitnall's tubercle. This tubercle is an attachment for:

- Lateral rectus check ligament
- Lockwood suspensory ligament[2]
- Lateral palpebral ligament
- Levator aponeurosis

In front of this septum is the palpebral part of the orbicularis oculi and superficial to this is the angular facial vein at the medial canthus. The eyelashes are adherent to the tarsal plates with the Meibomian modified sebaceous glands located here designed to waterproof the lid margins and to slow the evaporation of the tears.[3] At this medial point, the conjunctiva is adherent without redundancy during movement of the eyelids. The medial end houses the lacrimal papilla and at its apex the lacrimal punctum which opens into a lacrimal canaliculus that enters the lacrimal sac (Diagram 11.1). The blood supply to the lids is from the palpebral branches of the ophthalmic artery with the innervation from the lacrimal, supraorbital, supratrochlear and infratrochlear nerves. The lower lid is innervated by the palpebral branch of the infraorbital nerve [1].

As the lower lid has very little mobility gentle lid closure is performed by the palpebral fibres of the orbicularis oculi with a more forcible closure using the orbital fibres. The lids are opened by the *levator palpebrae superioris* muscle and the eyebrows are lowered by the orbital fibres of the orbicularis oculi with a support (sunvisor) effect brought into play by the medial corrugator supercilia muscles which draw the eyebrows together.

---

[2]Named after Charles Barrett Lockwood (1856–1914) who was a British surgeon also noted for his inguinal and femoral hernia repair techniques.

[3]Described by Heinrich Meibom (1638–1700) who held combined chairs in medicine, history and poetry at the University of Helmstedt. The glands had actually been described earlier by Galen in the first century AD.

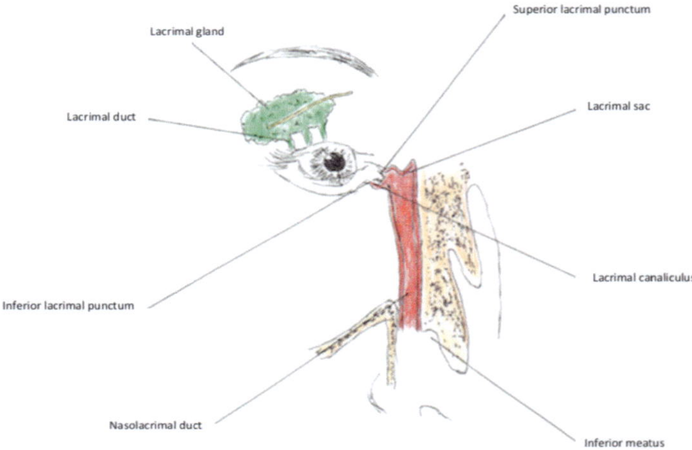

Diagram 11.1 The lacrimal apparatus. The lacrimal gland has about 15–20 lacrimal ducts which draw tears from lateral to medial. The gland has a palpebral and orbital part which is adherent to the levator palpebrae superioris muscle. Drainage is into the front of the inferior nasal meatus

The transparent conjunctiva is attached to the sclera at the corneal margins. The conjunctiva is reflected onto the inner surface of the eyelids and is firmly attached to the tarsal plates. The medial conjunctival fold (plica semilunaris) is considered in some textbooks as the homologue to the nictitating membrane (third eyelid) found in tailless amphbians, some reptiles and birds and in sharks which protects and moistens the eye whilst vision is maintained. At the medial canthus is the caruncle which is a small pimple of modified skin along with the *lacus lacrimalis* between the plica and the caruncle where excess tears accumulate before passing into the canaliculi. The *lacrimal glands* open via 12–15 separate lacrimal ducts through the tendon of the levator palpebrae superioris. Note too that the corneal nerve supply (via the short and long ciliary nerves) differs from the conjunctival nerve supply.

The neural arrangement of the orbit is shown in Diagram 11.2.

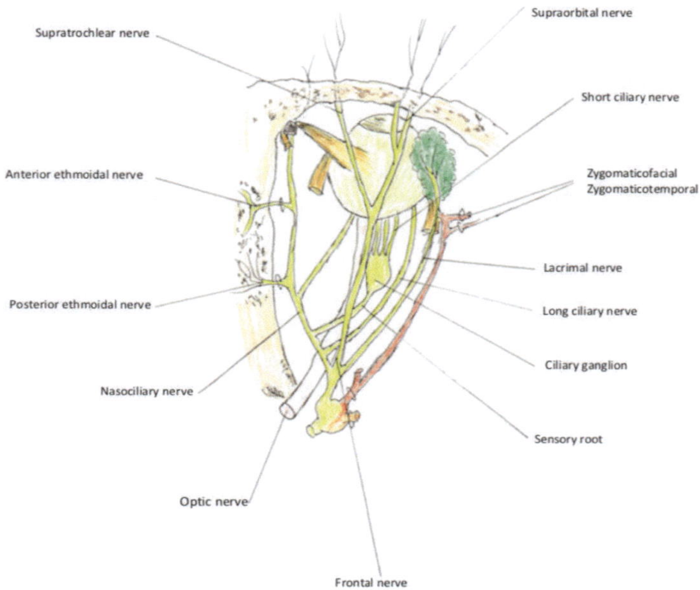

Diagram 11.2 Orbital dissection to display the nerves. The nasociliary, frontal and lacrimal are intraconal. V_2 is the maxillary nerve and V_3 is the mandibular nerve. There are usually 2–3 long ciliary nerves carrying sensory innervation to the eye along with SNS activity to the dilator pupillae. There are usually between 12 and 20 short ciliary nerves bringing PSNS and SNS fibres to the cornea, iris and ciliary body

Lacrimal Apparatus (Diagram 11.1)

The lacrimal apparatus comprises the lacrimal gland, the lacrimal canaliculi, the lacrimal sac and the nasolacrimal duct.

The lacrimal gland is a serous gland with a larger orbital and a smaller palpebral component. The orbital part is located at the outer edge of the eye supported by the aponeurotic part of the tendon of the levator palpebrae superioris which along with the orbital fat acts to stabilize the gland. The gland is visible through the superior conjunctival fornix. The lacrimal ducts lead from the palpebral part of the gland into the superior conjunctival fornix with those from the orbital part of the gland entering more deeply. Closure of the eyes moves tears from lateral to medial encouraging drainage. Reassess Chap. 5 for consideration of the autonomic control over tear flow.

Tear content is a mixture of sebaceous material from the Meibomian glands and the caruncle combined with an aqueous component derived from the lacrimal secretion and a deeper mucus element added from the few scattered goblet cells within the conjunctiva. The blinking reflex is produced by the palpebral fibres of the orbicularis oculi and is mediated by the afferent nasociliary branch of V_1 linked to the efferent limb via Cranial VII. The lacrimal sac removes excess tears with the lacrimal canaliculi leading from the puncta to the sac with fibres of the palpebral part of the orbicularis oculi inserted into the sac so that the puncta turn inwards with muscle activity so as to dip into the lacus lacrimalis. This effectively allows the tears to be sucked forwards by the canaliculi with the elastic tissue within the wall of the sac assisting in pumping tears into the nasolacrimal duct. The nasolacrimal duct is about 2 cm. in length sloping downwards and laterally alongside to open into the anterior part of the inferior meatus guarded by mucosal valves that prevent reflux when blowing the nose.

Eye Stability

The fascial sheath of the eye (fascia bulbi or Tenon's capsule) functions like a suspensory bursa or shock absorber running from the corneoscleral junction to the optic nerve. The recti insert into the outer sheath with the lateral part thickened for example as a lateral check ligament which attaches to Whitnall's tubercle. On the medial side over the medial rectus there is an homologous medial check ligament adherent to the posterior lacrimal crest. The effect created is for the region inferiorly to hold the eye up like a hammock (the suspensory ligament of Lockwood) which is a blend of the sheaths overlying the inferior oblique and the inferior rectus muscles. This leaves the eye nearer to the superior rather than the inferior orbital margin which is relevant clinically since the bone stock below the tubercle of Whittnall that preserves this suspensory mechanism allows removal of bone up to this point without disturbing the positioning of the globe.

As a consequence of this architecture, the eye rotates around a fixed geometrical centre to ensure that it is not displaced when moved either forwards or backwards. Posterior displacement is prevented by the bony attachments of the recti as well as by the large amount of orbital fat and the dynamics of the forward pull exerted by the oblique muscles. The attachments of the medial and the lateral recti to the check ligaments also discourages any posterior displacement of the eyeball.

Structure of the Eye (Diagram 11.3a, b)

The eye is not perfectly spherical with the anterior cornea having a smaller radius of curvature than the globe. Dissection of the fresh (as opposed to the formalinized) eye is actually quite difficult to appreciate. The venae vorticosae, the posterior ciliary arteries and the nerves all enter near the optic nerve.

There are three coats enclosing a cavity filled with light refracting media. The external fibrous coat, (sclera) has an anterior one-sixth which is the transparent cornea (Diagram 11.3a). A middle vascular and muscular coat comprises the iris anteriorly and the choroid posteriorly. Between these two lies the ciliary body. The internal coat is the retina with its light sensitive rods and cones along with the origins of the optic nerve. The uveal tract is the combined iris, ciliary body and choroid.

The refracting media are: the cornea, the aqueous humour (between the cornea and the lens filling the anterior chamber between the cornea and the iris) and the posterior chamber (between the iris and the lens). The two chambers (the anterior and the posterior) communicate via the pupil in the middle of the iris. The lens separates the posterior chamber from the vitreous body.

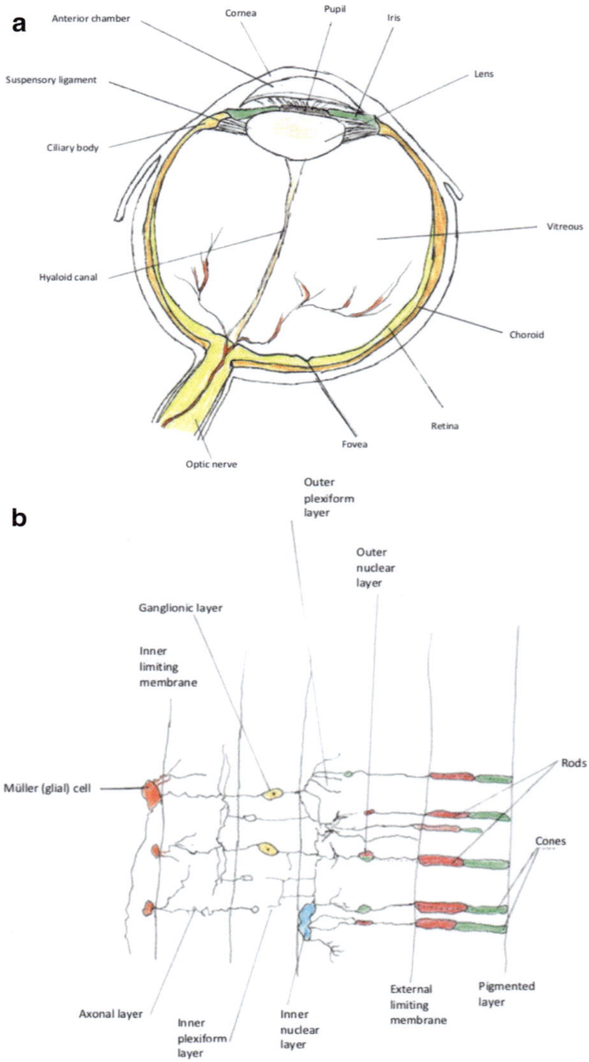

Diagram 11.3 Ocular structure
(**a**) shows the structure and chambers of the eye. The combined ciliary body, iris and choroid forms the uvea (middle vascular tunic)
(**b**) shows the division of retinal layers (*see main text*). Amacrine cells are inhibitory interneurons connecting ganglion and bipolar cells sending their dendrites into the inner plexiform layer

Like a camera, there is a light sensitive part (the retina) and a lens system for focusing (cornea, lens and refractive media) along with a means of controlling the amount of light admitted (the iris diaphragm acting like an aperture). Also similar to a camera, the inside is black in order to prevent internal reflections. The sclera is an expansion of the dura mater around the optic nerve with the choroid functioning like an expansion of the arachnoid and pia. The retina and its attachment to Cranial II is effectively an expansion of the brain. The ciliary zonule is a thickened part of the vitreous membrane that attaches to the posterior surfaces of the ciliary processes. Posteriorly lies the hyaloid fossa (*see below*) and anteriorly the suspensory ligament of the lens. When the ciliary muscle contracts the lens becomes fatter in shape pulling the ciliary processes and the zonule anteriorly and inwards medially to relax the suspensory ligament and to shorten the focal length in accommodation (and convergence).

The sclera remains densely adherent to the ciliary body but the inner choroid is readily stripped off during dissection. As the optic nerve breaks through it is at its thinnest point (lamina cribrosa) with at this point entry of the long and short posterior ciliary arteries, ciliary nerves and 4–5 venae vorticosae (choroidal veins). Near the corneoscleral junction there is a minute canal within the sclera (canal of Schlemm) which drains the aqueous humour.[4]

The middle (vascular) coat contains the choroid between the sclera and the retina consisting of two layers of blood vessels, a deep capillary net and a more superficial venous layer with the posterior ciliary arteries running between the layers. The middle coat is divided into an external part (ciliary muscle) and an inner part (ciliary processes). The ciliary involuntary muscle is arranged as radiating and circular fibres innervated by the short ciliary nerves with postganglionic PSNS supply synapsing in the ciliary

[4]The canal encircles the cornea connecting small canaliculi to blood vessels buried within the sclera. Named after Friedrich Schlemm (1795–1858) a Professor of Anatomy in Berlin. As a student Schlemm was briefly imprisoned for grave robbing in an attempt with others to study the anatomy of the corpse.

ganglion. The ciliary processes extend in a circular fashion from the choroid to the lens. The diameter of the pupil varies the amount of light that reaches the retina where a reduction in pupillary size occurs by contraction of the circular fibres of the sphincter pupillae (at the pupillary margin of the iris). Conversely, the pupil is dilated by the radial myoepithelial cells (the dilator pupillae). The nerve supply is therefore a mix of postganglionic PSNS (traveling in the short ciliary nerves) and postganglionic SNS fibres (traveling in the long ciliary nerves).

To summarize:

The short ciliary nerves form from the ciliary ganglion and pierce the sclera around the optic nerve as about a dozen fine filaments which break up into fine plexiform branches on the inner sclera that run to the ciliary muscle, iris and cornea. They contain:

1. Postganglionic PSNS to the ciliary muscle and the sphincter pupillae
2. Postganglionic SNS to the vessels of the eyeball
3. Sensory fibres from the nasociliary nerve

The long ciliary nerves transmit sensory and SNS fibres from the nasociliary nerve through the sclera.

At the back are the short posterior ciliary arteries which are branches of the ophthalmic artery ending in the choroid. These small vessels are distinct from the long ciliary arteries (also branches of the ophthalmic artery but which pierce the sclera some distance from the optic nerve and which run between the sclera and the choroid to anastomose with the anterior ciliary arteries). These latter vessels create a greater arterial circle at the periphery of the iris which is the blood supply to the iris, ciliary muscle and ciliary processes. The lesser arterial circle is a small anastomotic ring inside this greater arterial circle lying within the iris at the external border of the sphincter pupillae. The venae vorticosae arise from a large vein within the choroid which pierces the sclera just behind the equator with ultimate drainage into the superior ophthalmic vein.

Retina (Diagram 11.3b)

The retina has a complex structure consisting of three parts: an optic part (comprising the pigmented and nervous tissue arranged as ten discrete layers), a ciliary part and an iridial part. The layers of the retina include:

1. The pigmented layer is closest to the choroid providing nourishment support to the neural retina.
2. The layer of the rods and cones (inner rods and outer cones). Adults have approximately 7 million cones and 75–150 million rods. Rods are more primitive in development and only contain visual purple with sensitivity to dim light (scotopic). Cones are photoptic registering colour at higher thresholds. The retina in its periphery contains rods none of which are at the fovea. Cones are located at the fovea but not many peripherally. Cones are connected to single ganglion cells with rods connected to on average 80 ganglion cells.
3. The outer limiting layer (External limiting membrane) a row of junctional complexes which separates the photoreceptors from their cell nuclei
4. The outer nuclear layer (the cell bodies of the rods and cones)
5. The outer plexiform layer (synapsing with bipolar and horizontal cells)
6. The inner nuclear layer (amacrine, bipolar and horizontal cell bodies)
7. The inner plexiform layer (synapses between bipolar cells and ganglion and amacrine cells)
8. The ganglionic layer (the axons from these cells become the optic nerve)
9. The layer of nerve fibres (axons of the ganglion cells)
10. The inner limiting membrane (Müller glial cell basement membrane).[5]

[5]Named after Heinrich Müller (1820–1864) a German anatomist who discovered the neuroglia and the pigment rhodopsin.

Layers 2–10 comprise the neural layer.

Blood vessels are absent from layers 6 to 9.

In a retinal detachment the nervous layer (attached to the vitreous and pigmented layers) is stripped. The functional role divides the retina in four processing stages as: photoreceptors and then transmission to the bipolar cells, the ganglion cells and along the optic nerve. At each point of synapse there is a connection laterally to horizontal and amacrine cells. Cranial II connects to the lateral geniculate body in the diencephalon with projections to the superior colliculus, the suprachiasmatic nucleus and the nucleus of the optic tract.

The optic part of the retina extends to the *ora serrata* close to the posterior margin of the ciliary body with the two layers continued anteriorly over the ciliary processes (the *pars ciliaris retinae*) and the posterior surface of the iris (the *pars iridica retinae*). The back of these ciliary processes have a layer of pigmented cells which are continued forward from the retina (the pars ciliaris retinae). The optic part of the retina contains the outermost, (light-sensitive rods and cones) and the innermost (ganglion cells the nerve fibres of which become the optic nerve). This point of transmission leaves the white optic disc devoid of sensory retinal elements (blind spot).

The middle layer of the retina consists of bipolar cells connecting the rods and cones to the ganglion cells. The acuity is greatest at the point of the fovea centralis with the cones tightly packed and connected to individual ganglion cells. The outer retinal layers receives some choroidal blood supply however the central artery of the retina (reaching this region via the ophthalmic artery at the optic disc) is an end artery without collateral anastomosis. The central vein divides here into superior and inferior branches where it pierces the meningeal sheaths of the optic nerve and the subarachnoid space to drain into the superior ophthalmic vein.

The vitreous abuts against the retina, where the ciliary processes and the lens form the hyaloid fossa on its anterior surface filling 80% of the volume of the eyeball. The hyaloid canal (an embryological remnant of the central retinal artery supplying the foetal lens) extends from the posterior surface of the lens to the optic disc (Diagram 11.3a).

Extraocular Muscles: Anatomy, Function and Dysfunction

All of the extraocular movement is caused by a combination of the four recti and the two obliques. There is also the action of the levator palpebrae superioris and the small insignificant oribitalis muscle inferiorly. The orbit is unusual since the medial walls are parallel but the lateral walls slope away from one another so that the optic nerve and the muscles cone outwards laterally from the apex of the orbit. As a result, the orbital axis (apex to the mid-base of the orbit when viewed from above) is directed anterolaterally. This is naturally different from the optic axis (back to front of the eyeball) so that the optic axes (the eyes) are not aligned with the orbital axes.

The medial end of the retort-shaped superior orbital fissure has a tendinous ring attached which incorporates the optic foramen with the four recti arising from the ring. Diagram 11.4 shows the axial layout of the orbit with its musculature. Diagram 11.5 shows the appearance of the orbit and the disposition of the muscles seen during a deeper dissection. From above the levator palpebrae superioris is the first muscle seen. Nerves running via the superior orbital fissure are then considered as either intra- or extraconal (lacrimal, frontal and Cranial IV). (See also Diagram 6.5a; Chap. 6). The remainder of the lateral part of the superior orbital fissure is closed off with the dura mater of the middle cranial fossa. Those nerves destined for the eyeball or the muscles remain inside the cone with the only branches passing out through the cone being the posterior and the anterior ethmoidal nerves and the infratrochlear nerves (all branches of the nasociliary nerve) (Diagram 11.2).

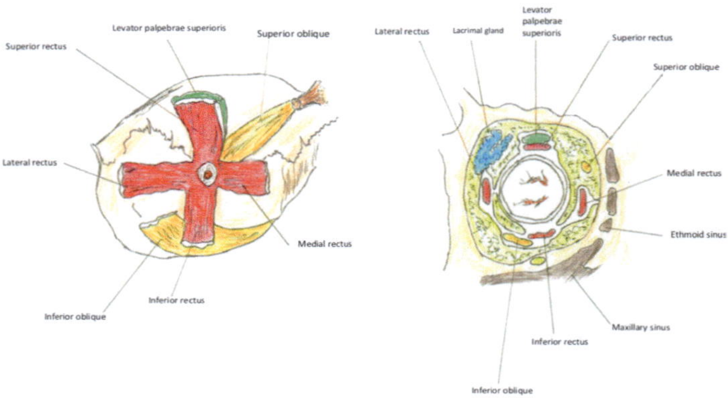

Diagram 11.4 The muscular layout of the orbit. The recti take origin from the common tendinous ring (annulus of Zinn). In dissection of the orbit from above the first muscle encountered is the levator palpebrae superioris. Running over this muscle is the large frontal nerve. Under the muscle is the superior rectus (inserting into the sclera in front the coronal equator) and under that is the superior oblique with a different line of pull inserting into the sclera behind the coronal equator

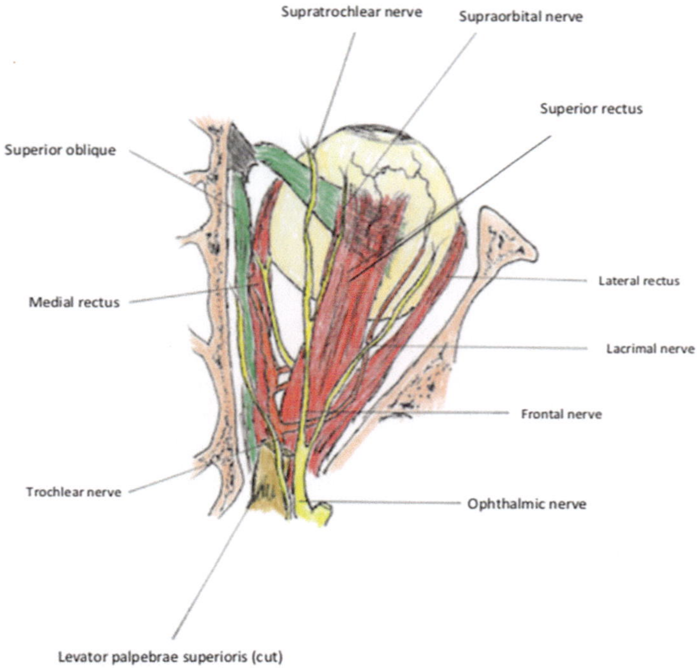

Diagram 11.5 Disposition of the neurovasculature and muscles in a deeper dissection of the orbit

Terminology

Let's define movement towards the nose as medial rotation, (nasal deviation, adduction or turn-in). Similarly, the opposite function is lateral rotation (abduction, turn-out). Upward movement is turn-up (superior, elevation) whereas downward movement is turn-down (inferior, depression).

The *levator palpebrae superioris muscle* arises from the under surface of the lesser wing of the sphenoid as a flat, rimmed muscle. The frontal nerve (which is quite large) lies on the top of the muscle with the muscle appearing like a ribbon which at its end has a crescentic horn that attaches to the superior tarsal plate and to the skin of the upper eyelid. This flange penetrates the orbital septum and the superior conjunctival fornix. The smooth muscle component of the levator is thin and innervated by the superior division of Cranial III which enters the lower part of the muscle on its medial side. There is a dual nerve supply (somatic and SNS) with the SNS fibres innervating the visceral muscle (cell bodies in the superior cervical ganglion). The muscle opens the eye and elevates the upper eyelid. The intact SNS supply does not, however, compensate for somatic loss so that in a IIIrd nerve palsy there is complete ptosis whereas in Horner's syndrome there is only partial ptosis. There is no ptosis with a Cranial VII palsy but the eye cannot be screwed tightly because the orbicularis oculi is denervated.

The *superior rectus muscle* (Diagram 11.5): This muscle arises from the upper part of the tendinous ring and also from the dural sheath of the optic nerve. The muscle passes beneath the levator and is inserted into the upper sclera anterior to the coronal equator of the eye. This insertion of the recti (in front of the equator) has particular anatomical significance for the line of pull of the recti and for the position of the eye where that line of pull is at its greatest advantage (*see below*).

The *medial rectus muscle* arises from the inner part of the tendinous ring and the dural sheath of the optic nerve, passing along the medial wall of the orbit below the superior oblique muscle to be inserted into the medial sclera **anterior to the coronal equator of the eye.**

The *inferior rectus muscle* arises from the lower tendinous ring and is inserted into the inferior sclera anterior to the coronal equator of the eye. There is an expansion from the sheath which inserts into the inferior tarsal plate.

The *lateral rectus muscle* arises from the lateral convexity of the tendinous ring but is longer in origin than the other recti to be inserted into the lateral sclera anterior to the coronal equator of the eye.

The *superior oblique muscle* arises from the inner tendinous ring and also from bone (the body of the sphenoid) to pass as a slender tendon under the trochlea lubricated where there is a synovial sheath. The superior oblique runs backwards under the superior rectus muscle to be inserted into the posteroinferior sclera **behind the coronal equator of the eye.**

The *inferior oblique muscle* arises from the bone of the floor of the orbit and is the only muscle not to arise from the back of the orbit like the other recti. The inferior oblique passes obliquely backwards below the inferior rectus and between the lateral rectus and the sclera inserts near the posteroinferior quadrant behind the coronal equator of the eye.

(Some use a chemical mnemonic formula in order to remember the nerve supply to the extraocular muscles such that: $LR_6SO_4O_3$ (which signifies that the lateral rectus is innervated by Cranial VI, the superior oblique by Cranial IV, and the others (the inferior oblique, inferior, superior and medial recti) by Cranial III).

It should be noted that as Cranial IV decussates in the midbrain that it controls the contralateral superior oblique.

Actions

- The medial rectus turns the eye in (as do the superior and the inferior recti).
- The lateral rectus turns the eye out (as do the obliques).
- The lateral rectus and the medial rectus have simple actions without secondary movements. Lateral rectus turning the eye out, medial rectus turning the eye in.
- The obliques are more complex because they insert behind the coronal equator of the eye so that their line of pull passes medial to the axis of rotation of the eye. (i.e. as their name suggests they pull obliquely).
- The superior rectus turns the eye up and in and the inferior oblique turns it up and out (i.e. the superior rectus and the inferior oblique act together to turn the eye up. Equally the inferior rectus turns the eye down and in and the superior oblique turns the eye down and out (i.e. these two muscles act together to turn the eye down). Pure up and down movement is therefore

the action of the relevant rectus with its oppositely named oblique.
- The elevating action of the inferior oblique or the depressing action of the superior oblique become progressively more pure (and hence more efficient) when the eye is turned inwards and the more the eye is turned outwards the less their contribution to ocular elevation or depression, respectively. Similarly, the more the eyes are turned outwards the purer the action of the superior and inferior recti to turn the eye up and down respectively.

It should be noted, however, that ocular movements are a little more complicated since the obliquity of pull of the muscles produces a wheel-like rotation (torsion) on the eye so that intorsion (viewing the right eye moving from 12 to 1 o'clock) is produced by the superior rectus and superior oblique. Extorsion of the eye (movement to the 11 o'clock position) is a result of action by the inferior rectus and the inferior oblique muscles. These torsion effects mean that in paralysis of one of these muscles, the resultant diplopia creates an oblique positioning of the second image above the first.

An appreciation of the anatomy of the extraocular muscles and their purist line of pull allows an interpretation of ocular palsy with a characteristic pattern of strabismus (squint) and diplopia (double vision).

The simplest lesion is Cranial VI palsy where the eye cannot look out because of paralysis of the lateral rectus. When looking straight ahead, the affected eye is intorted (turned in) because of the unopposed action of the medial, superior and inferior recti (Cranial nerve III).

A Cranial IV nerve palsy is a little more complex: In this case, when the eye is turned inwards it cannot look down affecting activity such as reading a book or walking down a flight of stairs. The superior oblique also normally produces a slight intorsion so that in these cases there is a subtle extorsion of the eye because of the unopposed action of the inferior oblique muscle. Often in these patients in order to compensate, they tilt their head towards the opposite shoulder in an attempt to counteract this extorsion (i.e. in a right IV palsy to bring the 11 o'clock up to 12 o'clock).

In addition the good eye tends to intort so as to align the oblique diplopia.

With a IIIrd nerve palsy there is complete ptosis of the eye lid. When the lid is held open, the eye looks down and out because of the unopposed action of the lateral rectus and the superior oblique muscles. In these patients, the diplopia improves looking laterally because the lateral rectus muscle is normal even though the eye cannot look inwards or upwards. The pupil is mydriatic and does not react to light or on accommodation because the PSNS fibres (transmitted in the inferior division of Cranial III) are lost. The consensual reflex in the opposite eye is, however, preserved.

Nerves of the Orbit: A Summary

- Seven nerves traverse the superior orbital fissure (Lacrimal, Frontal, Nasociliary, Trochlear, Abducent and the Superior and Inferior divisions of Cranial III). The lacrimal and frontal nerves and Cranial IV are extraconal. The lacrimal nerve is the most slender running on the lateral border of the lateral rectus muscle and innervating the periosteum and the orbital septum as well as being cutaneous for the outer upper eyelid. It is accompanied by the distal lacrimal artery supplying the conjunctival fornix. The frontal nerve lies between the levator and the orbital periosteum and is a large nerve innervating the mucous membrane of the frontal sinus and dividing into the supraorbital and supratrochlear nerves.
- The infraorbital and zygomatic branches of V_2 pass from the pterygopalatine fossa to the orbit via the inferior orbital fissure. The zygomatic nerve enters the zygomatico-orbital foramen as the zygomaticotemporal and the zygomaticofacial nerves before sending a communicating branch to the lacrimal nerve.
- The frontal and infraorbital nerves are cutaneous nerves using the orbit as a transit.
- The infraorbital nerve innervates the maxillary sinus and some upper teeth.

- The optic nerve is accompanied by the ophthalmic artery lying below and lateral to the nerve. It is covered with an extension of pia and subarachnoid and dura and is crossed from lateral to medial by the ophthalmic artery, the nasociliary nerve and the superior ophthalmic vein (Diagram 11.2). The ciliary ganglion lies lateral with the surrounding short ciliary nerves and vessels. The intracranial part of the optic nerve is supplied by the anterior cerebral artery with the posterior 2 cm of the nerve supplied in the orbit from the ophthalmic artery and the anterior 1 cm supplied by the central artery of the retina.
- The superior division of Cranial III innervates the superior rectus and the levator palpebrae superioris including SNS fibres from the cavernous plexus. The inferior division of Cranial III is much larger supplying the inferior and medial recti and the inferior oblique (the longest of the muscular nerves within the orbit). It transmits the PSNS root to the ciliary ganglion.
- The nasociliary nerve changes its official name twice becoming the anterior ethmoidal nerve (and then leaving the orbit to become the external nasal nerve). The nasociliary nerve crosses the optic nerve with the intervening ophthalmic artery and passes medially between the superior oblique and the superior rectus to enter the anterior ethmoidal foramen where it lies in the roof of the ethmoidal labyrinth. This nerve enters the nose at the side of the crista galli crossing the cribriform plate. Before entering this foramen, the nasociliary gives off the infratrochlear nerve just below the trochlea with a small accompanying artery supplying periosteum, the lacrimal sac and the conjunctiva and passing above the medial palpebral ligament to be distributed to the skin of the upper eyelid and the bridge of the nose. Within the cone of muscles the nasociliary gives off a number of branches:

  (a) Most distally is the posterior ethmoidal nerve which innervates the posterior ethmoidal and sphenoidal sinuses.
  (b) The sensory root of the ciliary ganglion leaves the nerve at the fibrous ring

(c) The long ciliary nerves pierce the posterior sclera (usually two in number) carrying the SNS fibres (and a few sensory fibres supplying the cornea with their cell bodies in the trigeminal ganglion). The long ciliary nerves run medial to
(d) The short ciliary nerves.

See Chap. 5 for discussion of the ciliary ganglion. To recap:

- The ganglion is minute (2 mm in diameter)
- It lies on the lateral side of the optic nerve in front of the ophthalmic artery about one third of the way from the apex of the orbit to the back of the eye.
- There are three roots which enter posteriorly:
  (a) A sensory root (a branch of the nasociliary nerve) innervating the eye, cornea, sclera, iris and ciliary body **but not the conjunctiva**.
  (b) The SNS root is a branch from the cavernous plexus with vasoconstrictor fibres to the vessels of the eye and with cell bodies in the superior cervical ganglion.
  (c) The PSNS root leaves the nerve to the inferior oblique and synapses in the ganglion (cell bodies in the Edinger-Westphal nucleus).

- Branches of the ciliary ganglion include:
  (a) Short ciliary nerves (usually >12 in number) containing fibres from all three roots to pierce the back of the sclera in the suprachoroidal space. Only the short ciliary nerves are concerned with accommodation.
  (b) Postganglionic fibres supplying the muscle of the ciliary body for accommodation with only about 3% innervating the sphincter pupillae (about 50 motor units in total). Sensory and SNS fibres supply the cornea, iris and ciliary body.

Vessels of the Orbit: A Summary

Ophthalmic artery: a branch of the ICA given off as the vessel emerges from the roof of the cavernous sinus with typically 10 (or more) branches accompanying all the branches of the naso-ciliary, frontal and lacrimal nerves supplying the ethmoidal air cells, the lateral wall of the nose, the external nose, the eyelids and the forehead. Anastomoses form with branches of the ECA (notably maxillary, facial and superficial temporal). Branches include:

- Anterior ethmoidal
- Posterior ethmoidal
- Lacrimal
- Supraorbital
- Supratrochlear
- Short ciliary
- Long ciliary
- Dorsal nasal
- Infratrochlear
- Posterior ciliary (choroid) and
- The Central Artery of the Retina

These last two vessels have no anastomoses.

Venous drainage is via the ophthalmic veins. The superior ophthalmic vein lies above the medial palpebral ligament with tributaries corresponding to the ophthalmic artery. This vein communicates with the angular facial vein and drains via the superior orbital fissure into the cavernous sinus. The inferior ophthalmic vein communicates with tributaries of the facial vein over the infraorbital margin running back to communicate with the superior ophthalmic vein to drain via the inferior orbital fissure into the pterygoid venous plexus.

Q & A: Chap. 11 (Answers at the End of This Chapter)

1. The orbit:
   (a) Is made up of 6 separate bones
   (b) Fractures of the floor are rare because of its thickness and orientation
   (c) Has an attachment of the lateral check ligament to Whitnall's tubercle
   (d) Has parallel lateral walls
2. The levator palpebrae superioris
   (a) Has no bony attachments
   (b) Attaches to the superior tarsal plate by penetrating the orbital septum
   (c) Is innervated by the inferior division of the oculomotor (III) nerve
   (d) The sympathetic supply comes from the superior cervical ganglion
   (e) Sympathetic supply to the visceral muscle compensates for somatic loss in a third nerve (Oculomotor) palsy
3. Regarding the nasolacrimal apparatus:
   (a) Some of the fibres of the levator palpebrae superioris are inserted into the lacrimal sac
   (b) Tearing is supported by the superior salivatory nucleus
   (c) The lachrymal gland is not visible through the conjunctiva
   (d) There is no mucus in the tears
4. In a trochlear nerve palsy
   (a) Patients typically have difficulty walking downstairs
   (b) The eye is neither extorted nor intorted
   (c) The unaffected eye may intort slightly
   (d) Diplopia is most commonly vertically disposed
5. Concerning the optical axes of the eye:
   (a) The visual axis connects an object in space with the fovea
   (b) The fovea lies in line with the pupillary axis
   (c) There is an angle between the optical and visual axes
   (d) There is no impact of differences in the optical and visual axis on the centralization of the cornea during refractive surgery

6. A blow-out fracture of the orbit
   (a) Commonly presents with diplopia on looking downwards
   (b) Commonly presents with diplopia on looking upwards
   (c) May present initially with enophthalmos
   (d) Does not have a maxillary sinus collection
   (e) Has a characteristic tear drop sign on CT scanning
7. The superior orbital fissure
   (a) Forms between the lesser and greater wings of the sphenoid
   (b) Transmits the ethmoidal vessels and nerve
   (c) Connects the middle cranial fossa with the orbit
   (d) Is a portal for cavernous sinus thrombosis
   (e) Transmits the postganglionic parasympathetic fibres for pupillary constriction
8. The optic canal
   (a) Traverses the greater wing of the sphenoid
   (b) Transmits the ophthalmic artery
   (c) May be duplicated
   (d) Is the widest part of the subarachnoid space surrounding the optic nerve

Answers

1. c
2. b, d
3. a, b
4. a, d
5. a, c
6. b, c, e
7. a, c, d
8. b, c

Reference

1. Shin K-J, Lee S-H, Park M-G, Shin HJ, Lee AG. Location of the accessory infraorbital foramen with reference to external landmarks and its clinical implications. Sci Rep. 2020;10:8566. https://doi.org/10.1038/s41598-020-65330-4.

The Nose and Paranasal Sinuses

12

Contents

Blood and Nerve Supply to the Lateral Nose and the Nasal Septum (Diagram 12.3) 262
Blood Supply 262
Nerve Supply 264
Paranasal Sinuses: (Diagram 12.4) 266
Maxillary Sinus 266
Ethmoid Sinus 267
Frontal Sinus 268
Sphenoidal Sinus 269
Waldeyer's Ring and the Adenoids (Nasopharyngeal Tonsil) 270
Anatomy of the Eustachian Tube 271
Q & A: Chap. 12 (Answers at the End of This Chapter) 274
Answers 275
References 275

The nose extends from the anterior nares to the posterior nasal septum, demonstrating a complicated nerve and blood supply and a particular relationship to the nasopharynx (opening via the posterior nasal apertures or choanae). Appreciation of its blood supply is of clinical importance in the management of severe epistaxis.

The nasal cavity is lined by respiratory (pseudostratified ciliated columnar) epithelium with a highly vascular mucosa which acts an air warmer and humidifier. The conchae increase

A. Zbar, *Anatomy--Head and Neck*,
https://doi.org/10.1007/978-3-031-69538-4_12

the overall surface area. As the inspired air is moistened, local mucus assists in particulate trapping. Note: the vestibule is located just inside the nostrils and is lined by stratified squamous epithelium. The olfactory area is evident in the roof and the upper nasal septum. The floor is the roof of the mouth (hard palate) and the lateral wall comprises (from above) the medial orbit (ethmoidal air cells) and the medial maxillary sinus (below). See Diagram 12.1.

In coronal section the nasal cavity is pear-shaped with the three conchae (or turbinates) projecting inwards, the largest of which is the inferior concha. The nasal septum has a particular framework incorporating the vomer, the perpendicular plate of the ethmoid and the septal cartilage. Most have a deviated septum which is evident on prosected specimens and dependent upon the precise nature of the sagittal split to demonstrate the conchae and meatuses. This effect is also noted on MRI images of the region.

The lateral wall of the nose is best appreciated in the dried skull where it curves inferiorly over the body of the sphenoid to become the nasopharynx. There are three conchae with the most inferior being the longest and broadest and the superior concha the smallest. The middle and the upper conchae are joined anteriorly and diverge posteriorly. The flat area in front of the conchae is called the nasal atrium.

- The space beneath each concha is the meatus and above and behind the superior concha the space is the *spheno-ethmoidal recess* (draining the sphenoid sinus).
- The posterior ethmoidal air cells drain into the superior meatus.
- The nasolacrimal duct opens into the front of the inferior meatus (about 2 cm behind the nostril).
- The sphenopalatine foramen lies just behind the posterior end of the middle concha.
- All the other openings of sinuses are into the middle meatus (which has the most complex internal structure).

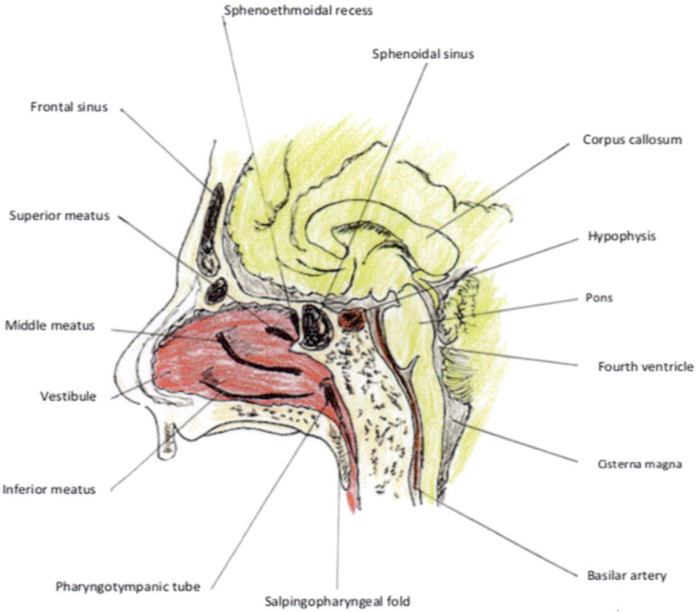

Diagram 12.1 Sagittal section through the nasopharynx. The Eustachian tube is superiorly limited by the *torus tubarius* and forms an inverted 'J-shape' because of the fold of the salpingopharyngeus muscle merging into the side wall of the pharynx. The soft palate closes against the pharynx at *Passavant's ridge*

Diagram 12.1.

Beneath the middle concha the middle meatus has a swelling (or convex bulge) called the *bulla ethmoidalis* (ethmoidal bulla) which accepts the drainage of the middle ethmoidal air cells. Beneath the bulla there is a distinct semicircular slit (*hiatus semilunaris*) which drains the remainder of the paranasal sinuses; the frontal sinus opening into the infundibulum at the anterior end of the hiatus, the anterior ethmoidal air cells opening nearby and the maxillary sinus which drains into the posterior end of the hiatus.

Despite the fact that the ostium is often duplicated it can readily be noted that the bulk of the maxillary sinus sits dependently in relation to the ostium (i.e. the floor of the maxillary sinus lies at a lower level than the floor of the nasal cavity). This anatomical relationship explains why maxillary sinusitis is most common. Nowadays this can be surgically relieved by functional endoscopic sinus surgical (FESS) drainage but in the past, the Caldwell-Luc operation was performed for treatment whereby the front wall of the maxillary sinus was opened into the mouth (behind the upper lip) and the mucosa of the mouth was sewn to the mucoperiosteum of the maxillary sinus so as to deliberately create a fistula for sinus drainage.[1] A second opening of the maxillary sinus may lead into the middle meatus just superior to the middle of the attachment to the inferior concha. Of interest, the position of the opening of the frontal sinus favours the flow of material towards the opening of the maxillary sinus. This design additionally permits infection to spread from the frontal to the maxillary sinus. The anatomy of the sinus drainage is shown in Diagram 12.2. The lower image of this Diagram shows detail of the middle meatus after the middle concha is cut off to show the hiatus semilunaris.

To summarize:

The nasal cavity is about 5 cm in height and 5–7 cm in length. It is narrow transversely (1.5 cm at the floor and 1–2 mm at the roof) with the width further reduced by the presence of the conchae. The middle part of the roof is the cribriform plate of the ethmoid with the anterior part formed by the nasal part of the frontal bone, the nasal bone and the nasal cartilage. The posterior roof is the anterior and inferior surfaces of the body of the sphenoid. The floor is formed by the palatine process of the maxilla and filled in by the horizontal process of the palatine bone.

The ethmoidal air sinuses include the anterior, middle and posterior cells which are squeezed into the space between the upper part of the nasal cavity and the orbit. The lateral wall of the nose comprises the vestibule (the area above the nostril with true skin and filtering vibrissae), the atrium of the middle meatus (just above the nostril internally) and the area in front of the middle meatus.

[1]Named after George W. Caldwell and Henri Luc who independently described this antrostomy in 1893 and 1897 respectively.

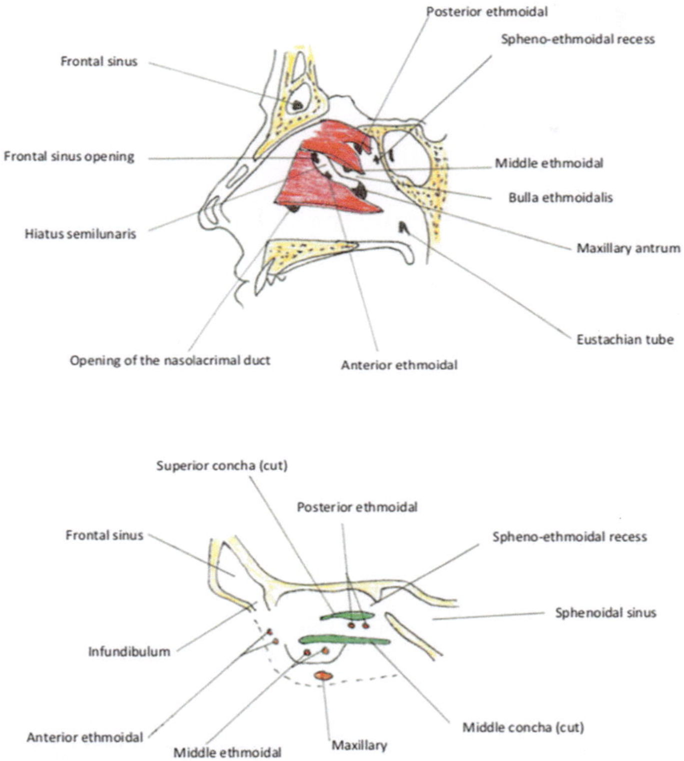

Diagram 12.2 Appearance of the nasal meatuses. The *top image* shows the complete arrangement with detail of the *hiatus semilunaris*. The *bottom image* focuses on the middle concha and meatus showing the entry points. The maxillary ostium is dependent with the flow from the frontal sinus running downwards via the infundibulum. The anterior ethmoidal sinuses can enter directly into the infundibulum on occasion rather than into the anterior middle meatus

An additional elevation is often noted here, the *agger nasi*, (also called the nasoturbinal concha) which is more prominent in some mammals (dogs and birds) where the continual humidification of air allows a greater running or flying endurance. The agger nasi may contain ethmoidal air cells that have arisen within part of the lacrimal bone and a large collection may interfere with adequate frontal sinus drainage. The nasal conchae (and meatuses) divide up the airway, forcing the air to flow around the largest possible surface area. The upper two conchae are processes of the ethmoid bone whereas the inferior concha is an independent bone.

Blood and Nerve Supply to the Lateral Nose and the Nasal Septum (Diagram 12.3)

Blood Supply

An appreciation of the blood supply is important in the control of epistaxis. The area represents a watershed of ECA (external carotid artery) and ICA (internal carotid artery) anastomosis.

- The main artery of the nasal cavity is the *sphenopalatine artery* (the terminal nasal part of the maxillary artery) which supplies the mucosa over the conchae and the nasal septum.
- For consensus and definition, the lower anterior part of the septum is called ***Little's area*** representing the anastomosis between the septal branch of the superior labial (a branch of the facial artery entering via the nostril) and the ascending branch of the greater palatine artery (which enters via the incisive canal). This area houses the **anastomotic plexus of Kiesselbach** (the commonest site for an epistaxis).[2]
- The roof and the anterior part of the lateral wall is supplied respectively by the posterior and the anterior ethmoidal arteries.

In simple terms the septum is divisible into quadrants of blood supply; namely, Anterosuperior and Postero-superior as well as Anteroinferior and Posteroinferior.

The Anterosuperior supply is provided by the anterior ethmoidal artery with the Posterosuperior supply from the posterior

[2]Named after James Lawrence Little (1836–1885) an American surgeon who described the area in 1879 and Wilhelm Kiesselbach (1839–1902) a German ENT surgeon who published an article on the anastomosis in 1884.

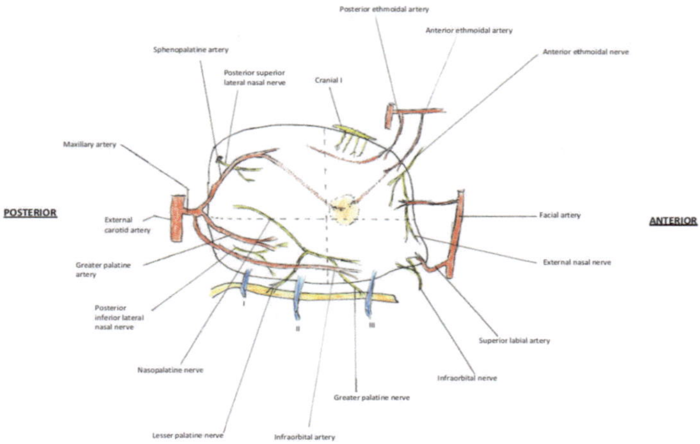

Diagram 12.3 Blood and nerve supply of the lateral nasal wall and the nasal septum. The lateral nasal wall can be divided into an upper and lower anterior and posterior segment. Kiesselbach's anastomosis represents the collateral connexion between the ophthalmic (ICA) and the maxillary (ECA) arteries. This is the commonest area of bleeding (Little's area) in epistaxis (*see text*). The nerve supply can be divided diagonally into an upper and a lower component. Specialized neuroepithelium in the roof of the nose leads via 15–20 *fila olfactoria* through the cribriform plate to the olfactory bulb. Venous drainage is into the facial vein and IJV (I), pharyngeal plexus (II) and the maxillary vein through to the pterygoid plexus (III)

ethmoidal artery. Both of these arteries are branches of the ophthalmic artery (ICA system).

Most of the Postero-inferior blood supply is via the sphenopalatine artery which is joined by the greater palatine artery (below the hard palate) that sends branches through the incisive canal into the Kiesselbach anastomosis. The Anteroinferior supply is largely from the superior labial branch of the facial artery entering through the nostril.

Examination of the lateral nasal wall shows slight differences from the septum in the posterior blood supply. The anterosuperior element is as for the septum (via the anterior and posterior ethmoidal arteries). Posteriroly the lateral nose is supplied by the terminal divisions of the maxillary artery (the sphenopalatine artery, the lateral posterior superior nasal artery and inferiorly from the infraorbital artery). Antero-inferiorly is the superior labial facial artery (*as per* the nasal septum).

Venous drainage is multiple and complex with drainage:

- Via the sphenopalatine foramen into the pterygoid plexus
- Anteriorly into the facial vein
- To the pharyngeal venous plexus
- Via the inferior ophthalmic veins, the inferior cerebral veins
- Via the ethmoidal foraminae and the cribriform plate and
- Rarely via the foramen caecum at the base of the crista galli (usually not patent) directly into the superior sagittal sinus.

Nerve Supply

This is equally best conceptualized in quadrants that somewhat mirror the blood supply. There is a specialized olfactory area in the roof including the olfactory bulb and the olfactory filaments (*fila olfactoria*). This area (near the superior concha and the corresponding septum) contains the olfactory receptors and the cell bodies of bipolar cells whose central processes coalesce as 20 or so olfactory filaments which pierce the cribriform plate to reach the anterior cranial fossa and synapse with the mitral cells of the olfactory bulb sitting on the under surface of the frontal lobe.

The vestibule is innervated by the infraorbital nerve.

The lateral wall of the respiratory area is innervated by the Anterior ethmoidal nerve (at the front), the Anterior superior alveolar nerve (Upper and Lower anterior), the Lateral Posterior Superior Nasal (Upper Posterior) and by the greater palatine (Lower Posterior).

In summary: The nerves supplying the lateral nasal wall are:

1. Anterior ethmoidal nerve (antero-superior)
2. Posterior ethmoidal nerve (Postero-superior)
3. Infraorbital nerve (antero-inferior—via the anterior superior alveolar branch of V_2)

4. Posterior lateral superior nasal (Postero-superiorly)
5. Posterior inferior nasal (a branch of the greater palatine nerve).

By contrast, the nasal septum is better conceptualized as a diagonal (above and below a line drawn across the septum) such that innervation is into a front and a back half.

1. In the part above and anterior is the anterior ethmoidal with the at the posterior superior nasal postero-superiorly.
2. Postero-inferior is the nasopalatine nerve grooving the vomer (This nerve used to be called the long sphenopalatine nerve as it traverses the sphenopalatine foramen). The nasopalatine nerve is a branch of the pterygopalatine ganglion which runs across the nasal septum to join the greater palatine nerve via the incisive canal (as well as the contralateral nasopalatine nerve). The nasopalatine nerve innervates palatal structures around the anterior maxillary teeth and the nasal septum.
3. Antero-inferiorly is the anterior superior alveolar nerve (whose continuation is the infraorbital nerve).

At this time it is best to examine a longitudinal section of a skull (if available) in order to note that the septum consists of the vomer, the ethmoid and the septal cartilage. The vomer is fixed to the rostrum of the sphenoid by alae forming the posterior border of the septum which slots into a groove on the palate and which extends forward to itself be grooved by the sphenopalatine artery on each side (See Diagram 6.4c; Chap. 6). The posterior bony septum can be seen to fall a little short of the anterior part of the vomer with this space being filled in by the septal cartilage. The roof is formed by the cribriform plate which is completed front and back by the sphenoid.

Laterally is the frontal process of the maxilla and below is the palatine bone which sends a vertical (perpendicular) plate across the posterior part of the maxillary hiatus. This palatal perpendicular plate bifurcates into an orbital and a sphenoidal process articulating with the maxilla (in the floor of the orbit) and with the body of the sphenoid. This arrangement encloses the sphenopalatine foramen as it leads away from the pterygopalatine fossa to the lateral wall of the nose just above the back end of the middle concha.

Paranasal Sinuses: (Diagram 12.4)

Each of the sinuses is lined by a respiratory (pseudostratified ciliated) epithelium.

Maxillary Sinus

This sinus is pyramidal with the roof formed by the orbital floor, and the floor the alveolar process of the maxilla lying below the level of the floor of the nose. There is some additional contribution by the lacrimal, ethmoid, inferior turbinate and the perpendicular plate of the palatine. The medial part abutting directly against the nasal mucosa is called the fontanelle, an area crossed

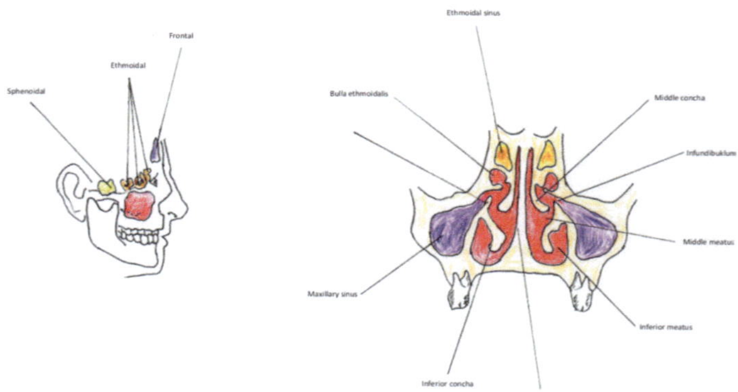

Diagram 12.4 Anatomy of the paranasal sinuses. The *left-hand image* shows the lateral sinus position and the *right-hand image* shows a coronal view of the drainage of the ethmoidal and maxillary sinuses. This appearance is evident in exquisite detail with CT scanning

and divided by the uncinate process. There can be a limited amount of bone against the molar teeth making dental extraction a risk for the formation of a sinus fistula [1]. The temporal fossa lies laterally and the pterygopalatine fossa medially. The location of a smaller accessory ostium (in about 15% of cases) is usually in the larger posterior fontanelle region and usually behind the natural ostium. The primary ostium lies well back and high up on the nasal wall. Recurrent sinusitis is more common in those with such an accessory ostium, likely a result of a circular flow of mucus between the two sites. This is usually managed by connecting the two ostia surgically. Occasionally extensions are noted infraorbitally (more an extension of the anterior ethmoidal sinus called a Haller cell) which may affect drainage.[3]

The rich blood supply is derived from the sphenopalatine, infraorbital, greater palatine, posterior lateral nasal, posterior superior alveolar and facial arteries. Venous drainage is via the pterygoid plexus. The V_2 divisional nerve supply is via the superior alveolar, (posterior, middle and anterior) as well as the greater palatine and infraorbital nerves with the greatest sensitivity around the ostium. Lymphatic drainage is to the submandibular nodes. The sinus is evident intra-utero and grows in size in the first 3 years of life and in a second phase between 7 and 12 years of age with full pneumatization and extension occurring at maturity.

Ethmoid Sinus

The ethmoidal sinuses are divided into anterior, middle and posterior elements lying between the orbit and the nose. The bone of this region comprises the crista galli, the cribriform plate, the perpendicular plate and the ethmoidal labyrinth. The lateral wall of the labyrinth is very thin (the *lamina papyracea*) forming part of

[3]Named after Albrecht von Haller (1708–1777) a renowned Swiss anatomist and polymath.

the medial orbital wall. The labyrinth comprises middle and superior turbinates and ethmoidal air cells. The anterior ethmoid has more air cells than the larger posterior ethmoid with the anterior (and middle) draining into the middle meatus and the posterior into the superior meatus (Diagram 12.2). The posterior ethmoidal air cells are closed by the fusion of the orbital process of the palatine bone with the sphenoidal concha and can extend as far backwards as to lie adjacent to the optic nerve (Onodi's cell).[4]

Blood supply to this area is from the anterior and posterior ethmoidal arteries, the supraorbital and the sphenopalatine (a collateral ICA/ECA network). The anterior ethmoidal foramen is within the lamina papyracea behind the anterior lacrimal crest whereas the posterior ethmoidal foramen lies further back. The nerve supply comes from the supraorbital, anterior and posterior ethmoidal and posterior lateral superior nasal nerves. Posterior ethmoidal air cells may be dually innervated (via V_1 and V_2 branches of the trigeminal) which may represent points of facial referral of pain during sinusitis. The sinuses are evident in foetal life and rapidly pneumatize after the first year of age until adolescence.

Frontal Sinus

These sinuses asymmetrically form within the squamous part of the frontal bone. The frontal sinus is the only sinus not evident at birth. The inner table of bone adjacent to the anterior cranial fossa may be very thin allowing infection to spread intracranially. This effect may be enhanced by the presence of a rich venous drainage channel network through small foramina (of Breschet) and which

[4]Named after Adolf Onodi (1857–1919), a Hungarian ophthalmologist who described this extension of the posterior ethmoid sinuses near the sphenoid and anterior clinoid process in 1904.

if not removed during frontal sinus obliteration may lead to postoperative mucocele formation.[5]

The ostium is located posteriorly and medially with the system forming an hour-glass drainage into the front of the middle meatus or against the uncinate process of the ethmoid and via the ethmoidal infundibulum. The blood supply includes the supratrochlear, supraorbital and anterior ethmoidal arteries and the nerve supply is derived from the supraorbital and supratrochlear nerves. Skin over this area drains into preauricular lymph nodes whereas the sinus itself drains to the submandibular lymph node group.

Sphenoidal Sinus

These are asymmetrical with a single medial ostium draining into the spheno-ethmoidal recess (usually just superomedial to the tail of the superior concha). It is a vital part of anatomy because of its relationship to the pituitary (for the conduct of a transsphenoidal hypophysectomy), the cavernous sinuses, the ICA and the V_2 nerves. The sinus has variable pneumatization creating a classification that includes:

A Conchal type (anterior part only pneumatized), a Presellar type (pneumatized up to the sella turcica) and a Sellar type (pneumatized as far as the pituitary fossa). The sellar variant is the most common (55–60%) with the conchal variant seen in about 5% of cases. The type of pneumatization affects the conduct of trans-sphenoidal skull base surgery. The sphenoid sinus is evident at birth with pneumatization beginning by the third year. The arterial supply is from the posterior ethmoidal artery and the posterior septal artery. The latter is a branch which traverses the back of the sphenoid sinus from lateral to medial between the ostium and the choana and which is at risk of injury in endoscopic sinus surgery [2, 3]. Venous drainage is to the superior ophthalmic vein and innervation is from the posterior

[5]Diploic veins named after Gilbert Breschet (1784–1845) a French anatomist who succeeded Jean Cruvelhier (1791–1874) as Professor of Anatomy at the Facultie de Médécine di Paris.

ethmoidal nerve with the orbital branch of the pterygopalatine ganglion (zygomaticofacial V_2). Lymphatic drainage is to the retropharyngeal nodes.

Waldeyer's Ring and the Adenoids (Nasopharyngeal Tonsil)[6]

This ring (part of the Mucosa Associated Lymphoid Tissue—MALT) is the collection of lymphoid tissue of the upper aerodigestive tract that coalesces into three main tonsillar groups, the palatine, nasopharyngeal and lingual tonsils. The nasopharyngeal tonsil (adenoids) are pyramidal in shape lying at the back of the nasopharynx with the apex of the pyramid directed forward to the nasal septum. These are removed mostly in children for adenoidal hypertrophy associated with Eustachian tube dysfunction or recurrent otitis media as well as sleep apnoea-related disorders. Techniques vary including curettage with an adenotome and laser adenoidectomy. The relevant nerve supply is principally via the pharyngeal plexus (Cranial IX), but also from the posterior palatine branch of the maxillary nerve and some lingual fibres from the mandibular nerve.

The blood supply is rich including the ascending pharyngeal, ascending palatine, the tonsillar branch of the facial, the pharyngeal branch of the maxillary, the artery of the pterygoid canal and the basisphenoid artery (a branch of the inferior hypophyseal). To get to the adenoid, the ascending palatine artery passes upwards between the styloglossus and the stylopharyngeus from the main facial artery and then runs between the upper edge of the superior constrictor and the medial pterygoid muscles. Venous drainage is into the paratonsillar veins which pierce the superior constrictor muscle to join the pharyngeal venous plexus on their way to the IJV. Lymphatic drainage is to the retropharyngeal nodes.

[6] Named after Heinrich Wilhelm Gottfried Waldeyer (1836–1921) a renowned German anatomist and pathologist who coined the terms 'neuron' and 'chromosome'.

Anatomy of the Eustachian Tube

View of the lateral wall of the nasopharynx (Diagram 12.1) is dominated by the conchae and the pharyngeal opening of the pharyngotympanic (Eustachian or auditory) tube. The opening has a superior bulbous area covering (*torus tubarius*) which is partly formed by a cartilaginous expansion but also with lymphoid tissue that creates an effective tubal tonsil. This tissue can be closely applied to the adenoids and may be removed in part during an adenoidectomy, sometimes compromising the integrity of the Eustachian tube.[7] There is an osseous posterolateral portion and a fibrocartilaginous anteromedial portion.

The Eustachian tube is about 3.5 cm long with a bony part lying between the tympanic and petrous portions of the temporal bone (See Diagram 6.6; Chap. 6) and a cartilaginous anteromedial two-thirds which lies between the petrous temporal and the posterior border of the greater wing of the sphenoid. By passing a probe into the pharyngeal orifice it can be appreciated that the tube runs superiorly and then posteriorly and laterally. A fold above the palate and below the opening of the tube is formed by the levator palati muscle with the tube running between this muscle and the tensor palati. This appearance gives the impression of the opening surrounded by a structure that looks like the letter 'j' where the long limb of the 'j' is formed by the salpingopharyngeal fold (mucosa overlying the salpingopharyngeus muscle). This fold can be seen to merge into the side of the pharyngeal wall.

The task of the tube is to equalize the pressure in the middle ear with the atmospheric pressure allowing freedom of movement of the tympanic membrane. This route also, however, permits infections to pass from the nasopharynx to the middle ear. The former function explains why the use of the Valsalva manoeuver (blowing the nose out against a closed glottis) increases (and equalizes) the pressures (as may occur in a commercial flight). This can be uncomfortable generating extra pressures in the system of between 20 and

---

[7]The tubal tonsil is also called Gerlachs' tonsil after Joseph Gerlach (1820–1896) a German anatomist.

40 mmHg. It will also explain why chewing and yawning are alternative methods successful in such pressure equalization where the tensor palati muscle attachment to the cartilaginous portion of the tube itself encourages opening.[8] The pharyngobasilar fascia is also attached to the lower end of the tube along with the tensor palati laterally (with an origin that is extrapharyngeal) and the levator palati (with an intrapharyngeal origin). Swallowing then pulls on the lower wall to open the tube and equilibrate the pressures.

The blood supply of the tube is from the ascending pharyngeal and middle meningeal arteries with the veins draining into the pharyngeal plexus. The nerve supply is via the pharyngeal branch of the pterygopalatine ganglion (at the ostium) and from the nervus spinosus (meningeal branch of V_3) innervating the cartilaginous part. The bony part is innervated by branches of the tympanic plexus (Cranial IX).

Diagram 12.5 shows greater structural detail of the Eustachian tube (modified after an illustration by Rüdinger) [4, 5]. The tubal lumen is separated into two parts, a Rudinger safety canal filled with mucus and air which tends to remain open in most adults and which is part of the equalization and ventilation function and a musculomembranous portion below called the auxillary gap which act as microturbinates assisting ciliary clearance. Between the tubal cartilage and the skull base lie suspensory ligaments which are surrounded by specialized fascia (a lateral fascia over the tensor palati separating it from the medial pterygoid) and a medial fascia (running from the lateral tubal lamina to the salpingopharyngeus). Closure of the tube is completed by a lateral fat pad (of Ostmann).[9]

There are four muscles around the tube that contribute to function; the tensor palati, the levator palati, the medial pterygoid and the salpingopharyngeus. The principal muscle is the tensor palati (see Chap. 13) which acts during swallowing and yawning the medial part of the

[8]Named after Antonio Valsalva (1666–1723) an Italian anatomist who also described the structure of the aortic and pulmonary vale cusps.

[9]Named after Paul Ostmann (1859–1945) a German otologist. The lateral fascia described is also called the Weber-Liel fascia and the medial fascia is referred to as the fascial plane of von Tröltsch named after Anton von Tröltsch (1829–1890) a German otologist.

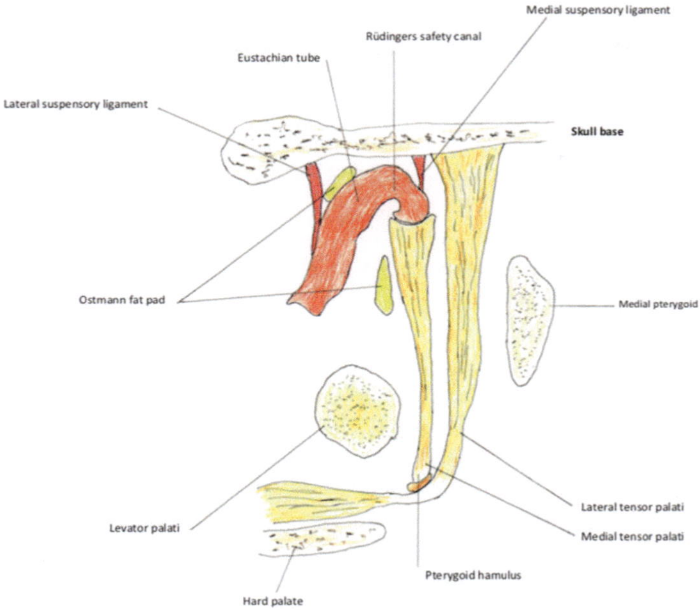

Diagram 12.5 Structural detail of the Eustachian tube (*after* Rüdinger). An Ostmann fat pad surrounds the tube which is suspended medially and laterally. The tube has a central safety canal bordered by medial and lateral tubal cartilage. The bottom of the pterygoid hamulus is protected by a small bursa. There are extensive mucosal folds in the lower part of the medial wall of the auxillary gap (between the medial tubal cartilage and the lateral Ostmann fat pad)

muscle arising from the tubal cartilage. Its action on the tube is complex with the medial part opening the tube by lateralizing the cartilaginous lamina (a ventilatory support mechanism). The lateral part of the muscle compresses the distal tube supporting protection. The medial pterygoid is a chewing muscle that closes the mouth which shifts the tensor palati and assists in tubal opening like a pivot point and acting as a mechanical functional unit. The levator palati has no direct attachment to the cartilaginous tube but indirectly moves the tube superomedially to assist in tubal drainage. The salpingopharyngeus is one of the three internal pharyngeal muscles (stylopharyngeus, salpingopharyngeus and palatopharyngeus discussed in Chap. 14). Each of these is a pharyngeal elevator with some of the attachments of the salpingopharyngeus to the floor of the tube as an antagonist to the tensor and levator palati actions. The salpingopharyngeus acts like an anchor chain to hold the tube in place as the palati muscles tend to roll the medial lamina of the tube forward.

Q & A: Chap. 12 (Answers at the End of This Chapter)

1. Little's area of the nasal wall
   (a) Is the commonest site for epistaxis
   (b) Is located in the posterosuperior part of the nasal cavity
   (c) Reflects the Kiesselbach anastomosis between the facial and the anterior ethmoidal arteries
   (d) The communicating greater palatine artery enters the region via the incisive canal
   (e) Is innervated by the posterior lateral superior nasal nerve and the middle superior alveolar nerves
2. In the nose, the bulla ethmoidalis
   (a) Is the opening of the posterior ethmoidal air cells
   (b) Is part of the middle concha which joins the upper concha posteriorly
   (c) Lies on top of the hiatus semilunaris
   (d) Has the maxillary sinus opening anteriorly
3. The nasal septum
   (a) Is supplied in its upper half by the anterior and posterior ethmoidal arteries
   (b) Is supplied in the lower half by the sphenopalatine artery
   (c) Has an identical blood supply with the lateral nasal wall
   (d) Has a venous drainage exclusively to the pterygoid plexus
4. The Eustachian tube
   (a) Is kept open by the Ostmann fat pad
   (b) Is innervated in its bony part by the pharyngeal nerve
   (c) Is normally collapsed
   (d) Is supplied by the middle meningeal artery in its bony part

5. The nasal septum is formed by:
   (a) The horizontal plate of the ethmoid bone
   (b) The vomer
   (c) The crest of the maxilla
   (d) The palatine bone
6. Concerning the conchae
   (a) The inferior concha is the smallest
   (b) The inferior concha is responsible for the largest amount of airflow direction and humidification
   (c) They do not alter the pressurization of airflow
   (d) The superior concha protects the olfactory bulb

Answers

1. a, d
2. c
3. a
4. d
5. b, c
6. b, d

References

1. Van den Bergh JP, ten Bruggenkate CM, Disch FJ, Tuinzing DB. Anatomical aspects of sinus floor elevations. Clin Oral Implants Res. 2000;11(3):256–65.
2. Lee JH. Endoscopic view of the posterior septal branch of the sphenopalatine artery. Ear Nose Throat J. 2013;92(4–5):170. https://doi.org/10.1177/014556131309200404.
3. Zhang X, Wang EW, Wei H, Snyderman CH, Gardner PA, Fernandez-Miranda JC. Anatomy of the posterior septal artery with surgical implications on the vascularized pedicled nasoseptal flap. Head Neck. 2015;37(10):1470–6.
4. Leuwer R. Anatomy of the Eustachian tube. Otolaryngol Clinics North Am. 2016;49(5):1097–106.
5. Rüdinger N. Vergleichende Anatomie und Histologie der Ohrtrompete. München: JJ Lentneŕsche Bucchandlung; 1870.

The Mouth and Palate 13

Contents

Brief Anatomy of the Teeth........ 278
Anatomy of the Palate and Palatal Musculature........ 281
Anatomy of the Soft Palate........ 282
Tensor Palati........ 284
Levator Palati........ 284
Palatoglossus........ 286
Palatopharyngeus........ 286
Musculus uvulae........ 288
Palatine Tonsil........ 288
Q & A: Chap. 13 (Answers at the End of This Chapter)........ 297
Answers........ 298
Reference........ 298

The region of the mouth extends backwards to the palatoglossal arches (the anterior pillars of the fauces). The area in front of the gums and cheeks is referred to as the vestibule and that area inside the teeth is the cavity proper. Visible is opening of the parotid duct (of Stensen) opposite the upper second molar and there may be additional openings of separate molar glands as well as numerous buccal and labial glands.

The nerve supply is the buccal nerve (the buccal branch of V_3), the mental nerve (from the inferior alveolar) and the infraorbital nerve (V_2). The upper gums are innervated by the leash of superior

A. Zbar, *Anatomy--Head and Neck*,
https://doi.org/10.1007/978-3-031-69538-4_13

alveolar nerves as well as by the greater palatine and nasopalatine nerves. The lower gums are innervated by the inferior alveolar, buccal and lingual nerves.

The *buccinator* forms the muscle layer of the cheek and follows the line of the teeth passing deep to the masseter muscle. Buccinator is continuous with the superior constrictor in origin from the pterygomandibular raphe (buccinator running forwards and the superior constrictor backwards). (See Diagram 8.1; Chap. 8). Buccinator lies between the buccopharyngeal fascia outside and the pharyngobasilar fascia inside (See Chap. 2) where in children this is filled with fat creating the infantile suctorial pad. The molar glands lie external to the buccinator near the entry of the parotid duct. The parotid duct itself passes above the buccal fat pad to pierce buccinator.

In the floor of the mouth there is the median fold of mucous membrane stretching to the tongue (the *frenulum*) which bulges upwards as the sublingual fold and which ends anteriorly as the sublingual papilla receiving multiple sublingual gland ducts. On the apex of the papilla is the submandibular duct (of Wharton).

The roof is the vaulted palate, the anterior 2/3 of which is the hard (bony) palate with the posterior 1/3 of soft palate. The uvula lies free posteriorly. Behind the incisive fossa is a midline raphe which can on occasion be visible in the living subject through the mucous membrane where the mucosa is thrown into 3–4 transverse palatal folds or ridges. Behind the third molar tooth is the pterygoid hamulus which is palpable.

The term fauces represents the region between the mouth and the pharynx containing the palatine tonsils (between the palatoglossal and the palatopharyngeal arches). The mouth joins the pharynx at the isthmus of the fauces and is so bound by the soft palate, the palatoglossal arches and the dorsum of the tongue.

Brief Anatomy of the Teeth

Outside of dentistry, this area of anatomy is infrequently considered (even though general anatomists and physicians often teach dental students). The bulk of the tooth consists of the dentine (a hard avascular calcified component penetrated by miniscule dentinal tubules). The part of the tooth that projects outwards is the crown which is covered by enamel (the crown is the functional component lying visibly above the gum). The root is held in the jaw (the unseen component fastening to the jaw) which is covered by the cementum so that the visible crown is less tissue than the anatomical crown. The root attaches to the tooth-bearing jaw (the alveolar processes) via the fibrous periodontal ligament. The neck forms at the junction of the enamel with the cementum so that at this point the dentine is not exposed. Inside the dentine lies the pulp cavity which connects to the outside via the root canal and the apical foramen with the cavity packed with dental pulp, nerves, blood vessels and lymphatics which enter via the foramen. To reiterate, the outer layer is inorganic enamel, the middle layer the dentine (similar to bone in its composition) and the innermost component is the pulp.

Of note:

- The shape of the teeth are functional so that incisors bite and cut (as well as pluck and tear), canines hold tightly and molars and premolars chew (and grind).
- There are the upper molars with three roots (two on the convexity and one on the concavity), the lower molars with two roots (one anterior and one posterior) and all the other teeth which usually have a single root. The incisor crowns are chisel-like and the canines pyramidal. The premolars have a lingual and a buccal cusp (hence bicuspids) with the upper molars possessing four and the lower molars five crown cusps.
- The pulp is sensitive but most of the dentine and all of the enamel and cementum are insensate. The innervation between the pulp and the periodontal ligament is shared but distinctly separate from that of the overlying gum. In the upper jaw:

  (a) it is the posterior superior alveolar nerve with the first molar and two premolars innervated by the middle superior alveolar nerve (also the two premolars).
  (b) The anterior superior alveolar nerve innervates the canines and incisors.

In the lower jaw the three molars and two premolars are innervated by the inferior alveolar nerve with some canine and incisors central overlap.

Knowledge of this anatomy is vital for dental anaesthesia:

For the bottom teeth an inferior alveolar blockade is needed often with associated infiltration of the buccal and lingual nerves. The inferior alveolar and lingual nerves are approached by inserting a needle through the buccinator (above the occlusal surface level of the molar) and in front of the pterygomandibular raphe. This is evident as a palpable ridge in the open mouth lying just behind the mandibular ramus. Supplemental anaesthesia is added just above the mandibular nerve in order to pick up the inferior alveolar nerve as it enters the mandibular foramen.

Note too that the attachment of the mylohyoid muscle to the mylohyoid line of the mandible lies below the apices of the teeth so that an apical abscess will point into the mouth. However, the second and third molar apices lie below this mylohyoid line and in these cases an apical abscess can dangerously point into the neck.

The adult has 16 permanent teeth in each jaw (2 incisors, 1 canine, 2 premolars and 3 molars). Milk dentition comprises 10 teeth in each jaw (2 incisors, 1 canine and 2 molars). In formation teeth develop as ectodermal buds where the enamel produced provokes a mesodermal reaction that differentiates into the dentine and the cementum. The growing tooth (primary enamel organ) consists of ameloblasts (enamel producing cells) and odontoblasts (producing dentine) These dental germ remnants may be the source of uncommon dental tumours and retention cysts. On average the timeline for deciduous teeth is such that:

Tooth	Eruption time (months)
Lower central incisor	6
Upper central incisor	7
Upper lateral incisor	8
Lower lateral incisor	9
First molars	12
Canines	18
Second molars	24

On average the timeline for permanent teeth is such that:

Tooth	Eruption time (years)
First permanent molars	6
Central incisor	7
Lateral incisors	8
First premolars	9
Second premolars	10
Canines	11
Third permanent molars (Wisdom teeth)	12

The usual chronology is for the lower teeth to precede their upper jaw fellow (opposite number) with the first permanent molar typically erupting before the deciduous are shed and with the second premolar coming in after deciduous shedding so that the order for replacement is: incisors, molars and then canines (*See Table above*). The decidua are smaller with a relatively large pulp chamber.

Anatomy of the Palate and Palatal Musculature

The hard palate comprises the palatal process of the maxilla and the horizontal plate of the palatine bone creating a mammalian premaxilla. The greater palatine foramen lies between these two bones with the lesser palatine foraminae behind this level (beyond the last molar tooth). The blood supply is by the greater palatine artery emerging from the greater palatine foramen lying lateral to the nerve and entering the incisive foramen. Venous drainage is towards the pterygoid and pharyngeal plexi. The palate is innervated by the greater palatine nerve as far forward as the incisive foramen and the anterior palate via the nasopalatine nerves.

Concerning bony structure, the palatine bone is located at the back of the nasal cavity squeezed between the maxilla and the pterygoid processes of the sphenoid bone (See Chap. 6). The palatine completes the floor of the nasal cavity, the roof of the mouth and a small sliver of the floor of the orbit. The connecting points include the pterygopalatine fossa and the inferior orbital foramen.

The bone itself has a horizontal and a perpendicular plate with the pyramidal process (or tubercle) directed backwards from the junction point of the two plates and then separate orbital and sphenoidal processes as part of the perpendicular plate. These two processes are separated by the sphenopalatine notch which completes the lower part of the sphenopalatine foramen (transmitting the sphenopalatine branch of the maxillary artery and the nasopalatine nerve).

The horizontal plate forms the back of the hard palate and has the tendinous tensor palati muscle stretched over it with the posterior limit of the bone forming the posterior nasal spine for attachment of the musculuus uvulae (*see below*). Anteriorly there is an articulation with the palatine process of the maxilla. The perpendicular plate forms part of the inferior and also the middle meatuses of the nasal cavity anteriorly. This section of bone also forms part of the medial wall of the pterygopalatine fossa as well as part of the medial wall of the maxillary sinus at the back end of the hiatus semilunaris. Posteriorly with the maxilla this part of the palatine bone completes the greater palatine canal for transmission of the descending and then greater palatine nerve and vessels. The sphenoidal process articulates with the root of the vaginal process of the medial pterygoid plate and so completes the formation of the palatovaginal canal transmitting the pharyngeal artery and nerve. The medial border of the sphenoidal process articulates with the ala of the vomer (Diagram 4c; Chap. 6).

Anatomy of the Soft Palate

The soft palate is a complex muscular structure which fuses at the side walls of the pharynx and which closes off the nasopharynx during swallowing. The soft palate is strictly an aponeurotic structure the shape and position of which changes by the muscular action of five paired muscles (Diagram 13.1):

1. Tensor palati (or tensor veli palatini) (*veli, velum* Lt: curtain).
2. Levator palati (or levator veli palatini)
3. Palatoglossus

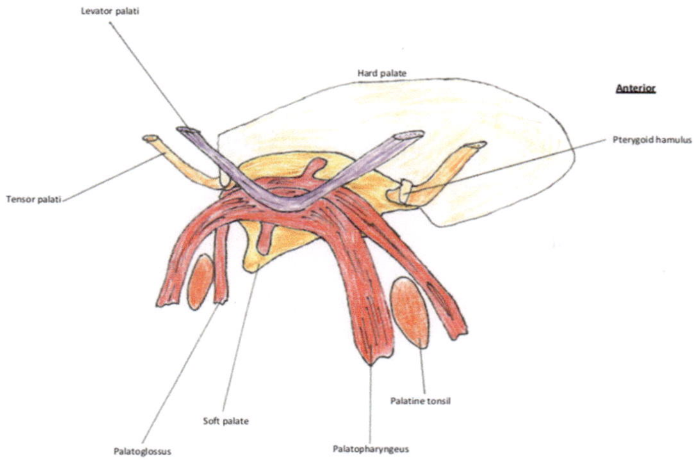

Diagram 13.1 The 3D anatomy of the palatal musculature. The diagram is shown with the front to the right and the soft palate to the left. The tensors run around the pterygoid hamulus to be splayed out into the palatal aponeurosis. The palatopharyngeus and palatoglossus form the posterior and anterior faucial pillars with the palatine tonsil between

4. Palatopharyngeus
5. Musculus uvulae

As previously mentioned in this book, the palatoglossus also belongs to the tongue with the palatopharyngeus also part of the pharyngeal musculature. The structure is such that competency of the soft palate as it pushes against the posterior pharyngeal wall, allows one to efficiently blow up a balloon, or to cough without nasal escape of air as well as to swallow without regurgitation into the nose. As the soft palate is pushed down against the tongue respiration can continue whilst sucking and chewing without any risk of inhalation. During coughing and sneezing the pressure differential between the naso- and the oropharynx is buffeted by the uvula which acts to prevent the soft palate from moving forcibly upwards. Tensing the soft palate also ensures that food is directed with the tongue towards the hypopharynx before the bolus is swallowed.

Tensor Palati

If available it is valuable at this time to examine the base of a dried skull.

The tensor palati is a thin strip of muscle that arises from a small but discrete area called the *scaphoid fossa* at the upper end of the medial pterygoid plate. The muscle also takes part of its origin from the cartilaginous portion of the pharyngotympanic tube as well as from the nearby spine of the sphenoid. The flat muscle converges towards the end of the pterygoid hamulus becoming tendinous and whipping around at this point (which is also part of the origin of the buccinator) so that the tensor palati twists around at a complete right angle to enter the pharynx and flatten out as an aponeurosis attached to the crest of the palatine bone.[1]

The posterolateral border of the tensor palati blends with the side wall of the pharynx (as do many muscles). Posteriorly, however, the tensor palati hangs downwards to form part of the edge of the soft palate with the uvula making up the remainder of the soft-tissues in the midline. In a child with a cleft palate the tensor palati does not insert into the palate. The task of the tensor palati is to maintain the palatal soft-tissue shape as other muscles exert their pull.

Levator Palati

This is a much rounder muscle mass arising from the quadrate-shaped area at the apex of the petrous temporal bone that lies in front of the carotid canal. Equally the muscle has origin from the medial part of the cartilaginous pharyngotympanic tube. The levator palati is inserted into the palatine aponeurosis by passing between the two heads of the palatopharyngeus muscle so that both levatores in running forwards and medially create a V-shaped sling that can elevate the palate and which can draw backwards to efficiently close off the nasopharynx. The recognizable point on the posterior pharyngeal wall which the soft palate abuts is *Pas-*

[1]This right angle is just as sharp as that subtended by the obturator internus muscle from its origin over the obturator foramen and its insertion into the greater trochanter of the femur (See Volume 2 of this series).

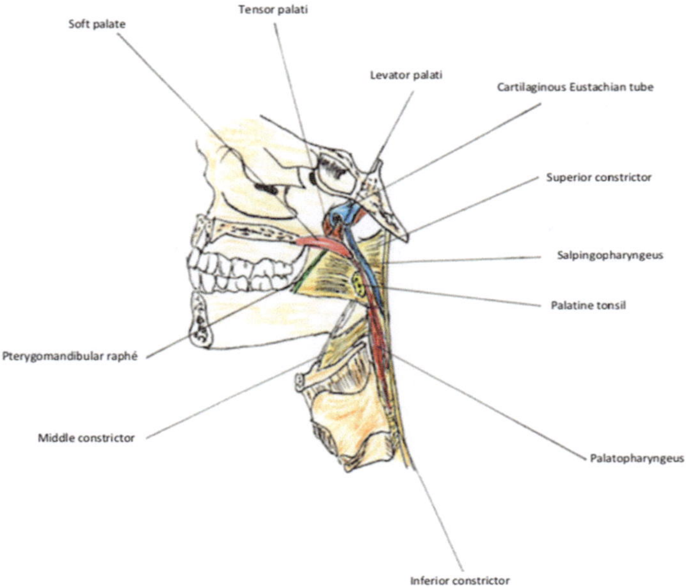

Diagram 13.2 Sagittal view of the palate designed to show the salpingopharyngeus (*blue*) and the palatopharyngeus lying inside the pharyngeal constrictors. The tensor and levator palati show partial origin from the medial side of the cartilaginous Eustachian tube

savant's ridge (at the level of the anterior arch of the atlas).[2] The ridge is demonstrable just inferior to the positioning of the palatine tonsil and inferior and posterior to the opening of the Eustachian tube. As stated previously the origin of this muscle is intrapharyngeal. The ridge of the levator palati is evident in a sagittal prosected specimen as an oblique line evident at the top of the soft palate extending to the skull base (See Diagram 8.1; Chap. 8). This differs from the tensor palati where the levator descends behind the auditory tube **inside the pharynx** against the free border of the superior constrictor Diagram 13.2 shows the anatomical relationship of the palatal and oropharyngeal muscles.

[2]Named after Gustav Passavant (1815–1893) a German surgeon who described this ridge in cleft palate cases in 1863.

Palatoglossus

The innervation exception of this muscle often causes confusion. This muscle arises at the undersurface of the palatine aponeurosis and passes downwards to interdigitate with the styloglossus muscle. It creates a raised palatoglossal fold in front of the palatine tonsil and is one of the tonsillar pillars (anterior pillar of the tonsillar fauces). This area represents a junction between the mouth and the oropharynx and is therefore a cross over between V_3 and Cranial IX innervation. The muscle raises the tongue and narrows the transverse diameter of the oropharyngeal isthmus. The point of confusion concerning its innervation is that it is the only extrinsic tongue muscle (muscle with the title 'glossus' in its name) NOT innervated by Cranial XII. If we consider palatoglossus more as a pharyngeal muscle (a depressor palati) then its innervation is more logically with the pharyngeal branch of the Vagus (X). In this way the palatoglossus functions more as a counterweight to the levator palati on the underside of the soft palate aponeurosis and meeting its opposite number in the midline.

Palatopharyngeus

This complicated muscle has two heads of origin, one bony and the other aponeurotic. The anterior head arises from the posterior border of the hard palate with the posterior head arising further back from the palatal aponeurosis. Both heads embrace the insertion point of the levator palati, arching downwards over the lateral edge of the aponeurosis behind the palatine tonsil so that the palatopharyngeus is the most internal of all of the pharyngeal muscles. The palatopharyngeal fold forms the posterior pillar of the fauces (enclosing the tonsillar fossa). The palatopharyngeus is inserted below into the posterior border of the thyroid lamina[3] where the

[3]As suggested in Last's *Anatomy Regional and Applied*, this muscle could also be renamed as the palatolaryngeus. 9th Edn p 494.

most posterior of the fibres merge with the inferior constrictor muscle.

The front part of the palatopharyngeus therefore elevates the larynx and the pharynx as well as bowing the palate upwards like a concave shell. But the back end of the muscle has a counteraction to depress the palate. As the muscle is a point of fusion (or intermingling) of the lateral and posterior pharyngeal musculature it is joined superiorly by the salpingopharyngeus and inferiorly by the stylopharyngeus (Diagram 13.2). This is because the palatopharyngeus inserts into the gap between the middle and the superior constrictor muscles and lies at the level of the body and the greater horn (cornua) of the hyoid bone.

It is also noted that a few of the muscle fibres of palatopharyngeus pass backwards horizontally with the superior constrictor muscle to narrow the pharyngeal isthmus. This region is greatly hypertrophied in patients with a cleft palate as a failed mechanism to compensate for a posterior soft-tissue deficiency.[4]

The functional effect of all of this is for the bulk of the palatopharyngeus to depress the palate onto the posterior part of the tongue and to prevent the soft palate from being forced into the nasopharynx when blowing forcefully through the mouth against resistance. In humans, Passavant's ridge has been evolutionarily drawn downwards. Here the muscles of the soft palate act as a functional palatopharyngeal (or velopharyngeal) sphincter. Passavant's ridge is then the combined activity of the palatopharyngeus, the superior constrictor, the salpingopharyngeus and the palatal musculature.

---

[4]The palatopharyngeus muscle is naturally quite large in those animals such as the rat (and other keen scented animals) where the laryngeal orifice sits high (almost at the nasopharynx) so that they are able to swallow and breathe simultaneously. In the rat for example the intranarial larynx is supported by the stylopharyngeus and the salpingopharyngeus both of which are far more comparatively developed than in humans. In these animals the palatopharyngeal 'sphincter' actually clasps the larynx and is even more appropriately considered a palatolaryngeus muscle.

Musculus uvulae

This is the last contributing muscle supporting the uvula with an origin from the posterior nasal spine and running through the swing of the levatores. Its function is to contract the uvula widening the mid-portion of the soft palate and assisting in maintaining competency between the naso- and oropharynx.

The blood supply of the soft palate include anastomoses between the lesser palatine and the ascending palatine (maxillary) and the palatine branches of the ascending pharyngeal (ECA) artery. The venous blood drains laterally through the pharyngeal wall into the pharyngeal and the pterygoid plexi with lymphatics draining into retropharyngeal and deep cervical nodes. The muscles of the soft palate are all innervated by the pharyngeal branch of Cranial X except for the tensor palati which is derived from a branch to the medial pterygoid nerve that has traversed the otic ganglion without synapse to supply both tensors (palati and tympani).

To recap, the somatic sensation of the soft palate is via V_2 (with some overlap of Cranial IX in the lateral pharynx). The V_2 nerves are the paired lesser palatine nerves and taste fibres from the greater petrosal nerve (with cell bodies in the geniculate ganglion). Remember that the greater petrosal nerve also carries a few sensate fibres running in the lesser palatine nerves for the intra-tonsillar cleft with their cell bodies also located in the geniculate ganglion.

Palatine Tonsil

The bed of the palatine tonsil is the superior constrictor muscle (overlain with a few of the fibres of the palatopharyngeus). Cranial IX crosses the lower part of this bed by passing under the lower border of the constrictor. The tonsil has discrete borders, poles and surfaces (Diagram 13.3a, b).

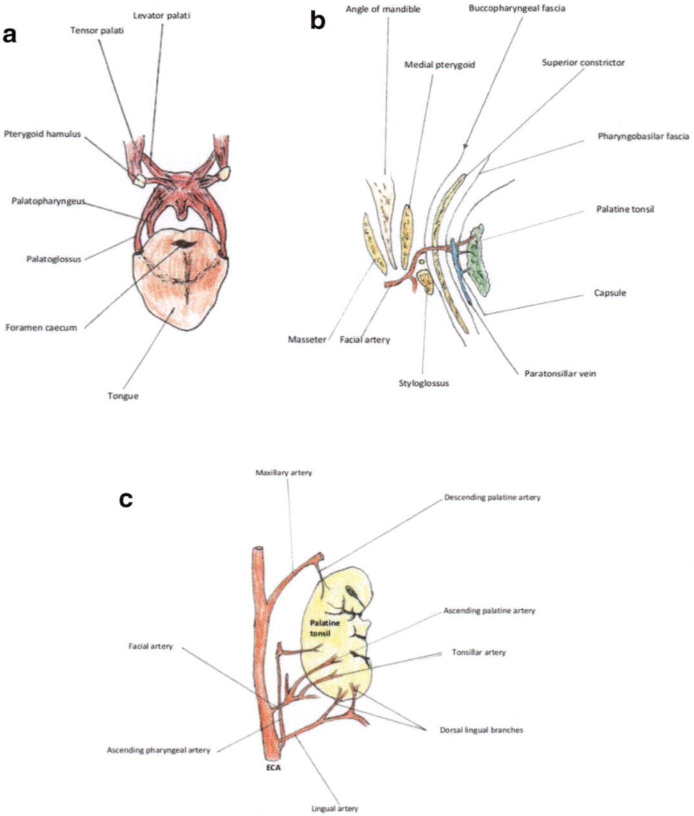

Diagram 13.3 (**a**) The oral appearance of the faucial pillars
(**b**) The soft-tissue layers of the tonsil and at tonsillectomy. The plane of tonsillectomy is a capsulectomy avoiding entry into the bed (superior constrictor) behind which lies the facial artery. Significant bleeding may occur from a confluent paratonsillar vein lying in front of the pharyngobasilar fascia
(**c**) The arterial blood supply of the palatine tonsil (divisible into upper, middle and lower thirds)

- The anterior and posterior borders lie adjacent to the palatoglossal and the palatopharyngeal folds respectively. The tonsillar fossa lies between these two (anterior and posterior pillars of the fauces)
- The upper pole of the tonsil extends to (and may even infiltrate) the soft palate with the lower pole reaching the dorsum of the tongue.
- There are about 20 tonsillar crypts that open on the medial surface with a large opening in the upper pole (the intratonsillar cleft) which is the embryological remnant of the second pharyngeal cleft.
- The lateral tonsillar surface forms the tonsillar capsule which is an extension of the pharyngobasilar fascia. As a consequence a peritonsillar abscess, (called a *quinsy*), is extracapsular.
- The superior constrictor muscle separates this capsular surface from the facial artery (and its relevant branches, the ascending palatine and the tonsillar branch).
- The tonsil is separated from the uvula by a mucosal semi-lunar fold which extends from the palatopharyngeal arch to the upper tonsillar pole. In foetal life there is also a similar fold that runs from the palatoglossal arch to the lower tonsillar pole. Although this is invaded by tonsillar lymphoid tissue, it tends to regress.

The blood supply of the tonsil is complex and extensive (Diagram 13.3c). The main arterial supply is:

1. The tonsillar branch of the facial artery (arching over the styloglossus and piercing the superior constrictor). This supplies the middle tonsil.
2. Lingual (lower tonsil)
3. Ascending pharyngeal (upper tonsil)
4. Descending palatine (upper tonsil).
5. Ascending palatine branch of the facial artery (lower tonsil)

Venous drainage forms a plexus around the capsule and also pierces the superior constrictor in order to drain into the pharyngeal plexus. There is often a large vein in the tonsillar bed, (often called the paratonsillar vein) and this is the usual culprit in a post-tonsillectomy bleed. The lymphatic drainage is into the deep cervical nodes but particularly the jugulodigastric lymph node which can be a harbinger presentation of a tonsillar carcinoma. (Most tonsillar carcinomas develop in the tonsillo-lingual sulcus which anterio-inferiorly separates the tonsil from the tongue). The tonsillar nerve supply is via the tonsillar branch of Cranial IX as well as via the lesser palatine nerves.

Given this anatomy a tonsillectomy usually commences at the arch margins starting at the upper pole with fine dissection keeping close to the capsule and working downwards. Arterial haemorrhage is uncommon but will occur when the bed is inadvertently penetrated. Arteries lie outside the superior constrictor. Most of the bleeding is venous from the paratonsillar vein lying in the tonsillar bed particularly if these small veins unite to form a potentially troublesome source of bleeding.

Brief Remarks on the Anatomy of Cleft Palate (See Chap. 17 for discussion of facial embryology).

In brief, the nasal cavities and the oral cavity are formed from the primitive stomodeum. Mesoderm forming the maxillary processes fuses with a frontonasal process which separates this stomodeum as an ectodermal pit from the developing brain. This separation then forms a shelf-like table, the palatal process, that is lateral to the tongue. Excavation of this part forms the nasal cavities and the nasal septum. Normally this entire area fuses (frontonasal process, maxilla and nasal septum) to form the palate explaining why from above and in front there is a V_1 nerve supply (as well as an ophthalmic blood supply) whereas behind it is V_2 with a maxillary artery supply.

Cleft palate (¬ 1: 2500 births) represents a failure of proper fusion of these palatal processes resulting in a variable cleft which can range from a simple bifid uvula to a complete anteroposterior defect (on one or on both sides). In effect, this represents a paramedian defect in the frontonasal process that runs forwards and lateral to the incisor teeth becoming continuous with a cleft lip (¬ 1: 1000 births) when also present. Because the incisive part of the maxilla (the pre-maxilla) forms separately, this explains why an off-midline split is present and why a bilateral cleft palate has a separate central piece. Cleft palate interferes with sucking and swallowing and presents with nasal regurgitation. As there is a separation of oral and nasal elements, there is a nasal escape-type speech pattern. The horizontal fibres of the palatopharyngeus and the superior constrictor hypertrophy markedly but are unable to compensate for the palatal deficiency. When there is a cleft lip only, this cleft lip runs down from the nostril laterally so that the median part of the lip is contributed to by the opposite maxillary process. When the cleft lip is bilateral, the central bridge of skin is derived from the frontonasal processes. Quite rarely, the lateral nasal and maxillary processes fail to fuse resulting in a lateral facial cleft formed along the line of the nasolacrimal duct.

The cleft lip repair is typically performed early at 3–6 months by a rotation/advancement flap. The cleft palate is repaired at about 12 months before speech development usually with a Z plasty style of palatal muscle realignment (intravelar veloplasty). More complex cases can require palatal expansion and bone grafting in order to create space for the permanent teeth. An orthodontic advancement osteotomy may be performed in adolescence for those where the maxilla is poorly formed behind the mandibular protrusion.

Anatomy of the Tongue (Diagram 13.4): The tongue has its regions (anterior two-thirds and posterior one-third) or its compo-

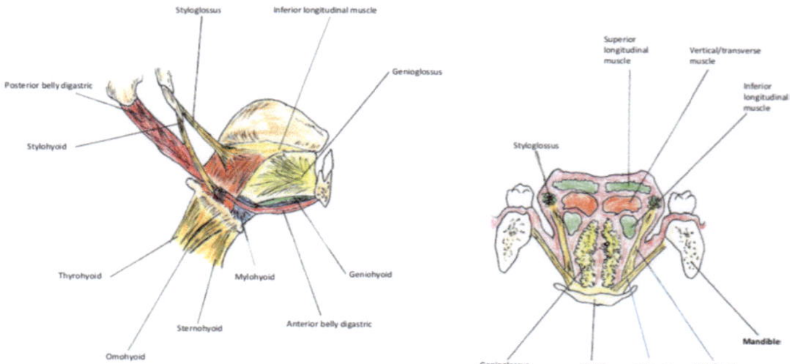

Diagram 13.4 Anatomy of the tongue. *Left-hand image* shows the extrinsic musculature (See also Diagram 2.4; Chap. 2 and Diagram 3.6; Chap. 3) *Right-hand image* shows the coronal view of the intrinsic tongue musculature divided into superior and inferior longitudinal and vertical and transverse elements

nent parts (tip, dorsum, ventral surface and root). The muscles are intrinsic (superior and inferior longitudinal, vertical and transverse) and extrinsic (genioglossus, geniohyoid, hyoglossus, styloglossus, palatoglossus). The intrinsic muscles are separated into symmetrical halves by its midline septum. The task of the intrinsics is to change the shape of the tongue (assisting in speech patterns, swallowing and eating). The role of the extrinsics is to change the position of the tongue.

The tongue forms early in development (fourth week) from a median bud and from the forming part of the first pharyngeal arch. This is supported a week later by two fusing lateral tongue buds forming the anterior two-thirds of the tongue and separated from the remainder by a V-shaped line of fusion (the *sulcus terminalis*) from the posterior one-third or *copula* (formed from the third and fourth pharyngeal arches). The *foramen caecum* forms at the tip of this V-shaped sulcus forming the thyroglossal duct and the line of development of the thyroid gland (See Chap. 3). The second pharyngeal arch is overtaken and the floor separates except at the frenulum.

The mucosa of the palatine part of the tongue is roughened by the papillae being smooth posteriorly with small lymphoid accumulations (lingual tonsil). This area continues posteriorly as the medial and lateral glosso-epiglottic folds around the vallecula and the epiglottis. In a carcinoma of the tongue, classification of region is made into the dorsum, the tip, the inferior surface and the root in accordance with the main anatomy but also in terms of anticipated lymphatic drainage.

Diagram 13.5.

There are 7–12 vallate papillae which are located immediately anterior to the sulcus terminalis. Each of these vallate papillae appears as a short stout cylinder with a peripheral deep trench with the ducts of the lingual (and salivary) glands (von Ebner's glands) emptying.[5] The fungiform papillae are smaller and more numerous appearing as bright red spots whereas the filiform papillae (also numerous) are minute and cover the palatine surface being laid out

[5]These are exocrine lipase-secreting glands named after the Austrian histologist Anton Gilbert Victor von Ebner (1842–1925).

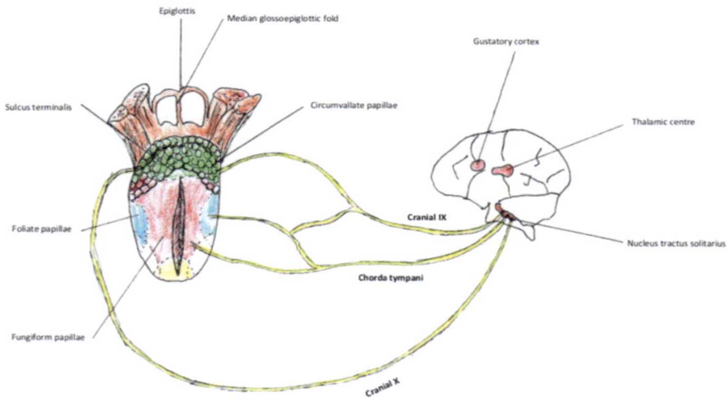

Diagram 13.5 Taste papillae of the tongue. The bulk are the fungiform papillae. The tip records sweet, (*orange*) the front sides salty, (*pink*) the true sides sour (*blue*) and the posterior part bitter (*green*). The foliate and fungiform papillae sensory afferents travel in the chorda tympani with the circumvallate papillae innervated by Cranial IX and the posterior elements traveling in the Vagus. These afferents synapse in the nucleus of the tractus solitarius before thalamic and gustatory cortical representation

in parallel rows alongside the sulcus. All of these (with the exception of the filiform papillae which are engaged in touch sensation) are taste buds for distinction of sweet, sour, bitter, salt and umami. The most abundant filiform papillae give the tongue its characteristic keratinized appearance. Despite the fact that the circumvallate papillae are located in front of the sulcus they are innervated by the nerve of the posterior one-third of the tongue (Cranial IX). The anterior two-thirds of the tongue is innervated by the chorda tympani (Cranial VII) and the lingual nerve.

In brief:

Genioglossus: forms the bulk of the tongue substance arising from the superior genial mandibular tubercle and fanning out into the tongue and with its inferior fibres inserting into the hyoid bone. The muscle is principally concerned with protrusion of the tongue although its action is complex (middle fibres depressing and lateral fibres deviating).

Hyoglossus: is a rectangular landmark surgical muscle originating from the body and the greater cornua of the hyoid bone. On its surface run the lingual nerve and the hypoglossal nerve. The muscle is exposed by retraction of the free edge of the mylohyoid posteriorly during a submandibular gland excision. The lingual nerve swerves around the submandibular secretory duct as the nerve attaches to the submandibular PSNS ganglion (See Chap. 3). Under the hyoglossus runs the lingual artery and the deep lingual vein. The muscle intermingles inferiorly with the inferior longitudinal muscle and supero-laterally with the styloglossus (Diagram 13.4). The muscle depresses and retracts the tongue.

Styloglossus: This narrow triangular muscle is the smallest of the styloid process and intermingles with the substance of the hyoglossus to retract and to elevate the tongue. The glossopharyngeal nerve running around the stylopharyngeus travels between it and the styloglossus. The styloglossus is considered a critical muscle in head and neck cancer where recent staging of lateral oropharyngeal cancer using MRI has upstaged those cases with styloglossus involvement [1]. The anterior two-thirds of the tongue drains into submental and submandibular lymph nodes with the posterior one-third draining into retropharyngeal and deep cervical nodal basins.

Diagram 13.6 is a recap of lingual innervation showing somatic, taste and motor elements. It should be remembered that there is a small component of the internal laryngeal nerve (Cranial X) that is sensory for the posterior one-third of the tongue.

Buccinator: The concluding part of the mouth to consider is the buccinator (See Diagram 8.1*;* Chap. 8 and Diagram 14.1*;* Chap. 14). This is a thin rectangular-shaped muscle filling the space between the maxilla and the mandible and forming the lateral cheek. The muscle has two discrete origins, one from the outer surfaces of the alveolar processes of the maxilla and the mandible (the last molar teeth) as well as from the front part of the pterygomandibular raphe. In insertion there is an intersection of fibres to support the orbicularis oris (as well as risorius, depressor anguli oris and above zygomaticus major) as well as to decussate into the upper and lower lips. This combination of muscles (orbicularis oris, buccinator, levator anguli oris,

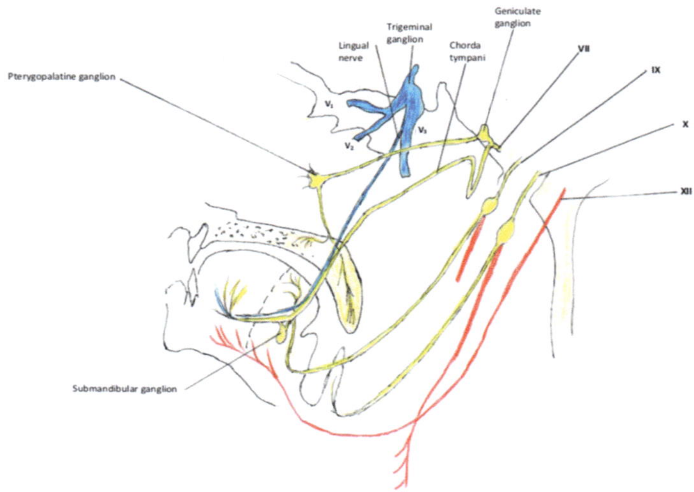

Diagram 13.6 Recap of the tongue innervation (somatic sensory, taste and motor). (See also Diagram 5.3b; Chap. 5 and Diagram 7.6; Chap. 7). GSA afferents of Cranial V are shown in *blue* including the lingual nerve that relays taste fibres via the chorda tympani. Cranial VII sends fibres via the geniculate ganglion and Cranial IX and X via their respective inferior ganglia (*yellow*). Motor fibres are shown in *red* including the XII nerve supply to all of the tongue musculature (except palatoglossus), the vagal fibres to the pharyngeal constrictors and Cranial IX motor fibres to the stylopharyngeus. Sensory elements to the epiglottis and the laryngopharynx from the Vagus are not shown

depressor anguli oris, zygomaticus major, zygomaticus minor, risorius, quadratus labii superioris, quadratus labii inferioris) forms the irregular fibromuscular mass of the *modiolus*, of importance as a landmark in prosthetic dentistry and lower denture stability.

The buccinator muscle is innervated by the buccal branch of Cranial VII with some proprioception via the buccal nerve (V_2). The muscle assists in holding the food bolus in place during mastication and in infants in suckling.

Q & A: Chap. 13 (Answers at the End of This Chapter)

1. The palatopharyngeus muscle
   (a) Merges in its insertion with fibres of the inferior constrictor muscle
   (b) Has a single origin
   (c) Flattens the palate
   (d) Is the innermost of the pharyngeal muscles
   (e) Has no connection with the salpingopharyngeus or the stylopharyngeus muscles
2. The buccinator:
   (a) Follows the line of the teeth in the same plane as the masseter muscle
   (b) Is continuous with the superior constrictor muscle
   (c) Lies on top of the buccopharyngeal fascia
   (d) Attaches ahead of the third molar tooth
   (e) Is innervated by the buccal nerve
3. The palatine tonsil:
   (a) Is located at the pharyngeal isthmus
   (b) Is innervated by V2 via the greater palatine nerves
   (c) Has a blood supply entirely from the lingual artery
   (d) Drains via a peritonsillar venous plexus into the lingual and pharyngeal veins
4. The palatopharyngeus
   (a) Has a posterior fasciculus which is separate from the contralateral side
   (b) Has an anterior muscular fasciculus lying between the levator and tensor veli palatini muscles
   (c) Inserts into the thyroid cartilage lamina with the stylopharyngeus muscle
   (d) Is innervated via the glossopharyngeal (IX) nerve
5. The palatoglossus
   (a) Takes origin from the palatal aponeurosis
   (b) Is separate from the intrinsic muscles of the tongue
   (c) Is innervated by the Hypoglossal (XII) nerve
   (d) Is a tongue depressor

6. Deciduous teeth
   (a) Form in embryonic life
   (b) Begins from backwards and runs forwards
   (c) Begin eruption usually after one year of life
   (d) Maintain the jaw arch length
   (e) Do not provide guidance for the eruption of the permanent teeth
7. Passavant's ridge
   (a) Is essential to normal speech (velopharyngeal closure) in both cleft and non-cleft individuals
   (b) Is a functional structure that projects along the lateral and posterior nasopharyngeal walls
   (c) May take part in whistling
   (d) Is video-endoscopically evident in less than half of examined cases
   (e) Is more frequently evident when the head is extended than when it is in the neutral position

Answers

1. a
2. b
3. a, d
4. b, c
5. a
6. a, d
7. b, c, d, e

Reference

1. Laccourreye O, Orosco RK, Rubin F, Holsinger FC. Styloglossus muscle: a critical landmark in head and neck oncology. Eur Ann Otorhinolaryngol Head Neck Dis. 2018;135:421–5.

The Pharynx 14

Contents

Q & A: Chap. 14 (Answers at the End of This Chapter).......................... 306
Answers.. 307
Reference.. 307

The adult pharynx is approximately 12 cm. in length and it extends as a tube from the base of the skull to C6 behind the nasal cavities (nasopharynx), the oral cavity (oropharynx) and the larynx (laryngo [or hypo] pharynx). It is widest at the base of the skull behind the Eustachian tube narrowing at the palate as the pharyngeal isthmus and then widening again before narrowing at the entrance to the oesophagus. Above the larynx the walls of the pharynx are not in contact but below the larynx they contact one another.

The pharynx is separated from the prevertebral fascia by a loose venous plexus which permits free gliding during swallowing. The main neck neurovascular bundle is positioned laterally along with the styloid apparatus. The mixed motor and sensory pharyngeal nerve plexus forms largely on the substance of the middle constrictor muscle. The basic structure of the pharynx is consistent throughout its four discrete layers. These include the *mucous membrane, the submucous layer, the muscular layer* and

A. Zbar, *Anatomy--Head and Neck*,
https://doi.org/10.1007/978-3-031-69538-4_14

the *buccopharyngeal fascia.* Some textbooks rather describe a five-layer system with the pharyngobasilar fascia the third layer lying between the submucosa and the muscles [1]. To recap, the buccopharyngeal fascia covers the exterior of the buccinator and the pharyngeal muscles with the pharyngobasilar fascia lining the interior of the muscular layer and attaching the pharynx to the base of the skull to fill in the space where the Eustachian tube enters and to adhere to the fixed part of the posterior nasal apertures (choanae).

The muscles of the pharynx include the three constrictors and the 'pharyngeus' group (stylopharyngeus, salpingopharyngeus and palatopharyngeus). The pharynx is remarkably thin at points with the three curved constrictor sheets supported internally by the three small vertical struts. The sagittal distribution and origins of the constrictors have been previously shown diagrammatically in other parts of this volume (See Diagram 2.7b; Chap. 2; Diagram 7.7; Chap. 7; Diagram 8.1; Chap. 8 and Diagram 13.2; Chap. 13).

The three constrictors originate in such a way that they overlap inferiorly appearing like three stacked flower pots. If you have access to a dried skull base, it is evident that the pharyngobasilar fascia starts at the pharyngeal tubercle where there is a midline pharyngeal raphé below which all of the constrictors insert (Diagrams 14.1 and 14.2). In examining the base of the skull one can appreciate the attachments of the pharyngobasilar fascia and how this maintains the nasopharynx open. The pharyngobasilar fascia passes over the longus capitis muscle and then towards the edges of the foramen lacerum to attach to the petrous temporal bone in front of the carotid canal. Here it is only attached to the cartilaginous part of the auditory tube (and not to the bony skull) and also to the sharp posterior edge of the medial pterygoid plate. This attachment extends down the plate to the rounded hamulus, swinging from there across the skull base to join its fellow on the other side. The fascia in this part is quite rigid creating a lateral recess for the origin of the levator palati.

Superior Constrictor Muscle: Continuing with our examination of the skull base, it is worth noting the shape and consistency of the medial pterygoid plate as an orientating landmark. Its upper part is soft and rounded to house the auditory tube but the lower

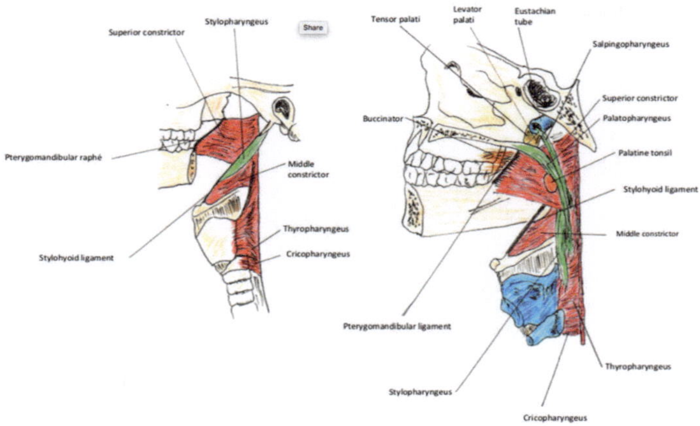

Diagram 14.1 Lateral views of the structure of the pharynx showing the exterior (*Left-hand image*) and interior (*Right-hand image*) of the pharynx and the disposition of the vertical muscles, salpingopharyngeus, palatopharyngeus and stylopharyngeus

end is very sharp. This sharp part down to the hamulus is the origin of the superior constrictor muscle which also takes origin from the pterygomandibular raphé attaching to the mandibular foramen. As already stated in Chap. 13, the buccinator runs in continuity forwards as the superior constrictor runs backwards. The effective shape of the superior constrictor results in vertical fibres running upwards to the pharyngeal raphé with transverse horizontally running fibres and lower descending fibres which extend inside the middle constrictor as far as the vocal folds (Diagram 13.2*;* Chap. 13). The gap between the superior and the middle constrictors is plugged by the back of the tongue and the structures that pass from outside the pharynx into the mouth; namely the stylopharyngeus, Cranial IX and the lingual nerve.

The *ascending* palatine artery and the levator and tensor palati muscles lie external to and above the superior constrictor.

Middle Constrictor Muscle: The gap between the superior and the middle constrictors is filled by the stylohyoid (attaching to the lesser cornua of the hyoid bone). This is deep to hyoglossus (See Diagram 3.6; Chap. 3). The middle constrictor arises between the

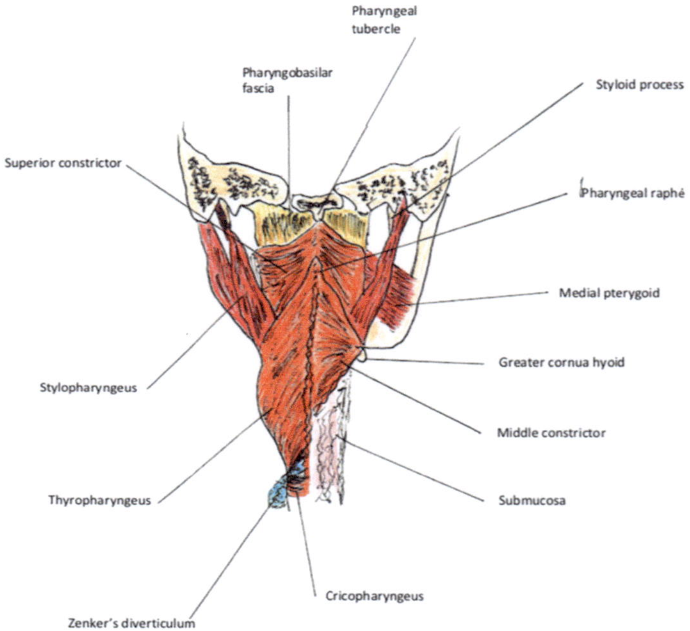

Diagram 14.2 Posterior aspect of the pharynx. The attachment of the superior constrictor to the skull base is shown with the fossa of Morgagni that is filled in with pharyngobasilar fascia. The image strips away the inferior constrictor to show how the muscles overlap internally. The attachment of the pharyngeal musculature to the pharyngeal tubercle and the pharyngeal raphé is evident from a posterior view

insertion of the stylohyoid (between the lesser and the greater cornua of the hyoid bone). Unsurprisingly, some textbooks include the origin of the middle constrictor as also from the lower part of the stylohyoid ligament. The middle constrictor appears as a flat sheet of thin muscle lying on its side but diverging backwards quite widely with vertically running fibres up and down the pharynx and horizontally running fibres between. These all simply end in the median pharyngeal raphé. The upper most fibres enclose the superior constrictor and the lowermost fibres reach down to the level of the vocal folds enclosed in their lower part by the overlapping inferior constrictor muscle. The natural gap between the middle and the inferior constrictors is closed by the thyrohyoid membrane with this area forming the piriform fossae (Diagram 14.1). Structures piercing the thyrohyoid membrane include the superior laryngeal vessels and the internal laryngeal nerve.

Inferior Constrictor Muscle: It is advised to consider this muscle as in two parts, both effectively named for their separate origin. The *thyropharyngeus* arises from the oblique lamina of the thyroid cartilage lying in series with the thyrohyoid. Inferiorly it is separate from the ring of the cricothyroid (*cricopharyngeus*) muscle. The inferior constrictor is the outside enveloping muscle of the pharynx and like the other two constrictors its fibres are divergent with some reaching nearly as high as the pharyngeal tubercle at the skull base. The lowermost fibres of the thyropharyngeus are almost horizontal and edge to edge with the cricopharyngeus. The latter is more rounded and thicker and a horizontal muscle that extends backwards from one side of the cricoid arch to the other around the pharynx. This is a point where there is no physical raphé so that its contraction at the top of the oesophagus acts as a functional sphincter. Continuation inferiorly is as the circular coat of oesophageal muscle. These muscle fibres are slow twitch without muscle spindles and are like those seen in the external urethral sphincter so that they are always closed except for momentary periods of relaxation (deglutition). This arrangement also explains why there is a different innervation from the other constrictor group.

This part is also the section where initial resistance is felt during oesophagoscopy, the region normally closing in order to stop air being sucked into the upper oesophagus as intrathoracic pressure falls. Beneath the cricopharyngeus is the recurrent laryngeal nerve (RLN) traveling with the inferior laryngeal vessels. As a reminder, the internal laryngeal nerve travels with the superior laryngeal artery (a branch of the superior thyroid artery). These pierce the thyrohyoid membrane. The RLN runs with the inferior laryngeal branch of the inferior thyroid artery and pierces the cricothyroid membrane. The inferior thyroid artery is the embryological vessel supplying the cervical tracheo-oesophageal anlage and so this is the principal blood supply to anastomoses of the cervical oesophagus. The latter form part of an anastomosis with the stomach that is typically pulled up into the neck in some cases of mid-oesophageal cancer. This procedure of oesophageal pull-up and anastomosis in the neck is often performed without thoracotomy (the transhiatal or Orringer oesophagectomy).[1]

The origin and formation of the inferior constrictor (in separate parts) results in a natural space between the horizontal 'ring pull' of the cricopharyngeus and the more oblique disposition of the thyropharyngeus. This triangle of Laimer (or Laimer-Hackermann) is also more often referred to as the dehiscence of Killian[2] through which a Zenker's pharyngeal pulsion diverticulum may appear.[3] The outer surface of the pharynx is covered by a rather delicate epimysium which allows it to expand and this is continued over the pterygomandibular raphe and the buccinator as the loose buccopharyngeal fascia. The vertical muscles of the pharynx (palatopharyngeus, salpingopharyngeus and stylopharyngeus) all lie inside the constrictors (Diagram 14.1).

The rich blood supply of the pharynx is contributed by the ascending pharyngeal, ascending palatine, lingual, tonsillar, greater palatine, artery of the pterygoid canal, superior laryngeal and inferior laryngeal arteries. The venous drainage forms a pharyngeal plexus on the substance of the middle constrictor and drains directly into the IJV with lower drainage into the inferior thyroid veins and upper drainage into the cavernous sinus. Lymphatics travel to the retropharyngeal and lower and upper

[1]Named after Mark Orringer a thoracic surgeon in Michigan who introduced the procedure for high-risk cases in 1976.

[2]Named after Gustav Killian (1860–1921) a German laryngologist who described the dehiscence in 1908 and who was the father of rigid bronchoscopy.

[3]Described in 1877 by Friedrich Albert von Zenker (1825–1898) a German pathologist and physician who also discovered the parasitic cause of trichinosis. To be pedantic an earlier description of Zenker's diverticulum was proffered at a postmortem performed by Abraham Ludlow (1737–1807) a Bristol surgeon in 1764. His findings were initially conveyed before publication to the great London anatomist William Hunter with drawings made by Hunter's in residence artist Jan van Rymsdyk (c. 1730–1790). Ludlow's dissection specimen is kept in the museum at the Glasgow Royal Infirmary.

deep cervical nodes. The nerve supply is via the pharyngeal plexus lying on the middle constrictor with the cell bodies of the plexus located in the nucleus ambiguus. The plexus is formed by the union of the pharyngeal branches of Cranial X, IX and XI (along). It is likely that this neural separation leads in some to crico-oesophageal incoordination and the formation of a pharyngeal pouch. Diagram 14.3 reiterates the anatomical make-up of the pharyngeal plexus reminding that the mucosa of the nasopharynx is supplied by V_2 (via the pterygopalatine ganglion), the oro- and laryngopharynx by Cranial IX and the vallecula afferently innervated by the internal and recurrent laryngeal nerves.

The exterior of this part of the pharynx (the laryngo- or hypopharynx) extends from the upper border of the epiglottis to the level of the cricoid cartilage (C6 vertebra) and ends at the com-

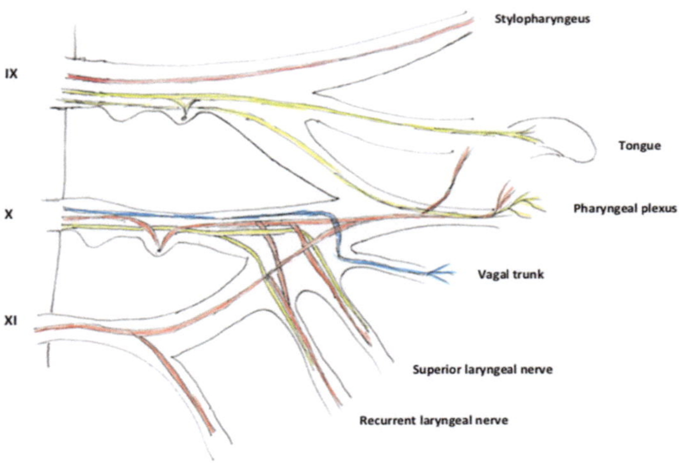

Diagram 14.3 Recap of the pharyngeal plexus. *Red* lines are motor and *yellow* lines are sensory. *Blue* are Vagal PSNS fibres to the heart and lungs. The plexus forms on the middle constrictor and is contributed to by the Cranial IX, X and XI. Cranial IX includes taste afferents with their cell bodies in the inferior IX ganglion and a motor supply to stylopharyngeus. The cranial XI provides a large amount of motor supply to the pharynx through its attachment to Cranial X as these three cranial nerves approach the jugular foramen

mencement of the oesophagus opposite the laryngeal inlet (aditus) forming the piriform recesses on either side. This area is best seen on a posterior pharyngeal prosected dissection if available (Diagram 14.2). The posterior wall here is formed by the three overlapping constrictors down as far as the level of the vocal folds (the upper border of the cricoid lamina) but mostly by the middle and inferior constrictors (with the stylopharyngeus internally extending to this level). The lateral glossoepiglottic fold separates the oropharynx from the laryngopharynx. Below this fold is the piriform recess (or piriform fossa) which is bounded medially by the laryngeal quadrangular membrane and below by the aryepiglottic fold (See Chap. 15). The lateral wall of this recess is formed by the thyrohyoid membrane above and by the lamina of the thyroid cartilage below.

Q & A: Chap. 14 (Answers at the End of This Chapter)

1. The pharyngeal plexus
   (a) Incorporates components of the superior cervial ganglion
   (b) Has no connexions with the lowermost cranial nerve (XII)
   (c) Enters at all cervical vertebral levels
   (d) Are anterior to the alar fascia
2. The middle constrictor
   (a) takes partial origin from the stylohyoid ligament
   (b) attaches to the greater and lesser cornua of the hyoid bone
   (c) Is separated from the superior constrictor by the stylopharyngeus muscle
   (d) Has the lingual artery lying deep to the muscle
3. The superior constrictor
   (a) Is partially supplied by the tonsillar artery
   (b) Has no mandibular attachment
   (c) Lies in front of the prevertebral muscles
   (d) Is separated from the middle constrictor by Cranial IX

4. The middle constrictor muscle:
   (a) Has a gap with the superior constrictor muscle filled by the styloglossus
   (b) Has its lowermost fibres extending as far as the vocal folds
   (c) Forms a gap with the inferior constrictor filled in by the thyrohyoid membrane
   (d) The gap with the inferior constrictor is pierced by the external laryngeal nerve
5. The pterygomandibular raphe:
   (a) Lies between the posterior tonsillar pillar and the retromolar trigone
   (b) Is a band of buccopharyngeal fascia
   (c) Attaches the lateral pterygoid plate to the mylohyoid line of the mandible
   (d) Can be absent with the superior constrictor and buccinator being continuous
6. The upper oesophageal sphincter
   (a) Prevents air insufflation during negative intrathoracic pressure
   (b) Is not supported anteriorly by the infrahyoid muscles
   (c) Is supported posteriorly by the pharyngeal muscles
   (d) Has as its primary motor nucleus the dorsal nucleus of the Vagus (Cranial X)

Answers

1. a, d
2. a, c
3. a, c, d
4. b, c
5. b
6. a

Reference

1. Romanes GJ, editor. Cunningham's manual of practical anatomy. 15th ed. London: Oxford University Press; 2013.

The Larynx 15

Contents

Laryngeal Skeleton (Diagram 15.1)........ 310
Thyroid Cartilage........ 312
Cricoid cartilage........ 312
Epiglottic cartilage........ 313
Arytenoid cartilages........ 313
Cavity of the Larynx (Diagram 15.3)........ 314
Arytenoid Movement and the Rima Glottidis........ 315
Joint Action........ 315
Ligaments and Membranes........ 316
Laryngeal Musculature (Diagram 15.4)........ 317
Q & A: Chap. 15 (Answers at the End of This Chapter)........ 323
Answers........ 324
References........ 325

The larynx (which becomes continuous with the trachea at C6) acts as a protective mechanism for the airway consisting of a cartilaginous and membranous skeleton. The support cartilages include the ring of the cricoid inferiorly, the V-shaped thyroid cartilage with its two laminae and the arytenoid and the epiglottic cartilages at the pharyngeal opening. The laryngeal cavity narrows at the arytenoids because of the projecting vocal and vestibular folds so that the lateral wall is then formed by the aryepiglottic fold and the piriform recess with the two small nodules of cartilage (the corniculate and cuneiform cartilages) embedded at the upper arytenoid margin.

A. Zbar, *Anatomy--Head and Neck*,
https://doi.org/10.1007/978-3-031-69538-4_15

Laryngeal Skeleton (Diagram 15.1)

The skeletal framework comprises *cartilages*, *joints*, *ligaments* and *membranes*.

- The single cartilages include the thyroid, the cricoid and epiglottic
- The paired cartilages include the arytenoid, cuneiform and corniculate
- The joints are paired, (cricothyroid, cricoarytenoid and aryteno-corniculate)
- The ligaments and membranes are
  - (a) extrinsic (thyrohyoid, crico-tracheal, hypo-epiglottic and thyro-epiglottic) and
  - (b) intrinsic (quadrangular and the crico-thyroid)

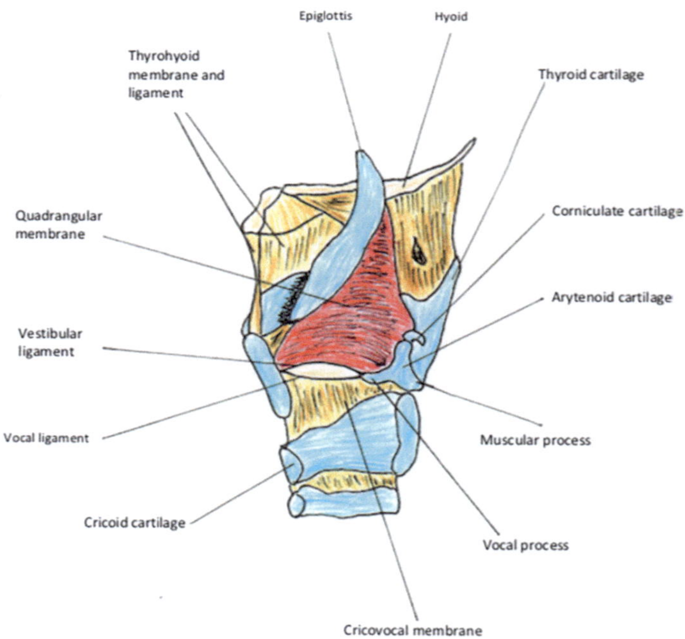

Diagram 15.1 The laryngeal skeleton

The upper cricothyroid ligament forms the vocal folds (crico-vocal membrane).

The thyroid, cricoid and arytenoid are all made of hyaline cartilage (they ossify over time). The epiglottic, corniculate and cuneiforms are made of elastic fibrocartilage.

Diagram 15.2 shows the typical appearance of a posterior dissection at the back of the tongue. This appearance and component parts should where possible be confirmed on a prosected specimen.

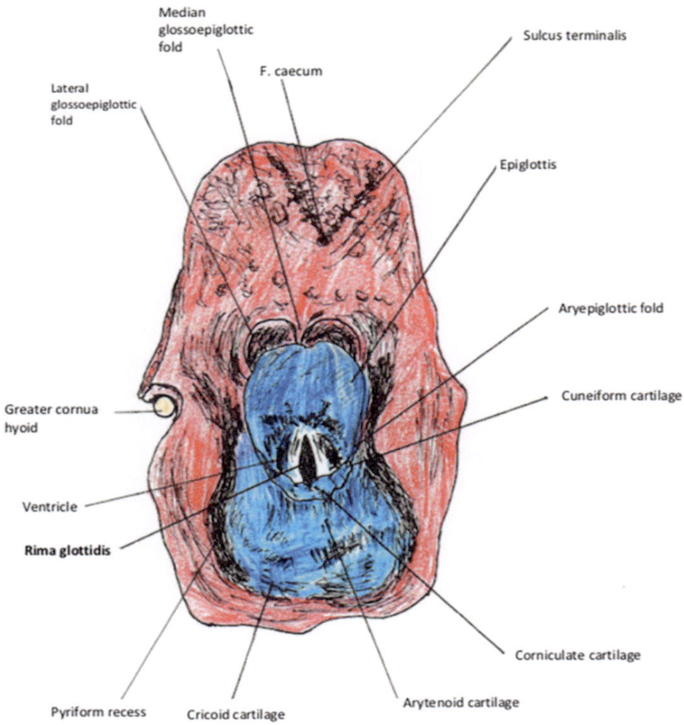

Diagram 15.2 Dissection of the glosso-epiglottic region showing the rima glottidis and the arytenoid cartilages as well as the cul-de-sac of the piriform recess

Thyroid Cartilage

The thyroid cartilage is the largest of the laryngeal cartilages comprising two conjoined laminae like a set of French doors where the posterior free border is projected upwards and downwards into a superior and inferior horns (cornua), respectively. The inferior cornua articulates with the cricoid at the cricothyroid joint. The laminae join at the laryngeal prominence (Adam's apple) with the notch above marking the level of the carotid bifurcation. The cartilage has a prominent oblique line for attachment of the thyrohyoid muscle above and the infrahyoid muscles below as well as for the inferior constrictor and the pretracheal fascia.

Thyrohyoid membrane and ligaments: At this point, these ligaments each contain a small cartilage nodule (*triticeal cartilage*) which is a thickened part of the posterior margin of the thyrohyoid membrane. This part is lined by the mucous membrane of the piriform recess which snakes its way up inside the hyoid and which is pierced by the internal branch of the superior laryngeal nerve (innervating the sensory supravocal mucosa) and by the superior laryngeal vessels. The anterior part of this membrane is defined as the median thyrohyoid ligament and is separated from the posterior part by a small bursa. This area is intimately related to the remnants of the thyroglossal tract which typically loop around the front and undersurfaces of the body of the hyoid bone and which necessitate removal of this central portion of the hyoid *en bloc* as part of a thyroglossal cyst/track excision (Cistrunk's operation, See Chap. 3).

Cricoid cartilage

This signet-ring cartilage articulates by synovial joints with the thyroid and arytenoid cartilages. The cricoid cartilage is the only complete airway cartilaginous ring forming an anterior part (arch) and a posterior projection (lamina). Above are the sloping facets for arytenoid articulation and between is a small ridge that takes the insertion of the posterior cricoarytenoid muscle. The cricothyroid joint allows movement of the lamina of the cricoid and the arytenoids to shift towards or away from the thyroid cartilage which can then either tighten or relax the elastic vocal ligament.

Epiglottic cartilage

The epiglottis is unique forming a leaf-like structure that overhangs the laryngeal vestibule. Posterior to the base of the tongue, the hyoid and the median thyrohyoid ligament the epiglottis tapers for attachment to the posterior thyroid cartilage in the midline at the thyro-epglottic ligament. The top of the epiglottis (its front and back) has modified stratified squamous epithelium, however, the remainder is covered by columnar ciliated (respiratory) epithelium. The anterior epiglottis is attached to the hyoid by a loose fibroelastic hyo-epiglottic ligament (that is separate from the thyro-epiglottic and median thyrohyoid ligaments). The central attachment of the epiglottis to the tongue is via the median glossoepiglottic ligament with lateral attachment via the lateral glosso-epiglottic ligaments on either side. Attachment to the arytenoids is via aryepiglottic folds (Diagram 15.2).

Arytenoid cartilages

The arytenoid cartilages articulate with the upper lamina of the cricoid and are the attachment points for the vocal folds. The right and left membranes form the *conus elsaticus* and are the attachment points for the laryngeal muscles The arytenoid cartilages are effectively like a three-sided pyramid that projects laterally as a **muscular process** for the attachment of the cricoarytenoid muscles and anteriorly as a **vocal process** for attachment of the vocal ligament. Superiorly is a gentle fold (corniculate cartilage) aligning the aryepiglottic fold. The posterior part of the arytenoid cartilage attaches the transverse arytenoid muscles with the thyroarytenoids and the vocalis muscles attaching anteroinferiorly. The space between the conus elasticus and the thyroid cartilage is filled in on either side by the cricothyroid, lateral cricoarytenoid and thyroarytenoid muscles and is represented posteriorly by the piriform recess. Inferiorly is the articulation of the cricoarytenoid joint.

Cavity of the Larynx (Diagram 15.3)

The laryngeal inlet (*aditus*) faces backwards and is tilted upwards to be bordered in front by the epiglottis and at the sides and the back by the aryepiglottic folds. The area below the inlet is the *vestibule* with the space between the vestibular and vocal folds the *ventricle* (*sinus*) of the larynx. A probe inserted here runs into the laryngeal *saccule*. The aryepiglottic folds separate the vestibule from the piriform recess and enclose the slender aryepiglottic and thyroepiglottic muscles as well as the corniculate and cuneiform cartilages.

Each vocal fold consists of the *conus elasticus*, the vocal ligament and vocalis muscle. The conus is a thin layer of fibroelastic tissue attached inferiorly to the upper border of the cricoid cartilage, terminating as the vocal fold and the thickened vocal ligament and passing from the thyroid cartilage to the vocal process of the arytenoid cartilage. The conus is continuous anteriorly with the cricothryroid ligament. The mucous membrane at this point is

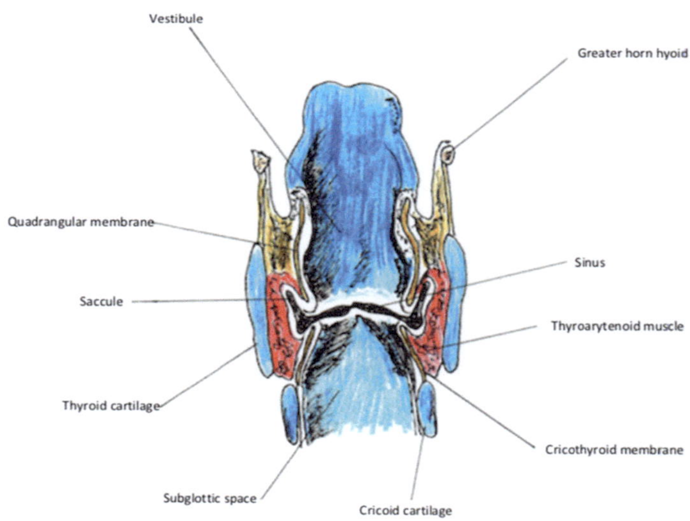

Diagram 15.3 Appearance of the laryngeal inlet

very tightly bound down and is stratified squamous epithelium unlike the remainder of the larynx which comprises ciliated columnar epithelium.

The vital rima glottidis (laryngeal airway) is about 23 mm in length in the adult male and 17 mm in the average adult female with a standard positioning of the vocal folds of about 8 mm in width separation (See Chap. 3 for the distinction between the position of the denervated and cadaveric vocal cords). The infraglottic part of the larynx down to the lower border of the cricoid continues into the trachea. The free margins of the vocal folds and the vocal processes of the arytenoid cartilages are the narrowest part of the laryngeal cavity.

Arytenoid Movement and the Rima Glottidis

As the arytenoids displace laterally on the cricoid, the posterior rima widens and the vocal process turns laterally. When the cricoid lamina tilts forward, the vocal ligaments become slackened and the opening is even wider. The rima closes if the arytenoid cartilages are rotated medially and drawn together as the vocal processes come into apposition. Tightening of the vocal ligaments results when the cricoid lamina tilts backwards at the start to coughing or sneezing.

The pitch and volume of the voice are a delicate interplay between the length and tension of the vocal cords, the width of the rima and expiratory effort. The lower male pitch correlates with the average increased length of the vocal folds in men.

Joint Action

The cricothyroid joint can be seen to act as a rocking joint which rotates around a horizontal axis passing between the two joints and displacing the arytenoid cartilages backwards and forwards. The inferior attachment is the cricothyroid ligament so important in emergency cricothryoidotomy. The mechanism of cricothyroid action is so that the arytenoids move in a way so as to either approximate or to separate the vocal processes (and the vocal ligaments). This action is actually a complex rotation around a vertical axis based on the cricoid lamina where there is a concomitant transverse sliding action with the strong posterior capsule of the joint preventing the arytenoids from slipping forwards on the cricoid lamina.

The RLN lies just immediately behind this joint. Rotation and lateral gliding at (and around) this joint allows the arytenoids to open the rima like a V-shape and further to open the airway into the shape of a diamond. The human larynx possesses more glide than rotation at this joint with some additional support from small synovial aryteno-corniculate joints. The effect of rotation is to swing the arytenoids around their longitudinal axis with the vocal processes rotating outwards to open the rima to a range of about 30° maximal rotation. The gliding action allows the arytenoids to approach one another or to move more distantly and inferiorly with movements at the cricothyroid joints altering the tension of the vocal cords. Diagram 15.4 shows different views of the intrinsic laryngeal musculature. Diagram 15.4a shows the muscles visible on the external laryngeal skeleton. Diagram 15.4b shows the internal dissection from this viewpoint. Diagram 15.4c shows dissection of the laryngeal inlet (*from above*) and Diagram 15.4d shows the posterior aspect of the larynx, epiglottis and aryepiglottic folds (*See below for description of the intrinsic laryngeal muscles*).

Ligaments and Membranes

Membranes include:

- Extrinsics –
  - (a) Thyrohyoid membrane (thickened in the midline as the median thyrohyoid ligament). The free posterior border contains the small triticeal cartilage with the thyrohyoid membrane forming the lateral wall of the piriform recess
  - (b) The epiglottis connects to the sides of the arytenoid cartilages as the *aryepiglottic folds* (Diagram 15.3) and to the

tongue as the *median glosso-epiglottic fold* and to the pharynx by the *lateral glosso-epiglottic folds*.
  (c) The epiglottis is attached to the hyoid and thyroid cartilages by the *hyo-epiglottic* and the *thryo-epiglottic* ligaments respectively.
  (d) The *cricotracheal ligament* connects the lower cricoid cartilage to the first tracheal ring.
- Intrinsics –
  (a) The *quadrangular membrane* runs between the arytenoid cartilage and the epiglottis (in profile) appearing as a thin fibroelastic connexion anteriorly which is attached to the side of the lower epiglottis. The posterior border attaches between the vocal process of the arytenoid and the corniculate cartilage.
  (b) The free lower border is the vestibular fold (false vocal cord)
  (c) The cricothryoid ligament is thickened in the middle as the *conus elasticus.* The lateral part attaching to the vocal process is often labelled as the *cricovocal membrane* (thickened and rounded as the cricovocal ligament *a.k.a.* vocal fold or true vocal cord). See Diagram 15.1.

Laryngeal Musculature (Diagram 15.4)

These small but important muscles move the different parts of the larynx with small alterations in the length and separation of the vocal cords to produce the voice and more importantly to change the size and shape of the rima glottidis and the passage of air.

Intrinsic muscles of the larynx are considered in two groups: those altering the size and the shape of the laryngeal inlet and those moving the vocal folds. The muscles creating a sphincter for the inlet are the aryepiglottic and oblique arytenoid muscles assisted by the transverse arytenoid muscle and sometimes by the thryroepiglottic muscle (particularly if the aryepiglottic muscle is poorly formed).

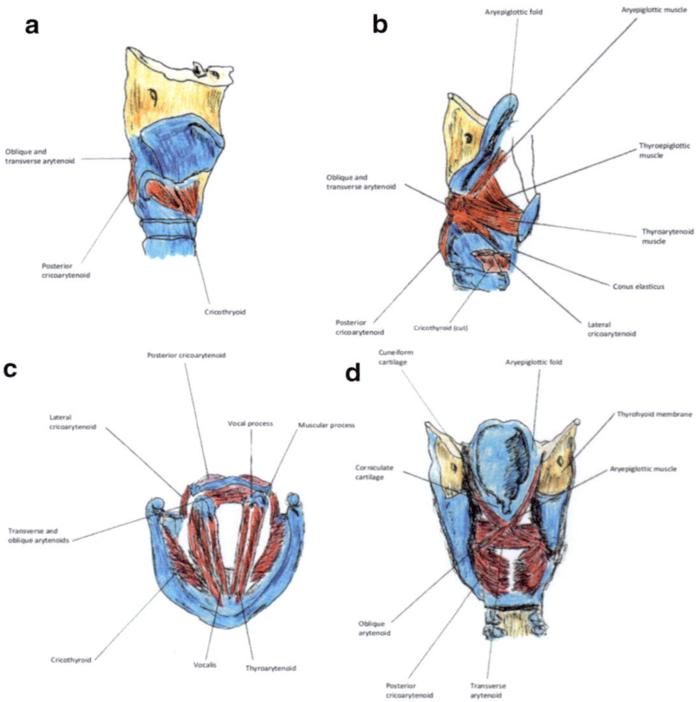

Diagram 15.4 The intrinsic musculature of the larynx
(**a**) External view
(**b**) Deeper dissection
(**c**) View from above
(**d**) Posterior dissection view

Those muscles involved in phonation and in moving the vocal folds include:

1. Posterior cricoarytenoid
2. Lateral cricoarytenoid
3. Thyroarytenoid
4. Vocalis
5. Transverse arytenoids and
6. Cricothyroid

The muscles of the inlet include:

Aryepiglottic muscle (Diagram 15.4b, d): This lies within the aryepiglottic fold and runs from the side of the epiglottis backwards to the muscular process of the arytenoid cartilage.

Oblique Arytenoid (Diagram 15.4d): This sends fibres to join the uppermost part of the aryepiglottic muscle passing from the muscular process of the arytenoid cartilage to the tip of the aryepiglottic muscle of the other side (this may actually attach to the contralateral corniculate cartilage). These two oblique arytenoids cross one another superficial to the transverse arytenoid muscle, acting as a sphincter of the laryngeal inlet. In effect, the aryepiglottic muscles and the oblique arytenoids appose the arytenoid cartilages drawing the epiglottis downwards to come into contact with the arytenoids.

Thyroepiglottic muscle (Diagram 15.4b): This arises from the upper thyroid lamina lying outside of the quadrangular membrane to be inserted into the side of the epiglottis. If the aryepiglottic fold is poorly formed then the oblique arytenoids and the thyroepiglottic muscle can take over this function to form the laryngeal sphincter. These muscles can compensate in this action even if the epiglottis is removed.

The muscles of the vocal folds are designed for opening and closing, lengthening and shortening acting in pairs as agonists and antagonists.

For the purposes of agreement opening is considered as vocal cord abduction and closure as vocal cord adduction. **Of major importance is that abduction is only produced by one muscle (regarded by otolaryngologists as the most important muscle in the body), the posterior cricoarytenoid muscle.** This muscle has two distinct actions each of which is opposed by a separate adductor muscle, the lateral cricoarytenoid and the transverse arytenoid. These muscles are named in accordance with their attachments and include:

Posterior Cricoarytenoid (Diagram 15.4d): This is the ONLY abductor of the cords (the only muscle capable of enlarging the rima). The muscle arises from the concavity of the back of the cricoid lamina and inserts into the muscular process of the arytenoid cartilage. Its upper part is horizontally disposed with the lateral fibres nearly vertical. Acting together the muscles pull (or rotate) the arytenoid cartilage laterally and also slightly tilts the vocal process laterally causing abduction of the vocal fold.

Lateral cricoarytenoid muscle (Diagram 15.4c) arises from the upper border of the cricoid arch and passes upwards to the muscular process of the arytenoid cartilage under the thyroid lamina. It draws the muscular process forwards but results in the vocal processes and folds approximating each other counteracting the cricoarytenoid rotation caused by the posterior cricoarytenoid muscle.

Transverse Arytenoid muscle is quite strong appearing as a transverse mass of muscle that connects the posterior and medial surfaces of the arytenoid cartilages to one another without any rotation (Diagram 15.4d).

The *Cricothyroid* is visible on the outside of the larynx (Diagram 15.4a) but also from the inside (Diagram 15.4c). In life this muscle is very evident during a thyroid lobectomy and it is the only laryngeal muscle that is visible in an anterior dissection of the neck running from the front of the cricoid arch and fanning out backwards on to the inferior and lower border of the thyroid lamina. When it contracts the arch of the cricoid and the tracheal notch are drawn together and as the cricoid is more of a fixed structure than the thyroid cartilage, the cricoid tilts downwards and backwards lengthening (and slightly adducting) the vocal fold. (This movement is a little easier to appreciate if one imagines the cricoid also moving).

The cricothryoid has as an antagonist the *thyroarytenoid muscle* which runs laterally from the saccule extending from the back of the thyroid lamina to the anterior part of the arytenoid cartilage.

As a rather flimsy muscle thyroarytenoid contraction shortens the vocal fold (Diagram 15.4c). The *vocalis muscle* pulls up part of the cricovocal membrane increasing the vertical depth of the opposing surfaces of the vocal folds and creating an action that is more complex than simple closure and opening by laterally augmenting the depth of the fold. These muscles act to oppose the cricothyroid effects on the tension and length of the vocal folds and their practical impact on voice pitch as well as intensity and quality (voice timbre). The length-tension changes induced by the thyroarytenoid and vocalis muscles can function independently.

To remind, the nerve supply of the cricothyroid is via the external branch of the superior laryngeal nerve which also innervates the thyropharyngeus component of the inferior constrictor. (See Chap. 3 including different classifications of the relationship of the external laryngeal nerve and the superior thyroid artery or the thyropharyngeus). The additional reminder is that all the intrinsic muscles of the larynx (except for the cricothyroid) are innervated by the recurrent laryngeal nerve, the continuity of which inside the larynx is as the inferior laryngeal nerve.

The intrinsic muscles of the larynx are particularly versatile and are also important in the activities of swallowing and respiration as well as phonation. In swallowing, the sphincter action of the aryepiglottic fold protects the airway, with the rima itself acting as a barrier, so that the larynx is hauled up beneath the tongue which bulges posteriorly. The epiglottis then tilts backwards and downwards like a lid to close over the laryngeal inlet. During phonation the voice intensity is dependent upon the air pressure and the timbre of the resonating chambers above in the vestibule, the pharynx, the mouth, the nose and the paranasal sinuses. This complex action is affected by the muscles of the soft palate and the tongue. The volume of these resonating chambers is increased by laryngeal depression.

Of importance:

1. The vocal folds form a dividing line or watershed into upper and lower laryngeal halves. The mucosa above the vocal folds is innervated by the internal laryngeal nerve and below by the RLN. The cell bodies of the afferent fibres of both of these

nerves lie in the inferior X ganglion. Secretomotor fibres lie in the dorsal vagal nucleus. The internal laryngeal is only sensory whereas the RLN is mixed. The SNS supply is with the STA and the ITA from the middle and the superior cervical ganglia.
2. Above the vocal folds are the superior laryngeal vessels (the superior thyroid artery entering the piriform recess with the internal laryngeal nerve by piercing the thyrohyoid membrane)
3. The lower half is supplied by the inferior laryngeal artery (a branch of the inferior thyroid artery which accompanies the RLN under the inferior constrictor muscle).
4. Lymphatics from the upper and lower laryngeal halves accompany the STA or the ITA to the deep cervical nodes with a few that travel directly to the pre-tracheal (Delphian) nodes [1].[1]
5. In RLN injury, the posterior cricoarytenoid muscle seems more vulnerable than the adductors. A partial lesion is more serious than a full paralysis and a bilateral partial lesion can be life threatening.
6. Paralysis of the external laryngeal nerve may go unnoticed but can cause some hoarseness of the voice which can recover with contralateral cricothyroid hypertrophy. When injured, it is difficult to produce higher frequencies with the affected vocal fold sitting slightly lower than its opposite number.

Concerning the extrinsic laryngeal musculature:

1. The larynx moves upwards during swallowing so that there are laryngeal elevators and laryngeal depressors.
2. Hyoid elevators transmit their pull to the thyroid cartilage through the thyrohyoid membrane so that the larynx cannot be depressed without an equivalent hyoid bone depression. Reversal of this function is via elastic recoil.
3. In swallowing the thyroarytenoid acts on a fixed hyoid bone and is assisted by the stylopharyngeus and the palatopharyn-

[1]This pre-cricoid lymph node may be involved in laryngeal and thyroid cancer and is not normally part of a lymphadenectomy. The prophetic role of the node as a sign of a more aggressive tumour biology has adopted the name Delphian after the Delphic oracle, a messenger of the Greek God Apollo.

geus so as to raise the larynx inside the hyoid and to compress the laryngeal orifice. The effect of the epiglottis tipping backwards is assisted by the bulging posterior surface of the tongue and by the aryepiglottic and thyroepiglottic muscles coming into contact with the elevated arytenoid cartilages.

Extrinsic elevators of the larynx include:

1. Those muscles *attaching to the hyoid that indirectly elevate the larynx*—mylohyoid, digastric, styloyoid, geniohyoid
2. Direct laryngeal elevators—thyrohyoid, stylopharyngeus, palatopharyngeus, salpingopharyngeus, thyropharyngeus. Note that salpingo, stylo and palatopharyngeus are laryngeal muscles that insert into the posterior lamina and horns of the thyroid cartilage (some preferring to refer to them as stylo, salpingo and palatolaryngeus muscles [2].

Extrinsic depressors of the larynx include:

1. Indirect depressors—the infrahyoid musculature; sternohyoid and omohyoid
2. Direct depressors—sternothyroid
3. Assistance in depression by oesophageal movement and the elastic recoil of the trachea

Q & A: Chap. 15 (Answers at the End of This Chapter)

1. The quadrangular membrane
   (a) Extends between the epiglottis and the arytenoids
   (b) Forms the vocal ligament inferiorly
   (c) Has a vestibular fold extending between the thyroid and cricoid cartilages
   (d) Superior and inferior borders that are not free

2. The thyroarytenoid
   (a) Takes origin between the thyroid and cricoid cartilages
   (b) Inserts posteriorly into the arytenoid cartilage
   (c) Inserts away from the posterior and lateral cricoarytenoid muscles
   (d) Tightens the vocal cords
3. Muscles of the vocal folds include:
   (a) Transverse interarytenoid
   (b) Oblique arytenoids
   (c) Cricothyroid
   (d) Aryepiglottic muscle
   (e) Thyroarytenoid
   (f) Thyroepiglottis
   (g) Lateral cricoarytenoid
4. Adductors of the cords include:
   (a) Posterior cricoarytenoid
   (b) Transverse and arytenoids
   (c) Lateral cricoarytenoids
   (d) Oblique arytenoids
5. A Unilateral vocal cord paralysis may be associated with:
   (a) Enlargement of the piriform sinus
   (b) No repositioning of the aryepiglottic fold
   (c) A normal laryngeal sinus
   (d) No atrophy of the thyroarytenoid muscle
   (e) Posterior cricoarytenoid atrophy
   (f) Compensatory bowing of the contralateral cord

Answers

1. a, c
2. a
3. a, e, g
4. b, c, d
5. a, e, f

References

1. Dy BM, Shaha AR, Tuttle RM. The Delphian node revisited: an uncommon site of recurrence. J Endocr Soc. 2017;1(12):1527–30.
2. Last RJ. In: McMinn RMH, editor. Last's anatomy regional and applied. 9th ed. London: Churchill Livingstone; 2019. p. 494.

The Ear

16

Contents

External Ear ~ (Diagram 16.1) 328
Middle Ear~ 330
Auditory Ossicles~ 334
Mastoid Bone, Antrum and Air Cells~ 336
Inner Ear ~ (Diagram 16.5) 337
Q & A: Chap. 16 (Answers at the End of This Chapter) 341
Answers 343

For the *purposes* of definition the *external ear* consists of the auricle (pinna), the external acoustic meatus and the outer aspect of the tympanic membrane. The *middle ear* comprises the tympanic cavity (tympanum) with the ossicles and the Eustachian tube. The *inner ear* lies inside the temporal bone housing the membranous labyrinth and the vestibule containing the semicircular canals, the cochlea and the vestibulocochlear neural receptors (vestibular and auditory nerves).

A. Zbar, *Anatomy--Head and Neck*,
https://doi.org/10.1007/978-3-031-69538-4_16

External Ear ~ (Diagram 16.1)

The particular landmarks of the pinna include the helix, the antihelix, the lobule, the tragus, the antitragus, the concha (behind the tragus), the scaphoid fossa and the triangular fossa. Two surfaces are also formed, the lateral and cranial surfaces. The cymba concha lying between the crus of the helix and the antihelix is the landmark for the mastoid antrum. Intrinsic muscles (helices major and minor, tragicus and antitragicus) are vestigial.

The cutaneous sensory supply is shown. This consists principally of the great auricular (entire cranial surface) and the auriculotemporal nerves (upper lateral and meatal surfaces). A small inner and insignificant aspect is innervated sensorily by Cranial VII (via tympanic plexus) and Cranial X (auricular branch innervating the posterior-inferior quadrant of the tympanic

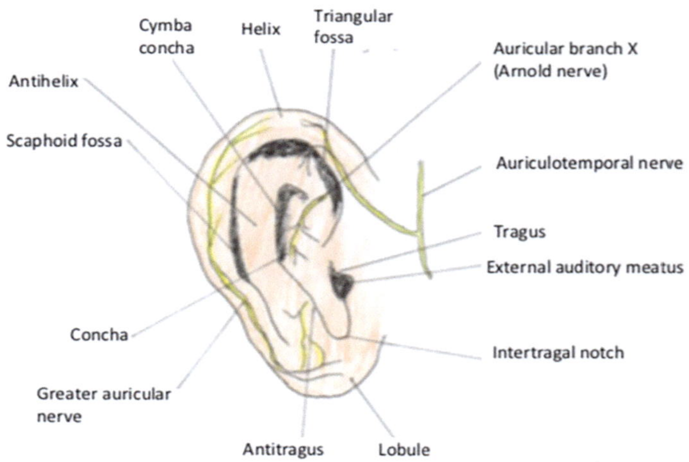

Diagram 16.1 The auricle and its components. The cutaneous nerve supply is derived from the auriculotemporal nerve (V_3), the great auricular nerve ($C_{2,3}$), the auricular branch of Cranial X (Arnold's nerve) and part of the tympanic plexus of Cranial VII

membrane).[1] This Arnold nerve may supply a similar part of the external meatal and postauricular skin. Cranial VII supplies a paucity of sensory tympanic branches running from the geniculate ganglion as representatives of the second pharyngeal pouch which join the tympanic plexus formed by Cranial IX. Evidence of this embryological connexion is shown in Herpes Zoster infection (shingles) which can show vesicles in this part of the external auditory meatus. The lesser occipital (C_2) has a small superior supply to the cranial auricular surface. The external acoustic meatus consists of an outer cartilaginous and an inner bony two-thirds. The canal has two main constrictions, one that is close to the cartilaginous portion and another just short of the tympanic membrane (isthmus) which is actually in the bony portion and not at the cartilaginous-bony junction. Because the floor (and the anterior wall) are longer than the roof (and the posterior wall) the tympanic membrane is obliquely positioned, necessitating the clinician to pull the pinna up and outwards so as to straighten the meatus for otoscopic visualization.

Blood supply to the auricle is via posterior auricular and superficial temporal arteries. The deep anterior part of the tympanic membrane has a supply from the deep auricular branch of the first part of the maxillary artery. The pinna of the ear forms from the first and second arch hillocks (of His)[1] and is completed by 20 weeks. The external auditory meatus forms from the dorsal part of the first arch along with the middle ear components (malleus and incus). The inner ear develops from the otic capsule.

[1]This auricular nerve is also known as Arnold's nerve after the German anatomist Friedrich Arnold (1803–1890). This nerve arises from the jugular X ganglion which is supported by a small twig from the petrous ganglion of Cranial IX. The nerve can supply part of the external auditory meatus and the tragus. Of clinical relevance is that this can be part of a glomus jugulare tumour of the superior X ganglion. In laryngeal cancer pain can be referred to the ear via Arnold's nerve. Wilhelm His Sr. (1831–1904) was a Swiss anatomist who worked with Rudolf Virchow (1821–1902) and who described the foetal tubercles (the His hillocks) which colaesce in the formation of the ear. He invented the microtome in pathology designed to cut tissues evenly and his son Wilhelm His Jr. (1863–1934) described the bundle of His as part of the conduction system of the heart.

Middle Ear~

This is a transmission chamber designed to increase the kinetic energy from the outer ear acoustic vibrations. The tympanum is part of the blind diverticulum connected to the nasopharynx via the Eustachian tube. Consideration of the complex includes an appreciation of the anatomy of the Eustachian tube (See Chap. 12), the mastoid antrum and the mastoid air cells. The tympanic cavity running from the tympanic membrane to the medial wall (lateral wall of the inner ear) is tilted at the same angle as the membrane (set at 55° obliquely to the external auditory meatus). The *umbo* in the membrane is formed by the impression of the handle of the malleus which also leaves two visible mallear folds extending to the membrane edge (Diagram 16.2). The area above is the *pars flaccida*[2] which has a close internal relationship to the chorda tympani (and which may be visible on well illuminated otoscopy). The remainder of the drum below is the *pars tensa*. Maintenance of the position of the tympanic membrane is kept by the pull of the tensor tympani. Blood supply outwards and inwards is via the deep auricular and anterior tympanic branches of the maxillary artery (See Chap. 8). The latter branch is supported on the mucosal side by the stylomastoid artery (a branch of the facial). Innervation on the meatal side is via the auriculotemporal nerve (with Cranial VII and X support) whereas the mucosal side is supplied by the tympanic plexus of Cranial IX. Lying between the neck of the malleus and the pars flaccida and bounded above by the lateral malleolar fold is *Prussak's space* which is the commonest site for formation of a cholesteatoma.[3]

Diagram 16.3 shows the anatomy of the middle ear.

This anatomy of the middle ear may be considered by its walls. The medial wall is mainly formed at a central bulge, the

---

[2]Also known as Shrapnell's membrane after the English anatomist and physician Henry Jones Shrapnell (1792–1834) a work colleague of the father of vaccination Edward Jenner (1749–1823).

[3]Named after Aleksandr Federovich Prussak (1839–1897), a Russian otologist who first described the anatomy of this space in 1867.

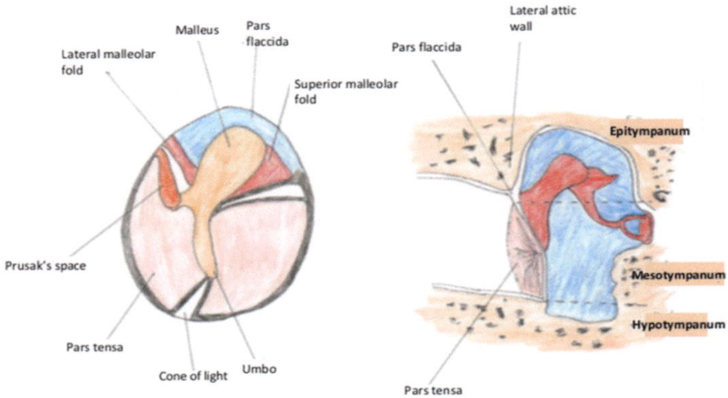

Diagram 16.2 The tympanic membrane. The *left-hand image* shows Prussak's space which is part of the epitympanic space and which is bordered laterally by the pars flaccida, superiorly by the lateral malleolar fold, medially by the neck of the malleus and inferiorly by the short process of the malleus (Diagram 16.4)
The *right-hand image* shows the relationship of the auditory ossicles and the tympanic membrane and the boundaries of the epitympanum, mesotympanum and hypotympanum

promontory which is created by the first turn of the cochlea. In this wall there are two openings connecting the middle and inner ears (oval and round windows). The oval window (*fenestra vestibuli*) is located above and behind the promontory (and is closed by the footplate of the stapes). The round window (*fenestra cochleae*) lies below and behind the promontory and is closed by the secondary tympanic membrane. The canal for the facial nerve (Cranial VII) lies just above the oval window (Diagram 16.4).

The roof (superior or tegmental wall) of the tympanum (the tegmen tympani part of the petrous temporal bone internally) attaches the tensor tympani (See Diagram 6.6; Chap. 6). This has

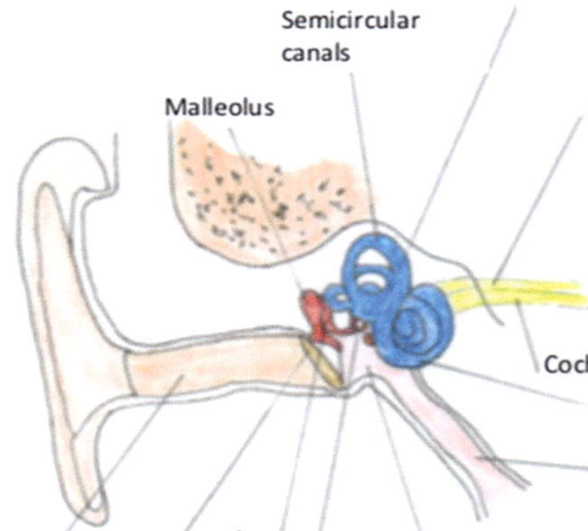

Diagram 16.3 The anatomy of the middle ear and tympanic cavity

important clinical significance since at this point the bone is a very thin plate separating the temporal lobe of the brain (and the middle cranial fossa) from the mastoid antrum posteriorly. The floor is separated from the jugular fossa and the bulb of the IJV by a thin bony plate. Anteriorly lies the tympanic canaliculus housing the tympanic branch of Cranial IX. The anterior wall is perforated by the bony Eustachian tube, the canal for the chorda tympani and the tensor tympani muscle canal along with a leash of caroticotympanic branches of the ICA, the anterior tympanic artery and by SNS fibres traveling with the artery (internal carotid nerve). This wall separates the middle ear from the ICA.

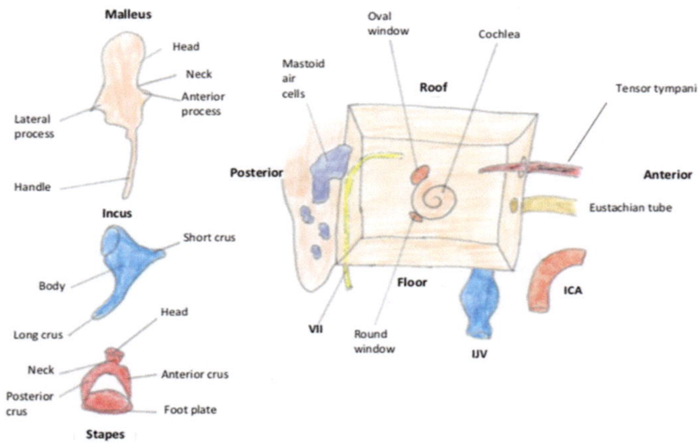

Diagram 16.4 The auditory ossicles and the 3-dimensional relationship of the middle ear to the mastoid antrum and air cells, the cochlea and the round and oval windows. Note the anterior connection to the tendon of the tensor tympani muscle and the close relationship to the internal jugular vein (IJV) and the internal carotid artery (ICA). The facial nerve is seen posteriorly and deeply. In this locale it gives off the chorda tympani and a branch to stapedius

The posterior wall separates the middle ear from the mastoid. It is deficient above to form the aditus opening which connects the attic of the middle ear (epitympanum) with the mastoid antrum. The ridge of the VII nerve canal passes here along the medial wall of the aditus with the lateral semicircular canal causing a bulge above, the incus forming a bulge below and below further still an area called the pyramid projects out conically where it is perforated by the tendon of the stapedius. Appreciation of the anatomy here is of clinical significance since a facial recess is created (also called the suprapyramidal recess) between the Cranial VII and the pyramid which is a point of surgical access to the middle ear where a posterior approach is possible without disturbing the posterior wall of the meatus. The facial recess is also a waek area that is a recognized site of recurrence of a cholesteatoma after mastoid surgery.

Vascular anastomosis for the middle ear is particularly complicated and implicates: the anterior tympanic, posterior tympanic (a branch of the posterior auricular), superior tympanic (a branch of the middle meningeal), inferior tympanic (a branch of the ascending pharyngeal), petrosal (a branch of the middle meningeal), caroticotympanic ICA branches and the stylomastoid artery.

Auditory Ossicles~

The task of the auditory ossicles is to transmit and modify vibrations of the tympanic membrane to the inner ear via synovial joints. The first of these the malleus is club-like in shape, with its convex head lying in the epitympanic recess (Diagram 16.4) and with a posterior articular facet for the incus (incudomalleolar joint) so that the neck lies against the pars flaccida with the chorda tympani crossing medial to the malleus neck. The lower end of the handle is the visible umbo so that the upper part of the handle forms a lateral process. The incus is formed by a body and two slender limbs and has a long posteriorly located limb for articulation as the lentiform nodule with the stapes (incudostapedial joint). The stapes has a neck which forms slender anterior and posterior limbs which attach to a foot piece fitting into the oval window (tympanostapedial syndesmosis). These articulations increase the force of transmitted vibrations but reduce their amplitude.

The muscles attached to the ossicles dampen the vibrations from low-pitched sound waves. The tensor tympani arises from the superior part of the cartilaginous Eustachian tube and attached petrous temporal bone and the greater wing of the sphenoid passing to the tympanic cavity in the middle ear in a small canal. The muscle gives way to a slender tendon that inserts into the upper part of the handle of the malleus. It has a blood supply from the superior tympanic branch of the middle meningeal artery and is innervated by the mandibular nerve through the nerve to the medial pterygoid. This little nerve runs through the otic ganglion without synapse. The task of the muscle is to pull the handle of the malleus medially tensing the tympanic membrane to dampen the oscillations with some secondary tightening of the footplate of the stapes against the oval window. The stapedius arises from the pyramidal process of the petrous temporal bone to enter the mesotympanum and attach to the posterior part of the stapedial neck. It has a multiple blood supply (posterior auricular, anterior tympanic and middle meningeal) and is innervated by Cranial VII to dampen oscillations passing through the oval window to the cochlea. A lower motor neuron VII palsy combined with hyperacusis (noise hypersensitivity) places the facial nerve lesion in the middle ear (See Chap. 7). Arterial supply may be from the anterior tympanic artery (via the squamotympanic fissure) and the stylomastoid artery (via the posterior auricular or the occipital and passed through the stylomastoid foramen).

The venous drainage is clinically important since small tributaries can pass via the squamotympanic fissure to the pterygoid venous plexus or through the petrous temporal to the superior petrosal sinus. If a septic thrombophlebitis spreads to this area from middle ear infection this can lead to direct formation of a temporal lobe abscess. The main sensory supply of this region is via the tympanic branch of Cranial IX (Jacobson's nerve) which enters the petrous temporal via the tympanic canaliculus in the thin plate of bone between the carotid canal and the jugular foramen. This is joined by minute caroticotympanic branches coming from the carotid sinus nerve.

This sensory nerve supply may hook up with a small component of Cranial VII whose cell bodies lie in the geniculate ganglion so that otalgia may have an origin in the draining areas of Cranial V, VII, IX and X (as far afield as the teeth, the larynx and pharynx and the posterior one-third of the tongue). The lesser petrosal nerve (formerly the lesser superficial petrosal or Jacobson's nerve) emanates from the tympanic plexus and runs across the middle cranial fossa lateral to the greater petrosal nerve to pass via the foramen ovale to the otic ganglion for synapse (containing the preganglionic fibres from the inferior salivatory nucleus destined for parotid sudomotor activity).

Diagram 16.4 shows the ossicles separately and the orientation in the middle ear cavity of the round and oval windows.

Mastoid Bone, Antrum and Air Cells~

Behind the epitympanic recess and communicating with the middle ear (Diagram 16.4) lies the mastoid antrum which has a spherical-shaped connecting aditus near the upper and outer margin of the external auditory meatus. The antrum is variably sized and is filled in by the tegmen tympani part of the petrous temporal bone which gradually becomes pneumatized by mastoid air cells with completion of this process by the age of 6 years. This variability can provide separate or connected groups of cells (squamosal, periantral, perisinus, peritubal, retrofacial, zygomatic, petrous apical etc.). Of importance is the venous drainage via a mastoid emissary vein linking the sigmoid sinus to the posterior auricular veins. Chronic infection here can lead to sigmoid sinus thrombophlebitis and even to an occipital lobe cerebral abscess. There are some clinical landmarks: suprameatal triangle (bounded by the temporal line, the bony meatus wall and a line connecting the two) or by the sinodural angle or by a thin bony plate of the petrosquamous fissure which extends posteriorly from the epitympanum to divide the mastoid air cells into separate lateral and medial compartments (Koerner septum).[4]

The Eustachian tube has already been considered in Chap. 13. In brief, the proportions of the bony and cartilaginous portions are the reverse of the external auditory canal with the shorter bony part narrowed at the isthmus near the posterior and lateral part of the spine of the sphenoid. The longer cartilaginous part is snug inside the groove between the greater wing of the sphenoid and the apex of the petrous temporal bone. The disposition of the cartilages creates a long posterior end and a tubal torus which is

[4]Named after Otto Körner (1858–1935), a German otorhinolaryngologist who described the plate (also called the petrosquamous lamina) in 1926.

clearly evident in the lateral nasopharynx (See Diagram 12.1; Chap. 12). The cartilaginous portion of the tube is dually innervated by the pharyngeal branch of the pterygopalatine ganglion as well as by the nervus spinosus (the meningeal branch of V_3). The sensory innervation of the bony portion is via the tympanic plexus (Cranial IX).

Inner Ear ~ (Diagram 16.5)

The inner ear is carved into the petrous temporal bone and includes the osseous labyrinth, the membranous labyrinth, the cochlear canal, the vestibule and the semicircular canals. This system supports the functions of hearing and balance with development from an otic placode that has vestibular formation occurring before cochlea development and that is complete before birth.

The *membranous labyrinth* includes the cochlear duct and the semicircular canals (Diagram 16.6). This part is closed but filled with endolymph. It comprises three layers, an outer vascular element, an intermediate cellular layer and an inner layer which contains receptors of sound, static balance and kinetic balance. This area is served by both the vestibular and cochlear nerves which are distributed in the walls of the membranous labyrinth. The membranous and bony labyrinths are separated by the perilymph and there is no communication between endolymph and perilymph. The membranous labyrinth forms the vestibule which houses the *utricle*, *saccule* and *semicircular ducts*. The semicircular ducts open via five separate ampullae into the utricle as shown in Diagram 16.6. These areas contain the sensory receptors (hair cells) for kinetic balance. Each of these (hair cells of the *maculae* of the utricle, and the saccule and the transverse crest, the crista on the medial surface of the semicircular duct ampullae) is stimulated by movement of the otolithic membranes, sensitive to the movement of endolymyph that occurs with head movement or change in position. The maculae respond to gravitational changes. The saccule is connected to the utricle lying under the petrous dura mater with an inferiorly passing *ductus reuniens* which joins

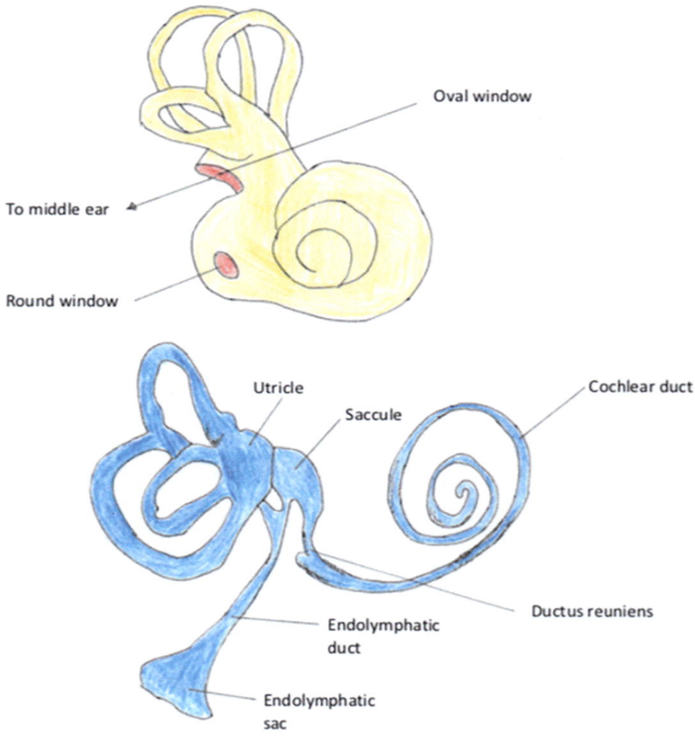

Diagram 16.5 The osseous and membranous labyrinth. The *top image* shows the connexion between the semicircular canals and cochlea and the middle ear
The *bottom image* shows the components of the membranous labyrinth and circulation of the endolymph

the lower end of the saccule to the base of the cochlea. The connecting endolymphatic duct projects as a blind *endolymphatic sac* and is a point of absorption of the endolymph lying under the posterior cranial fossa dura mater. The medial wall of the saccule is thickened as a macula and houses the sensory receptors for static balance.

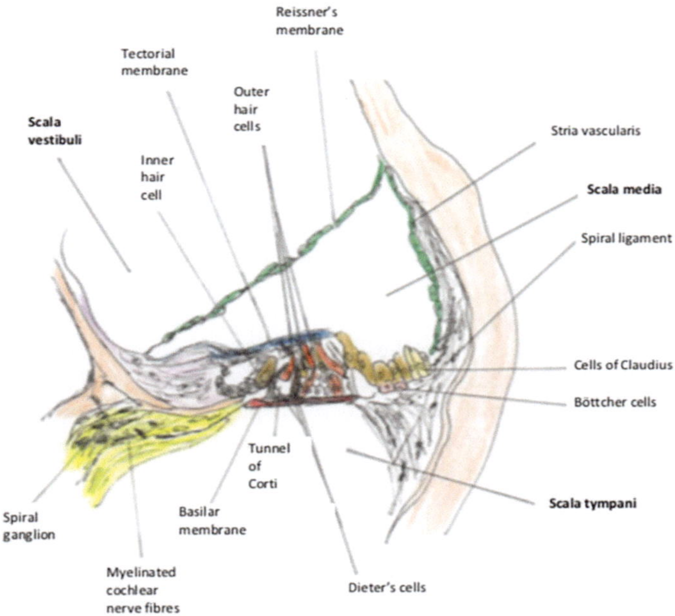

Diagram 16.6 The Organ of Corti. The area above is the scala vestibuli and the area below is the scala tympani. The scala media lies between. There are a range of supporting cells including the Dieter's cells (outer pharyngeal cochlear supporting cells), Böttcher cells (basal cells that may possibly alter the composition of the endolymph) and larger supporting cells of Claudius

Otto Friedrich Karl Dieters (1834 – 1 863) a German neuroanatomist described these cells along with the first description of the axonal and dendritic components of a basic neuron. He died at 29 from typhoid fever. Arthur Böttcher (1831 – 1 889) was an Estonian anatomist and Friedrich Matthias Claudius (1822 – 1 869) was Professor of Anatomy at Marburg University Germany who described these supporting cells of the Organ of Corti in 1856

The blood supply of the membranous labyrinth is via the labyrinthine vessel spreading along the vestibular and cochlear nerves. The labyrinthine artery is a branch of the anterior inferior cerebellar artery (basilar; Diagram 9.4; Chap. 9) and divides into a cochlear and a vestibular branch with additional contribution from the stylomastoid artery. The venous drainage is via the inferior petrosal sinus.

The cavity of the osseous labyrinth opens into the medial wall of the middle ear via the oval window and the round window. The former is guarded by the footplate of the stapes and the latter by the secondary tympanic membrane (Diagrams 16.2 and 16.4). There is an opening via the aqueduct of the vestibule and the aqueduct of the cochlea into the posterior cranial fossa for drainage of the perilymph into the cerebrospinal fluid. The cochlear canal is that part of the petrous temporal bone containing the cochlear duct appearing as a spiral shell turn. The whole spirals around an axial stem the *modiolus* attaching the membranous cochlear duct. The modiolus is perforated by twigs of the cochlear nerve passing towards the spiral ganglion.

The cochlear duct is a spiral anterior part of this membranous labyrinth containing the sound receptors. This cochlea duct connects the scala vestibuli (the top part of the cochlea communicating with the subarachnoid space) and the scala tympani, the most inferior part of the cochlea (hence the cochlear duct is also known as the scala media). The cochlear duct contains the sensory organ of Corti which in cross-section appears triangular. This area is formed by a basilar membrane supporting the spiral organ, the vestibular (Reissner's) membrane passing across the apical side of the basilar membrane and the sensory apparatus hair cells. The latter are supported by phalangeal cells arranged in rows all overlain by a tectorial membrane.[5]

The semicircular canals lie in the 3-dimensional planes. The anterior is placed vertically in the plane of the petrous temporal

[5]Named after Alfonso Giacomo Gaspare Corti (1822–1876) an Italian anatomist whose father knew the famous Pavian anatomist Antonio Scarpa (1752–1832). Ernst Reissner (1824–1878) was a Latvian anatomist who was Professor of Anatomy in Estonia.

with its convexity facing upwards and its ampulla laterally disposed. The posterior canal is vertically placed in the long axis of the petrous temporal (convexity lying backwards and the ampulla below). The ampullated end of this canal has a separate nerve supply from the inferior division of the vestibular nerve. The lateral canal is obliquely off the horizontal plane (ampulla anterior with convexity backwards). The upper division of the vestibular nerve supplies the macula of the utricle and the ampullae of the anterior and lateral semicircular canals. Cell bodies of the cochlear fibres are located in the spiral ganglion at the modiolus with those of the vestibular fibres lying in the vestibular ganglion inside the internal acoustic meatus. Cranial VIII divides in the internal acoustic meatus into an anterior cochlear nerve and a posterior vestibular nerve.[6] The cochlear nerve ramifies at the modiolar base and terminates in the inner and some outer hair cells. The vestibular nerve divides into superior, inferior and posterior branches distal to the ganglion, the superior nerve innervating the utricular macula and the ampullae of the anterior and lateral semicircular canals. The inferior branch innervates the saccular macula in the 3-dimensional planes. The anterior branch is placed vertically and the posterior branch in the ampulla of the posterior semicircular canal.

Q & A: Chap. 16 (Answers at the End of This Chapter)

1. In the ear drum:
   (a) Sensation of the outer surface is via the auriculotemporal nerve
   (b) Part of the inner surface sensation comes from the Vagus
   (c) The pars flaccida lies below the lateral process of the malleus
   (d) The pars tensa is the usual site of perforation

[6] An anastomosis between these two nerves is referred to as Oort's anastomosis joining the saccular nerve before it ramifies to the cochlear nerve and before it penetrates the cochlea.

2. The auricle:
   (a) Is solely supplied by the posterior auricular artery
   (b) Is supplied on its deep aspect of the external acoustic meatus and in the tympanic membrane by the maxillary artery
   (c) Is innervated entirely by the great auricular nerve
   (d) Has some innervation via the lesser occipital nerve
   (e) Has lymphatics draining to the parotid and mastoid group of lymph nodes
3. The organ of Corti:
   (a) Converts the movement of hair cells into electrochemical signals
   (b) Has its scala media lying between the tympanic and vestibular ducts
   (c) Does not have stereocilia
   (d) Is unable to amplify the auditory signal
4. The semicircular canals:
   (a) Has a posterior component detecting rotation in the coronal axis (sagittal plane)
   (b) Has a posterior component that is operative when the head nods
   (c) Has an anterior canal that detects rotation in the sagittal plane (lateral axis).
   (d) The anterior canal is operative when one's head touches the shoulders or in performing a cartwheel
   (e) Has a lateral component is the longest of all the canals.
   (f) The lateral canal operates when the head moves around a vertical axis (rotation in the transverse plane on the neck and in turning the head from side to side).
5. Considering the ossicles:
   (a) The incus is adherent to the eardrum
   (b) The incudostapedial joint involves the short crus of the incus which moves independently from the head of the stapes
   (c) Develops separately from Meckel's cartilage
   (d) Transmit vibrations to the round window
   (e) Transmit vibrations to the oval window

6. The round window:
   (a) Is sealed by the secondary tympanic membrane
   (b) Vibrates with an same phase to that of the oval window
   (c) Lies anteriorly to the oval window
   (d) Is located near the basal turn of the cochlea in the meso-tympanum

Answers

1. a, b, d
2. b, d, e
3. a, b
4. f
5. e
6. a, d

Relevant Developmental Embryology: An Overview

17

Contents

Pharyngeal Arches ~ (Diagram 17.1a–d) ... 347
Pharyngeal Pouches ~ ... 351
Pharyngeal Clefts~ ... 351
Development of the Tongue~ ... 352
Thyroid Development ~ (See Chap. 3) ... 352
Development of the Face ~ ... 354
Q & A: Chap. 17 (Answers at the End of This Chapter) ... 354
Answers ... 355

It is relevant to complete this volume after an appreciation of the basic head and neck anatomy by adding an understanding of the embryology of head and neck and craniofacial development. Embryology is not usually formally considered in many anatomical textbooks and when it is the relevant information is often placed at the commencement of studies without any contextual understanding or before there is a complete grasp of the germane anatomy.

In broad terms, the formation of the head and neck structures is from specialized mesenchyme. This is divisible into paraxial and

A. Zbar, *Anatomy--Head and Neck*,
https://doi.org/10.1007/978-3-031-69538-4_17

lateral plate mesoderm, the neural crest and the ectodermal placodes. The paraxial mesoderm (also referred to as the somites) forms the voluntary craniofacial musculature and the soft-tissues and part of the meninges (caudal to the prosencephalon or forebrain). The lateral plate mesoderm is responsible for the laryngeal cartilages and the local connective tissue. The migration of neural crest tissue into the pharyngeal arches forms the arch skeletal constructs with a rostral migration around the forebrain and the optic cup to form mid-facial structures. This is a highly mixed area that differentiates into whatever is needed (bone, cartilage, dentin, meninges etc.). The ectodermal placodes form neurons that lie in the sensory ganglia of cranial nerves V, VII, IX and X.

One major area of head and neck development is via the pharyngeal (branchial) arches which are paired structures that form the face, jaw, ear and neck, forming early at the fourth or fifth week of development (there are five arches by the end of the fourth week with the fifth arch regressing and leaving ultimately arches 1, 2, 3, 4 and 6). Between these arches lie the pharyngeal (branchial) clefts and specific outpouchings the pharyngeal (branchial) pouches (thus five pharyngeal arches and four pharyngeal pouches). The entire area consists therefore of arches, clefts (or grooves), pouches and membranes so that each arch consists of a core of somatic mesoderm and neural crest mesenchyme.

The somatic mesoderm forms the arch artery and the skeletal arch musculature. The neural crest mesenchyme forms the bone, cartilage and connective tissue applicable to each arch. Each arch also has a discrete cranial nerve: Arch 1 (Trigeminal), Arch 2 (Facial), Arch 3 (Glossopharyngeal), Arch 4 (Superior laryngeal branch of the Vagus) and Arch 6 (Recurrent laryngeal branch of the Vagus). The inner part is lined by endoderm and the outer part (four pharyngeal clefts) are covered by ectoderm.

These pharyngeal arches are also important in facial structure where the initial stomodeum is surrounded by the pair of first pharyngeal arch mesoderm. In effect each pharyngeal arch has its own particular muscular, arterial and neural component.

Pharyngeal Arches ~ (Diagram 17.1a–d)

- The first pharyngeal arch: has a dorsal maxillary process and a ventral mandibular process (Meckel's cartilage). Much of Meckel's cartilage (See Diagram 7.1; Chap. 7) degenerates leaving only the malleus and the incus and the mandible. The maxillary process forms the premaxilla, the maxilla, the zygomatic bone, the palatine bone, the vomer and part of the squamous temporal bone. Muscles of this first arch include:
  (a) Muscles of mastication (pterygoids, masseter, temporalis)
  (b) Anterior belly of digastric
  (c) Mylohyoid
  (d) Tensor tympani
  (e) Tensor palati

The *nerve of this arch* is $\mathbf{V_3}$. The *artery* is part of the first aortic arch (**maxillary artery**)

- Second Pharyngeal arch: (Reichert's cartilage) forms the stapes, the styloid, the stylohyoid ligament and the lesser cornua of the hyoid bone and the upper segment of the body of the hyoid bone. Muscles of the second arch include:
  (a) Stapedius
  (b) Stylohyoid
  (c) Posterior belly of the digastric
  (d) Muscles of facial expression
  (e) Auricular muscles

The *nerve of the arch* is **Cranial VII**. The *artery* is part of the second aortic arch, the **stapedial artery**.

- Third Pharyngeal arch: This third cartilage forms the lower part of the body of the hyoid bone and the greater cornua. *There is only one muscle*, the **stylopharyngeus**.

Diagram 17.1 Basic foetal structure of the pharyngeal arches, pouches and clefts
(**a**) Neural crest cells migrate into the pharyngeal arches and face from the forebrain, midbrain and hindbrain (*arrows*). The arches (I, II, III, IV and VI) are shown as are the relevant cranial nerves (VII, IX and X)
(**b**) Pharyngeal arches. Each arch comprises a cartilage element, a cranial nerve, an artery and a muscular component
(**c**) Pharyngeal pouches: are shown as connected to the foregut with segmental arterial supply from aortic arches
(**d**) Pharyngeal clefts and pouches: The first pharyngeal pouch becomes the primitive tympanic cavity and the first pharyngeal cleft forms the external auditory meatus. Components of the second pharyngeal pouch form the palatine tonsil and the third pouch forms the inferior parathyroids III and the thymus (explaining their connexion and the path of an ectopic lower parathyroid adenoma). The fourth pharyngeal pouch forms the superior parathyroid (IV) and the ultimobranchial body. The primordial thyroid does not form from pouch tissue

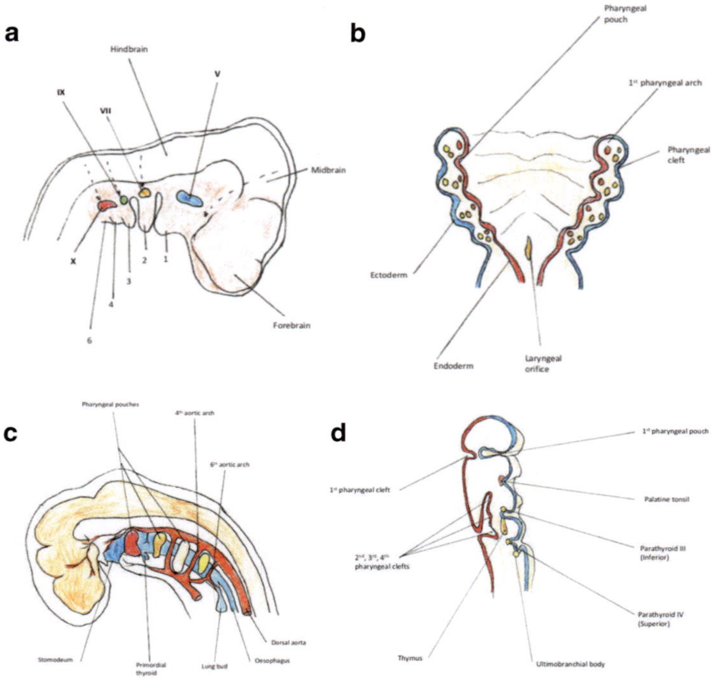
a
Hindbrain
V
IX
VII
Midbrain
X
2
1
3
4
6
Forebrain
b
Pharyngeal pouch
1st pharyngeal arch
Pharyngeal cleft
Ectoderm
Endoderm
Laryngeal orifice
c
Pharyngeal pouches
4th aortic arch
6th aortic arch
Stomodeum
Primordial thyroid
Lung bud
Oesophagus
Dorsal aorta
d
1st pharyngeal pouch
1st pharyngeal cleft
Palatine tonsil
2nd, 3rd, 4th pharyngeal clefts
Parathyroid III (Inferior)
Parathyroid IV (Superior)
Thymus
Ultimobranchial body

The *nerve of this arch* is the **Glossopharyngeal (Cranial IX)**. The artery is associated with the third aortic arch forming part of the common carotid artery and the initial part of the ICA. It explains why Cranial IX and the stylopharyngeus run between the ECA and the ICA.

- The fourth and sixth Pharyngeal arches: fuse in the formation of cartilages (thyroid, cricoid, arytenoid, corniculate and cuneiform). Muscles of this region include:
  (a) fourth arch musculature—cricothyroid, levator palati, pharyngeal constrictors, salpingopharyngeus, muscles of the soft palate (except for the tensor palati)
  (b) Intrinsic laryngeal muscles

The *nerve supply of the* four*th arch musculature* is via the **superior laryngeal nerve**. The *nerve supply of the sixth arch musculature* is via the **recurrent laryngeal nerve**. The fourth pharyngeal arch is associated with the fourth aortic arch forming the proximal part of the right subclavian artery. Another way of remembering the fourth arch musculature is as: muscles of the soft palate (excluding the tensor palati) and muscles of the pharynx (excluding the stylopharyngeus) and the cricothyroid. In thinking of the sixth arch separately, the artery associated with the sixth aortic arch contributes to the formation of the proximal part of the pulmonary arteries and the ductus arteriosus territory. This area contributes to all of the laryngeal intrinsics (excluding the cricothyroid) and part of the skeletal (striated) musculature of the upper oesophagus.

In addition, aside from these branchial arches there is somatic musculature from the paraxial mesoderm that does not migrate into the arches and which forms the extraocular muscles (Cranial III, IV and VI). The somitic paraxial mesoderm migrates into the tongue to form the extrinsic and intrinsic tongue muscles (Cranial XII). The lateral plate occipital mesoderm develops into the sternocleidomastoid and trapezius muscles (Cranial XI).

Pharyngeal Pouches ~

- The first Pharyngeal pouch: as the *tubotympanic recess* comes into contact with the first pharyngeal cleft (which forms the external auditory meatus). The distal part of the pouch forms the middle ear (tympanic) cavity and the proximal part forms the primitive Eustachian tube. Soft-tissue differentiation forms the tympanic membrane.
- The second pharyngeal pouch: forms the primordial palatine tonsil.
- The third pharyngeal pouch: separates into ventral and dorsal wings. The dorsal wing of the third pouch forms the inferior parathyroid with the ventral wing forming the thymus (See Diagram 3.2; Chap. 3 and also Diagram 17.1c). These separate completely from the pharyngeal wall and migrate inferiorly. This can explain the low position of an ectopic parathyroid gland adenoma which can be difficult to locate in a patient with hypercalcaemia from hyperparathyroidism. This also explains why the tail of the thymus can be adherent to the lower part of the thyroid gland in so-called thyrothymic tissue (See Chap. 3).
- The fourth pharyngeal pouch: forms the superior parathyroid gland which separates from the pharynx and adopts an association with the upper pole of the thyroid gland. The ventral part of the fourth pouch forms a diverticulum (the ultimobranchial body) which migrates into the substance of the thyroid gland as the parafollicular (C-or calcitonin-producing cells that form medullary thyroid cancers).

Pharyngeal Clefts~

These are ectodermally lined and are evident on the outside of the pharynx. The dorsal part of the first cleft contributes to the external auditory meatus. The remainder of the clefts move internally and normally merge and become obliterated.

Development of the Tongue~

The tongue appears very early (4 weeks) as two lateral lingual swellings and a median *tuberculum impar* all originating from the first pharyngeal arch. The other arches (second, third and fourth) contribute to an additional midline swelling the *copula* and there is a third median swelling which forms from the back of the fourth arch that is destined to form the epiglottis. The lateral swellings and the tuberculum all merge to form the anterior two-thirds of the tongue explaining how Cranial V_3 is sensory. The posterior part is separated by the *sulcus terminalis* and arises from the second, third and fourth arches so that the sensory innervation is via Cranial IX. The separation of first arch structures from the other arches explains why the sulcus represents a developmental watershed. The Cranial IX representation of the posterior tongue is a measure of the overgrowth of this region by elements of the third arch.

This pattern of development also shows how the developing epiglottis is innervated by the superior laryngeal nerve as part of the fourth arch. The Cranial XII innervation of the tongue musculature shows its development from occipital somites whose myoblasts invade this first pharyngeal arch mesoderm. Differentiation of taste at the circumvallate papillae has the chorda tympani as the anterior nerve supply (hitchhiking fibres along the local part of V_3 the lingual nerve) and Cranial IX behind this line.

Thyroid Development ~ (See Chap. 3)

The gland forms in the floor of the pharynx (between the tuberculum impar and the copula) and not from a pharyngeal pouch as such. The thyroid forms from the area of the *foramen caecum* (the endodermal pit in the floor of the pharynx just caudal to the first pharyngeal arch). This tissue descends in front of the gut as a bilobar diverticulum (Diagram 3.2; Chap. 3) so that it is connected to the tongue base by the thyroglossal duct. It lies in its normal pretracheal position by week 7 but the thyroglossal tract (with its *levator glandulae thyroidea muscle*) has an intimate association with the body of the hyoid bone running adherent in front and around the top and bottom of the bone. This intimate connection is important in removal of a thyroglossal cyst or fistula in order to ensure eradication of cystic and epithelial remnants (the latter fistula usually a recurrence after an incomplete Sistrunk's operation). Rudimentary thyroid function begins at 3 months (Diagram 17.2). Most thyroglossal cysts are infrahyoid but on the same principle, aberrant thyroid tissue (which may be functional or subject to any type of thyroid disease) may be found anywhere along this migration-development pathway (e.g. lingual thyroid).

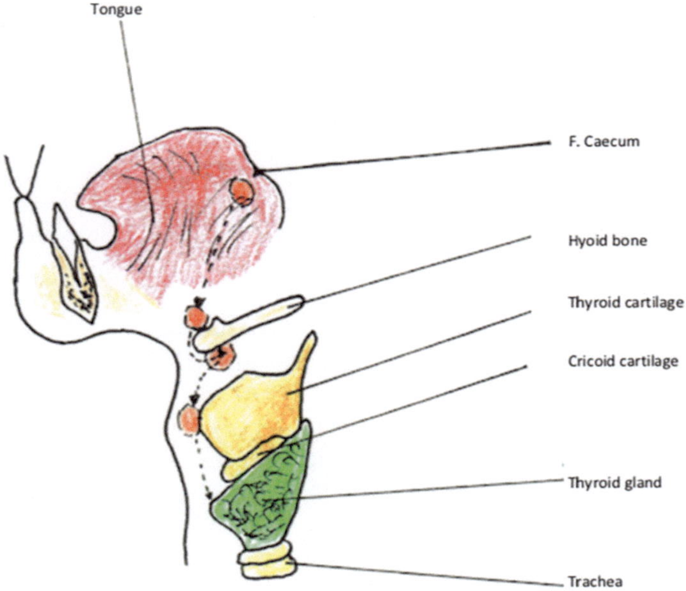

Diagram 17.2 Pathway of the thyroglossal duct. This moves distally from the foramen caecum and travels in intimate association with the body and undersurface of the hyoid bone. Most thyroglossal cysts are subhyoid in position but their removal necessitates removal of the central portion of the hyoid body. Muscular tissue in the tract is the levator glandulae thyroideae

Development of the Face ~

In brief, this forms from the fusion of five discrete mesenchymal swellings (also known as processes or prominences); two maxillary, a frontonasal and lateral and medial nasal. The separation between the lateral nasal and the maxillary prominences forms the track of the nasolacrimal duct. There is a primary palate (intermaxillary segment) formed by part of the medial maxillary prominences and the medial nasal processes with a labial, upper jaw and palatal element attached rostrally to the nasal septum. This premaxillary segment houses the five incisors and the incisive canal. The secondary palate form two discrete palatine shelves which fuse with the incisive canal the boundary in fusion between the secondary and primary palates. The shape of the face has a contribution by the shape and formation of the paranasal sinuses but also by the dentition and growth of the maxillary and mandibular processes. The common defects are the cleft lip and palate with both anterior and posterior defects of varying severity. The rare oblique facial clefts result from a failure of fusion of the lateral nasal and maxillary processes with a split around the exposed nasolacrimal duct.

Q & A: Chap. 17 (Answers at the End of This Chapter)

1. During development, the paraxial mesoderm forms:
   (a) The occipital bone
   (b) The tongue musculature
   (c) The pharyngeal musculature
   (d) The extraocular musculature
2. The thyroid gland forms principally from:
   (a) The first pharyngeal pouch
   (b) The third pharyngeal arch
   (c) The foramen caecum
   (d) The dorsal part of the fourth pharyngeal pouch

3. The second pharyngeal arch
   (a) Forms the mandible
   (b) Is innervated by the glossopharyngeal nerve
   (c) Contributes to the stapes and stapedius
   (d) Has derivatives innervated by Cranial III (Oculomotor)
   (e) Has derivatives innervated by Cranial XII (Hypoglossal)
4. If there is a congenital problem with pharyngeal arches 1 and 2 you would expect to find:
   (a) palatal anomalies
   (b) A potential problem in maxilla formation and/or fusion
   (c) Hearing loss
   (d) A thyroglossal cyst
   (e) A branchial fistula
5. Concerning cleft lip and palate:
   (a) A cleft lip results from a failure of fusion of the maxillary prominence and the medial nasal process
   (b) With a cleft palate dental problems usually occur before the permanent teeth erupt
   (c) Dental problems with a cleft palate may include fused, missing or extra teeth
   (d) Cleft palate affects tooth enamel and is associated with a higher incidence of caries

Answers

1. a, b, d
2. c
3. c
4. a, b, c
5. c, d

18 Closing Remarks and Introduction to Volume 2

In this first volume I have tried to compartmentalize what I regard as probably the most intricate part of the study of human anatomy from a complex relational standpoint. An appreciation of the fasciae, viscera, neurovascular arrangement, osteology and specialist soft-tissue spaces and sense organs allows one afterwards to integrate these areas. This integration is an essential element for understanding operative surgical approaches and in an appreciation of the anatomy of compartment infiltration in head and neck cancer. The approach I have adopted uses simple line drawings which the reader can trace or copy. Each of these images is designed to shore up or elucidate one or two discrete points of anatomy. More complicated images in anatomy textbooks require the reader to decipher the picture and frequently to find the answers to specific anatomy questions. Our approach here has been to limit the information provided by the image with the view that if you can draw it, you understand it. Further, if you understand the anatomy concerned you are more likely to remember it.

In Volume 2, we examine the anatomy of the upper and lower limbs. If the reader can appreciate the compartmental design of the limbs, it becomes evident that there is considerable homology between the upper and lower limbs and in their neurovascular arrangement. The brachial and lumbosacral plexi will be covered in detail pointing out the similarities and differences between the two main areas. The approach is also designed to appreciate the osteology and developmental aspects of the limbs in a way that informs clinical examination and surgical practice.

A. Zbar, *Anatomy--Head and Neck*,
https://doi.org/10.1007/978-3-031-69538-4_18

Index

A
Abducent nerve, 155
Abducent nerve lesion/palsy, 155
Accessory nerve, 167
Accessory nerve injury in neck, 168
Accessory nucleus, 164
Accessory phrenic nerve, 86
Agger nasi, 262
Alar fascia of neck, 28
Anterior cranial fossa, 115, 121
Anterior jugular veins (AJV), 34
Arachnoid granulations, 114
Arterial circulation
 ascending pharyngeal artery, 193, 194
 basilar artery, 202, 203, 205
 carotid bifurcation, 187
 carotid body, 192
 carotid body tumour, 188
 CCA, 191
 ECA, 187, 188, 190–193
 facial artery, 196, 197
 ICA, 187, 191
 IJV, 188
 lingual artery, 195, 196
 occipital artery, 197, 198
 posterior auricular artery, 198, 199
 STA, 194, 195
 thyroid cartilage, 192
 vertebral artery, 199, 200, 202
Aryepiglottic muscle, 320
Arytenoid cartilages, 314
Arytenoid movement, 316, 317
Asterion, 113
Auditory ossicles, 334–336
Auriculotemporal nerve, 154
Autonomic nervous system (ANS), 91, 92, 94–98, 100, 105–107

B
Basilar artery, 202, 203, 205
Basilar sinuses, 219
Brachial plexus injury, 16
Brains stem orientation and cellular structure, 138
Brainstem nuclei, 140
 cell subtypes, 138
Branchial fibres, 159
Branchial motor function, 138
Buccal nerve, 154
Buccinator forms, 278
Buccinator muscle, 295, 297
Buccopharyngeal fascia, 23, 27
Bulla ethmoidalis, 259

C
Calvarium, 134
Cardiorespiratory fibres, 142

A. Zbar, *Anatomy--Head and Neck*,
https://doi.org/10.1007/978-3-031-69538-4

Carotid sheath, 22
Carotid sinus nerve, 159
Carotid triangle, 11, 13, 29
Cavernous sinus, 219, 221–224
Central relay for taste, 160
Cerebellopontine angle tumour, 168
Cerebellopontine tumour, 185
Cervical fascia, 4, 7
  investing layer, 29, 30
Cervical oesophagus, 304
Cervical plexus, 82, 86, 87
Chorda tympani, 158
Clavipectoral fascia, 7
Cleft palate, 291, 292
Cochlear duct, 340
Cochlear nerve, 158
Common carotid artery (CCA), 191
Conjunctiva, 236
Conus elasticus, 315
Cranial IX, 161
Cranial nerves, 168
Cranial nerves, brain stem, 142
Cranial vault, 113
Cribriform, 115
Cricoid cartilage, 313
Cricoid lamina, 316
Cricopharyngeus, 303
Cricothyroid, 163, 194, 304, 314, 321–323, 350
  joint, 313, 316
  muscle, , , , , , , 320, 35, 38, 43, 50, 162, 163

D

Danger space, 24
Deep cervical fascia, 7, 20
  investing layer, 19
Descendens hypoglossi, 38
De Sedibus et Causus Morborum per anatomem indigatis, 26
Digastric triangle of neck, 28, 29
Diploic veins, 223
Dysphagia lusoria, 50

E

Ear
  auditory ossicles, 334–336
  definition, 327
  external ear, 328, 329
  inner ear, 337, 340, 341
  mastoid bone, antrum and air cells, 336
  middle ear, 330, 332–334
Ectopic thyroid tissue, 41
Embryology, 1
  face, 354
  head and neck structures, 345, 346
  pharyngeal arch, 347, 350
  pharyngeal clefts, 351
  pharyngeal pouches, 351
  somatic mesoderm, 346
  thyroid development, 352, 353
  tongue, 352
Emissary veins, 224
Epiglottic cartilage, 314
Ethmoid air cells, 234
Ethmoidal sinuses, 268
Eustachian tube, 271, 272, 274
External carotid artery (ECA), 12, 187, 188, 190–193
External jugular vein (EJV), 34
Eyelids, 234–236
Eye stability, 238, 239

F

Face, 354
Facial artery, 196, 197
Facial nerve, 155, 157
Facial nucleus, 157
Farabeuf's triangle, 11, 13
Fine-needle aspiration cytology (FNAC) for neck masses, 15
Foramen lacerum, 118, 134
Foramen of Vesalius, 118
Foramen rotundum, 117
Foramen spinosum, 118
Frontal nerve, 150

G
General somatic afferents (GSA), 159
General systemic efferents (GSE), 142
General visceral afferents (GVA), 142
General visceral efferents (GVE), 142
Geniohyoid, 67
Glossopharyngeal (IX) nerve, 167
Glossopharyngeal nerve, 159
Greater petrosal nerve, 157

H
Head and neck cancer, 357
Hyoid musculature, 1
Hypoglossal nerve, 164, 167

I
Inferior alveolar artery, 177
Inferior alveolar (dental) nerve, 154
Inferior constrictor muscle, 303–305
Inferior oblique muscle, 249
Inferior petrosal sinus, 119
Inferior thyroid artery (ITA), 44
Infrahyoid muscles, 38
Infrahyoid musculature, 35, 37, 38, 86, 324
(the strap muscles), 35, 37–39
Infraorbital nerve, 152
Infratemporal fossa, 170
Internal acoustic meatus, 119
Internal carotid artery (ICA), 187, 191
Internal jugular vein (IJV), 34, 209–211

J
Jugular foramen, 119

L
Lacrimal apparatus, 237, 238
Lacrimal gland (zygomatic and lacrimal nerves), 184
Lacrimal nerve, 150
Laryngeal skeleton, 310, 311
Larynx
arytenoid movement and rima glottidis, 316, 317
cartilaginous and membranous skeleton, 309
cavity of, 314–316
laryngeal musculature, 320–324
laryngeal skeleton, 310, 311
ligaments and membranes, 317, 318
thyroid cartilage, 313, 314
Lateral cricoarytenoid muscle, 321
Lateral pterygoid, 179
Levator palati, 284, 285
Levator palpebrae superioris muscle, 248
Limbs, 357
Lingual artery, 195, 196
Lingual nerve, 155
Local chewing reflex, 186
Long sphenopalatine nerve, 152
Lymphatic drainage, 51

M
Mandibular nerve, 153, 173, 174
Masseter muscle, 178
Mastication muscles, 186
Mastoid bone, antrum and air cells, 336
Mastoid process, 20
Maxillary artery, 174, 176, 185
Maxillary nerve, 151–153, 181, 183
Meckel's cartilage, 1, 139
Meckel's cave (*Cavum trigeminale, cisterna trigeminalis*), 117
Medial foramen rotundum, 117

Medial pterygoid, 179
Medial rectus muscle, 248
Membranous labyrinth, 337
Meningeal veins, 223
Middle cervical sympathetic ganglion, 51
Middle constrictor muscle, 302, 303
Middle cranial fossa, 115, 117, 185
Minimally invasive thyroidectomy (MIVAT) approaches, 49
Mouth and palate
- buccinator, 278, 295, 297
- cleft palate, 291, 292
- fauces, 278
- genioglossus, 294
- hyoglossus, 295
- incisive fossa, 278
- levator palati, 284, 285
- musculus uvulae, 287, 288
- nerve supply, 277
- palatal musculature, 281, 282
- palatine tonsil, 288, 290, 291
- palatoglossal arches, 277
- palatoglossus, 285
- palatopharyngeus, 285, 287
- soft palate, 282, 284
- styloglossus, 295
- teeth, 278–281
- tensor palati, 284
- tongue, 292, 293
- vallate papillae, 293, 294

Muscular Triangle, 13

N

Nasociliary nerve, 150
Nasopalatine nerve, 152
Nasopharyngeal carcinoma, 26, 168
Neck
- anterior triangle, 7
- triangles and spaces, 4, 6, 7

Neonatal skull, 121
Nerve Supply, 51
Non-recurrent nerve, 49
Nose and paranasal sinuses
- agger nasi, 262
- air warmer and humidifier, 257
- blood supply, 262, 264
- bulla ethmoidalis, 259
- ethmoidal air sinuses, 260
- ethmoidal sinus, 268
- ethmoid and septal cartilage, 258
- Eustachian tube, 271, 272, 274
- frontal sinus, 269
- maxillary sinus, 260, 266–268
- nasal atrium, 259
- nerve supply, 264–266
- ostium, 259
- sphenoidal sinus, 269, 270
- Waldeyer's ring and adenoids, 270, 271

NRLN, 49

O

Oblique arytenoid, 320
Occipital artery, 197, 198
Occipital bone, 134
Occipital sinus, 219
Occipital triangle, 15, 16
Oculomotor nerve, 146
Oculomotor nerve palsy, 168
Olfactory nerves, 143
Olive and inferior cerebellar peduncle, 160
Omohyoid, 37
Ophthalmic division, 150–151
Optic nerve, 143, 145
Orbit
- actions, 249–251
- ethmoid air cells, 234
- extraocular muscles, 245
- eyelids, 234–236
- eye stability, 238, 239
- eye, structure of, 239, 241–243
- inferior orbital fissure, 232, 233
- lacrimal apparatus, 237, 238
- lacrimal bone, 232

lacrimal sac, 233
nerves and vessels, 251–254
osteology, 231
palatine bone, 234
retina, 243–245
smooth roof, 232
terminology, 247–249
Orbital walls, 135
Osseous labyrinth, 340
Osteology of skull, 133
Ostium, 259

P
Palatal musculature, 281, 282
Palatine tonsil, 288, 290, 291
Parathyroid glands, 51, 52
Parotid fascia, 7
Parotid gland, 53, 56, 57, 59, 60
Parotid gland, secretomotor function, 60
Pars flaccida, 334
Pelizzo grading, 48
Petrotympanic fissure, 134
Pharyngeal arch, 347, 350
Pharyngeal clefts, 40, 351
Pharyngeal groove, 40
Pharyngeal nerve, 184
Pharyngeal pouches, 351
Pharyngobasilar fascia, 26, 29, 300
Pharynx
Eustachian tube narrowing, 299
inferior constrictor muscle, 303–305
middle constrictor muscle, 302, 303
pharyngobasilar fascia, 300
sagittal distribution and origins, 300
structure of, 299
superior constrictor muscle, 300, 302
Phrenic nerve, 86
Platysma, 73
Posterior auricular artery, 198, 199
Posterior auricular nerve, 158
Posterior cranial fossa, 119
Posterior cricoarytenoid, 321
Posterior triangle of neck, 14, 15
Postganglionic secretomotor fibres, 61
Preganglionic PSNS fibres, 161
Pretracheal and prevertebral fasciae, 27
Pretracheal fascia, 7, 22, 27
Prevertebral fascia, 21
Pterion, 113
Pterygoid hamulus, 134
Pterygoid laminae, 112
Pterygoid plexus of veins, 174
Pterygomaxillary fissure, 112
Pterygopalatine fossa (PPF), 170, 171, 177, 180, 181, 183–185
Pterygopalatine ganglion, 177

R
Recurrent laryngeal nerve (RLN), 39, 46–51, 303–304, 317
Reichert, K.B., 139
cartilage, 139
Retina, 243–245
Retromandibular vein, 60
Right subclavian artery (RSA), 49
Rima glottidis, 316, 317
RLN palsy, 50, 51

S
Saccule, 337
Salivary glands, 53
Scalenus medius, 81
Scalenus minimus, 81
Scalenus posterior, 81
Secretomotor supply, 159
Semicircular canals, 340, 341
Sensory peripheral ganglion, 161

Sigmoid sinus, 219
Sinus of Morgagni, 26, 168
Skull
  component parts, 111
  ossification, 121, 122
  osteology, 133
  sutures and points, 113
Sleep apnoea-related disorders, 270
Small tympanic branches, 157
Sphenoid, 122, 124, 126, 134
Sphenoidal sinus, 269, 270
Spinal accessory nerve, 76, 77, 79–81
Stapedius, 335
Sternoclavicular joints, 34
Sternocleidomastoid (SCM), 34, 74, 75
  piercing, 60
Sternohyoid, 37
Sternothyroid muscle, 34, 38
Straight sinus, 219
Stylohyoid muscle, 64–68
Styloid process, 161
Subclavius, 82
Submandibular (digastric) triangle, 8, 11
Submandibular gland (suprahyoid region), 62–64
Submental triangle, 14
Superficial temporal artery, 133
Superior constrictor muscle, 300, 302
Superior oblique muscle, 249
Superior orbital fissure, 117
Superior rectus muscle, 248
Superior sagittal sinus, 217
Superior thyroid artery (STA), 41–43, 194, 195
Supraclavicular triangle, 16, 18, 19
Suprasternal incision, surgical approach, 33
Systemic visceral efferents (SVE), 142

T
Teeth, 278–281
Temporal bone, 126, 128–132
Temporalis fascia, 132, 133
Tensor palati, 284
Tensor tympani, 334
Thyroepiglottic muscle, 320
Thyrohyoid, 37
Thyrohyoid membrane and ligaments, 313
Thyroid cartilage, 39, 192, 313, 314
Thyroid development, 352, 353
Thyroidea ima artery (TIA), 45
Thyroidectomy, 33
Thyropharyngeus, 39
Tongue, 292, 293, 352
Transverse arytenoid muscle, 321
Transverse sinus, 217, 218
Trapezius, 75
Trigeminal nerve, 147, 150
Trochlear (IV) nerve, 167
Trochlear nerve, 147
Trotter's triad, 26
Tympanic nerve or Jacobson's nerve, 61

V
Vagal nuclei, 161, 162
Vallate papillae, 293, 294
Vascular anomaly, 50
Venous drainage, 45, 46, 209–230, 254, 263, 264, 267, 269, 270, 281, 290, 305, 335, 336, 340
  ear, 335
  and sinuses
    basilar sinus, 219
    cavernous sinus, 219, 221–224
    CSF dynamics, 226, 228
    features, 215
    IJV, 209–211

occipital sinus, 219
overview, 213–215
sigmoid sinus, 219
straight sinus, 219
superior sagittal sinus, 217
transverse sinus, 217, 218
vertebral venous plexi, 225, 226
of thyroid gland, 45
Vertebral artery, 199, 200, 202
Vertebral venous plexi, 225, 226
Vestibulocochlear nerve, 159
Vital rima glottidis, 315

W
Waldeyer's ring and adenoids, 270, 271

Z
Zenker's diverticulum, 304
Zenker's pharyngeal pulsion, 304
Zygomatic bone, 111
Zygomatic nerve, 152
Zygomatic process of frontal bone, 132, 133

MIX
Papier aus verantwortungsvollen Quellen
Paper from responsible sources
FSC® C105338

If you have any concerns about our products,
you can contact us on
ProductSafety@springernature.com

In case Publisher is established outside the EU,
the EU authorized representative is:
Springer Nature Customer Service Center GmbH
Europaplatz 3, 69115 Heidelberg, Germany

Printed by Libri Plureos GmbH
in Hamburg, Germany